The Jossey-Bass Health Series brings together the most current information and ideas in health care from the leaders in the field. Titles from the Jossey-Bass Health Series include these essential health care resources:

Strategies for the New Health Care Marketplace

Strategies for the New Health Care Marketplace

Managing the Convergence of Consumerism and Technology

Dean C. Coddington, Elizabeth A. Fischer,

Keith D. Moore

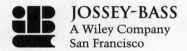

JOSSEY-BASS
A Wiley Company
San Francisco

Jossey-Bass books and products are available through most bookstores. To contact Jossey-Bass directly, call (888) 378-2537, fax to (800) 605-2665, or visit our website at www.josseybass.com.

Substantial discounts on bulk quantities of Jossey-Bass books are available to corporations, professional associations, and other organizations. For details and discount information, contact the special sales department at Jossey-Bass.

 Manufactured in the United States of America on Lyons Falls Turin Book. This paper is acid-free and 100 percent totally chlorine-free.

Library of Congress Cataloging-in-Publication Data

Coddington, Dean C.
    Strategies for the new health care marketplace: managing the convergence of consumerism and technology / Dean C. Coddington, Elizabeth A. Fischer, and Keith D. Moore.
        p.; cm.—(The Jossey-Bass health series)
    Includes bibliographical references and index.
    ISBN 0-7879-5593-0 (alk. paper)
    1. Medical care—Forecasting. 2. Medical innovations. 3. Consumers. 4. Medical economics.
5. Medical technology. [DNLM: 1. Delivery of Health Care—organization & administration—United States. 2. Consumer Satisfaction—United States. 3. Marketing of Health Services—methods—United States. 4. Technology—United States. W 84 AA1 C613s 2001] I. Fischer, Elizabeth A. II. Moore, Keith D. III. Title. IV. Series.
RA427 .C56 2001
362.1—dc21   00-012247

FIRST EDITION
HB Printing   10 9 8 7 6 5 4 3 2 1

Contents

Foreword

Leading health care organizations in today's environment is akin to leading a forced march across a bog. Each step is precarious, the reference points keep changing, and just when you think you have secured a foothold, the ground shifts. Some of the troops, intent on preserving their own interests and safety, break rank and pursue another course. Others retreat to the shore you just left behind. Those who continue the journey are tired and disillusioned, their energy consumed by the immediate need to stay afloat. There is not much reserve available to plan for what awaits us on the other side of the bog.

For those leading the expedition, the destination is not fully visible, but it is taking shape. *Strategies for the New Health Care Marketplace* is concerned with living in the present yet keeping an eye toward several possible futures. The book begins with an overview of *why* we need to change, but the main focus of the book is on *what* we need to change. It represents a realistic assessment of the broad range of challenges we face. The book includes a great deal of practical information about what needs to be done to develop the organizational characteristics and competencies required to be successful players in a new marketplace shaped by the forces of consumerism and technology. Although its overall message is one of optimism, it does not minimize the scope of change that will be required in our industry—and in the thinking of those who will lead it.

I am a physician, and I admit to feeling chastened by the authors' assessment that many of us have become so immersed in the immediacy of the current environment that we have not given adequate weight to the profound shift that is already under way in health care. I, too, find myself mourning the passing of the "Golden Age" of medicine and can conjure up fond memories of simpler times when health care and medical care were virtually synonymous. However, I wholeheartedly agree with the authors' point that health care is becoming more about quality of life and less about traditional medical care. Consumers have driven this shift, and the rate of change has been accelerated by technology.

Most of us have had at least one awakening jolt in regard to our ability to comprehend the transforming power of a new technology, but it is the long-term impact that we need to understand better. In my own experience nothing has made this point more clearly than the lessons learned in implementing an electronic medical record (EMR).

We began using an EMR on a limited basis at several clinical test sites three years ago. Initial attention focused on the technology itself—how it worked and how it fit into everyday practice. A fair amount of resistance surfaced over the disruptions in daily routines that made the physician-patient interface less efficient. Many of the disruptions had to do with gaps between the new technology and old systems (such as scheduling) or with misalignment between systems (such as compensation). This first pilot project underscored the need to examine change systemically and to understand the relationship between new technology and the processes that support it. Our initial failure to recognize this meant that we had to make our way through a great deal of resistance to changing the here and now.

Subsequent EMR implementation sites were selected with physician groups that volunteered to be part of the test. Greater attention was given to aligning support systems and taking deliberate steps to create readiness among users. As a consequence, the second pilot group was able to embrace the EMR technology as a means of changing the way they do their work (how they refer patients or write prescriptions, for example) and the way they interact with patients. Their use of information technology resulted in fundamental changes in their work processes—in the way they sign charts and orders, order lab tests and receive lab results, use guidelines, provide follow-up care, and communicate with their patients. As a result of technology and the type of interaction their patients are demanding, these physicians have learned to use their time in new ways. Their practices operate much differently from those in the first pilot.

Marshall de Graffenried Ruffin, M.D., captured the essence of our experience when he said, "We tend to overestimate the immediate consequences of new technologies and underestimate their long-term effects" (1999, p. iv). Not only will care delivery be different, but all supporting systems will require change as well. If we accept that consumerism is a force driving future change, we must be equipped to understand what consumers want and need. Once we understand this, we must be able to act on their demands and help shape their expectations. This means providing more convenience, greater access, and better service. In order to be responsive, health care's traditional approach to marketing, strategic planning, human resources, compensation, financing, and facility development needs to reach a higher level of sophistication and achieve a greater degree of alignment with the goals we are trying to achieve.

The authors of this book present the health care marketplace from a comprehensive perspective, and I find their work thought-provoking and useful in a very practical sense. The authors' expertise in the health care arena comes through in their overall assessment, and their depth of understanding allows them to challenge the status quo. There is much about the book that is unsettling. There are no global answers, but there are numerous insights and options for those seeking the right questions to pursue in developing new strategies. Therein lies its value for those of us who could use some help out of the bog.

In addition to a wealth of information, there are two main messages in this book. One is that the entire construct of health care has already changed as a result of the intertwined forces of consumerism and technology, and we have not yet grasped the extent of the change. The second is that the opportunity to serve is not diminished by this construct—in fact, it is expanded. A new marketplace is emerging, and within it there are many opportunities to serve people in ways that make their lives better.

It is this belief that compels me to stay in this profession and in this business.

Roger L. Gilbertson, M.D.
President and CEO, MeritCare Health System

In loving memory of E. C. Coddington,
father, husband, teacher, and school administrator.
A person of integrity, humor, faith, and discipline
with a profound interest in others.
He is sorely missed.

Preface

We have been through physician bonding, continuous quality improvement, owning primary care practices and health plans, and now we are being told to get back to the basics. How should we be positioning our organization for the future? What evidence do we have that investments in anticipation of a future dominated by consumerism and technology will pay off?
PHYSICIAN EXECUTIVE OF A LARGE WEST COAST HEALTH SYSTEM

Thus far, we've known what to do—cut costs and consolidate. However, pretty soon we're going to need a new vision. What do we do after we've achieved acceptable financial performance?
HOSPITAL SYSTEM EXECUTIVE IN THE MIDDLE OF A SUCCESSFUL "TURNAROUND" (FROM UNPROFITABLE TO PROFITABLE)

These are challenging times for health care organizations. On one hand, reduced reimbursement for services is prompting unprecedented cutbacks in hospital operating budgets and in physician and health plan revenues. On the other hand, the convergence of two powerful forces—more assertive, empowered health care consumers and rapid advances in both medical and information technology—may well make this one of the most innovative and progressive periods in the history of health care. Together, these factors create formidable problems for health care leaders, who must decide when to be aggressive and when to be conservative, when to act independently and when to partner with others, where to cut costs and where to invest.

Here is an exchange that took place during a strategy retreat of the forty-two-physician Dawson Clinic (clinic and speaker names are fictitious), located in a Chicago suburb:

George Jensen (internist): How are we going to position our clinic to be successful when employers and managed care plans don't recognize that we are cost effective and produce higher quality than other physicians in our service area? You can talk about consumers playing a bigger role in health care decision making, and the impact of the Internet and health care information technology, but I'm concerned about making sure we are recognized—and paid appropriately—for what we do for our patients.

John Melrose (cardiologist): I think we need to quit focusing our attention on managed care and Medicare and what they want out of us. More and more, I see patients calling the shots. Have you all listened to the radio for all of the ads for ultrafast CT scanning for heart disease? This procedure is not covered by most insurance companies, but consumers, including some of our patients, are spending $500 a crack out of their own pockets for these scans.

What are we going to do in the future to make the clinic more patient friendly? Are we willing to spend the money to market directly to consumers? Is that what it is going to take to be successful? I think it is.

Janice Borden (pediatrician): It's interesting to talk about all the new developments in health care, but I'm concerned about the increasing number of my patients whose parents don't have health insurance. It has gotten to the point where one out of three kids whom I see lacks insurance; and their parents either pay out of their pockets, or we get nothing.

It seems to me the biggest problem for the future is pretty basic: getting universal coverage. The government's program for low-income kids has been slow to get off the ground. If we have an economic downturn and some employers stop providing health insurance, we're in big trouble.

Jason Martin (general surgeon): I agree with Jan, but when I think about the future of our clinic, I'm concerned about a number of additional factors. How are we going to handle the increasing number of patients who show up having done their own searches on the Internet? How are we going to compete with the hospital-based clinic two miles down the road that has been spending millions on its new clinical information system and electronic medical record? And what about the big boys downtown who are advertising directly to consumers about their advanced technology and superior clinical outcomes? Where are we going to get the money to invest in the new technology that we need to stay competitive?

David Johnson (urologist and clinic president): I see a different future for our clinic. We've been complaining for years about managed care and how these big health plans are trying to push us around and cut payments. The fact is, hard-core managed care hasn't really worked, at least not in this community. And I don't think managed care will be the dominant force in the future that it has been in the past.

At the same time, I see consumers, especially younger women and the baby boomers, stepping forward to take control of their families' health. The drug companies must know something we don't. Have you seen the number of full-page health-related ads in *Time* and *Newsweek* or the huge number of ads on TV?

I believe that we are entering a new era in health care where demand for drugs and medical services is going to explode. I think we, as a multispecialty group, are ideally positioned to take advantage of the opportunities over the next five years. Rather than being defensive or thinking of ourselves as victims, I think we should get aggressive and position ourselves to become a metro-wide leader in medicine. This is not the time to be fainthearted. Let's look into a health care future that is far different than what we have experienced over the past few years.

For the first time in several years, the annual retreat ended on a positive note. Task forces were formed to investigate how the clinic might capitalize on the Internet (such as through increased use of e-mail and the creation of a first-class Web site) and accelerate development of its clinical information system. Other task forces focused on how to enhance marketing, improve convenience and services, increase product differentiation (for example, by measuring and reporting clinical outcomes and using patient satisfaction surveys), and, most important, develop a long-term financial plan.

Strategies for the New Health Care Marketplace

This book is the second in a planned trilogy. Our previous book *Beyond Managed Care* (Jossey-Bass, 2000), the first in the series, was our attempt to assess the health care marketplace and environment of the future. That book focused on the growth of consumerism and technology and on factors likely to shape health care during the first five years of the twenty-first century. *Strategies for the New Health Care Marketplace* identifies and assesses strategies that health care organizations should consider as they position themselves for the future. Although we have included a limited discussion of management issues, the focus is on strategy. Management of health care in the new marketplace is the third leg of the stool, and perhaps the most important. One of our reviewers said, "Don't overlook the difficulty of implementing the strategies you propose." We have not, but the subject of strategies is sufficiently complex to warrant a book of its own. Perhaps others will also accept our reviewer's challenge to write a book about managing in the new health care marketplace.

Part One of this book begins with a summary, in Chapter One, of the health care marketplace and environment as we anticipate it to develop between now and 2005. Chapters Two through Five discuss what consumers want out of their health care system. The nine value-added characteristics discussed in these four chapters include quality, information, service, convenience, access, affordability, choice, personal relationships with physicians, and innovation.

In Part Two we identify and assess strategies for various types of health-related providers and payers and explain how these strategies will enable health care organizations to better meet the needs of the new marketplace. For example, a movement toward consumer-dominated health care would have profound implications for health plans—instead of directing their marketing efforts at employers, they would have to target consumers and purchasing alliances.

In Part Three we discuss management, governance, and marketing issues that will be increasingly important for health care organizations as they prepare for the new health care marketplace. We examine questions such as these: What management styles are likely to be successful for health care executives in the future? How should hospitals, medical groups, and integrated systems change the ways they govern themselves? What is the potential of mass customization and branding as marketing strategies?

Part Four concludes the book with two chapters, one that describes successful health care organizations of the future and another that presents what we consider to be several myths and economic realities concerning health care. These last two chapters summarize the insights we have gained in performing the research and analysis that underlie this book.

Research Approach

We used a number of research methodologies in preparing this book. In part, we digested what others have written about the future of health care and what it will take to be successful. We also relied very heavily on interviews with leaders of medical groups, physician networks, integrated systems, hospitals, multihospital systems, academic medical centers, specialty hospitals, health plans, and other health-related organizations. Many of the strategies described in Part Two emerged from our interviews. Our colleagues at McManis Associates have had many years of experience in assisting various types of health care organizations in developing management and process improvement strategies; their input, too, was invaluable.

The Acknowledgments section, which follows, identifies the many contributors to this book. We thank all of them for their help.

Denver, Colorado   DEAN C. CODDINGTON
January 2001   ELIZABETH A. FISCHER
                                                      KEITH D. MOORE

Acknowledgments

This book involved a large number of interviews, a literature review, and the collaboration of a number of colleagues at McManis Associates.

Interviews

In formulating the strategies health care organizations can use to prepare for a future dominated by the convergence of consumerism and technology, we relied on interviews with a number of key individuals in different types of health care organizations. Our interviewees included the following people.

Physicians, Group Practice Administrators,
and Others with a Physician Perspective

Robert Bohlmann, senior consultant, Medical Group Management Association (MGMA), Englewood, Colorado

Jerry Buckley, M.D., chief executive officer, Copic Insurance Company, Englewood, Colorado

Barry Greene, professor and deputy director, CHP&R, University of Iowa, Department of Health Management Policy, Iowa City

Patrick Hinton, executive director, Jacksonville Orthopedic Institute, Jacksonville, Florida

Gigi Hirsch, M.D., chief executive officer, IntelliNet, Brookline, Massachusetts

Allan Kortz, M.D., Denver

Mark Levine, M.D., associate medical director, Colorado Foundation for Medical Care, Aurora

Acute Care Hospital Sector

Reginald Ballantyne, III, president, PMH Health Resources, Phoenix, Arizona

Richard Batt, chief executive officer, Franklin Community Health Network, Farmington, Maine

Robert Burn, president and chief executive officer, Washoe Health System, Reno, Nevada

Larry Griffin, vice president, VHA Mountain States, Denver

Richard Henley, senior vice president, operations, Vassar Brothers Hospital, Poughkeepsie, New York

Fred Linville, senior vice president, VHA Mountain States, Denver

Pete Tucker, director of community relations, Franklin Community Health Network, Farmington, Maine

Larry White, president, St. Patrick Hospital, Missoula, Montana

Don Wilson, president, Kansas Hospital Association, Topeka, Kansas

Specialty Hospitals

Dennis C. Brimhall, president and chief executive officer, University of Colorado Hospital, and associate vice chancellor for Fitzsimons University of Colorado Health Sciences Center, Aurora

Robert Dickler, senior vice president for health care affairs, Association of American Medical Colleges, Washington, D.C.

Larry McAndrews, president and chief executive officer, National Association of Children's Hospitals and Related Institutions, Alexandria, Virginia

Dennis O'Malley, president, Craig Hospital, Englewood, Colorado

Donna Shelton, director, child health financing, National Association of Children's Hospitals and Related Institutions, Alexandria, Virginia

Raymond Uhlhorn, president and chief executive officer, Moss-Rehab, Albert Einstein Healthcare Network, Philadelphia

Integrated Health Systems

J. Lindsey Bradley, Jr., president and chief administrative officer, Trinity Mother Frances Health System, Tyler, Texas

William Corley, chief executive officer, Methodist Community Hospitals, Indianapolis

Kevin Fickenscher, M.D., senior vice president, CareInsite, Tiburon, California, and former medical director, Catholic Healthcare West, San Francisco, California

John Koster, M.D., vice president, clinical and physician services, Sisters of Providence Health Systems, Seattle

Maynard Oliverius, president and chief executive officer, Stormont-Vail Healthcare, Topeka, Kansas

Robert Parker, M.D., Carle Clinic Association, Urbana, Illinois

Rob Rosenbaum, Dartmouth-Hitchcock Medical Center, Lebanon, New Hampshire

Thomas Royer, M.D., former senior vice president for medical affairs and chairman of the board of governors, Henry Ford Health System, Detroit

Robert Waller, M.D., chief executive officer emeritus, Mayo Foundation, Rochester, Minnesota

Health Plan Executives and Managed Care Advisers

Chris Binkley, regional president, Kaiser Permanente, Denver

Max Brown, senior vice president, network management, WellPoint Health Networks, Thousand Oaks, California

James Hertel, president, Healthcare Computer Corporation of America, Denver

Dennis Horrigan, vice president, managed care development, Independent Health, Williamsville, New York

Lee Newcomer, M.D., former medical director, UnitedHealth, Minneapolis

Kate Paul, former western region president, Kaiser Permanente, Denver

Greg Van Pelt, administrator of system development, Sisters of Providence Health System, Portland, Oregon

Robert Vernon, senior vice president, Aon Managed Care, Fort Worth, Texas

Other Individuals Interviewed

Jock Bickert, president, Looking Glass, Denver

Patrick Gross, founder and chairman, executive committee, American Management Systems, Fairfax, Virginia

James Fisher, director, PPO sales and marketing, The Alliance, Denver, Colorado, and former director, managed care and provider relations, Rocky Mountain Vision Service Plan, Denver, Colorado

Rufus Howe, former vice president, product integration, Access Health, Broomfield, Colorado

Thomas Oberle, general manager, Equity Link, Westminster, Colorado, and former executive director, Colorado Dental Association, Denver, Colorado

Thomas H. Hansen, president and CEO, HealthCare Colorado, Denver, Colorado

Mary K. Wakefield, director, Center for Health Policy and Ethics, and professor, College of Nursing and Health Science, George Mason University, Fairfax, Virginia

Steve Wetzell, executive director, Buyer's Health Care Action Group, Minnetonka, Minnesota

Collateral Research

We also conducted case studies of a number of integrated health care systems. These included Mayo Foundation, Scott & White, Henry Ford Health System, Dartmouth-Hitchcock Medical Center, MeritCare Health System, HealthSystem Minnesota, Carle Clinic Association, Aurora Health Care, Moses Cone Health System, Scripps Health, and Trinity Mother Frances Health System. The thinking of physician leaders and other executives of these systems influenced our analysis, particularly Chapter Ten. The case studies were sponsored by MGMA, and the results have been published in a two-volume book, *The Changing Dynamics of Integrated Health-care.* We thank Kerstin B. Lynam, operations manager of MGMA's center for research, and all of the participating integrated systems for their contributions.

Special Thanks

We wish to give special thanks to a number of health care specialists and colleagues for their particular insights and guidance.

Roger L. Gilbertson, M.D., president and chief executive officer of MeritCare Health System in Fargo, North Dakota, wrote the Foreword. We have always valued Roger's insights into where health care is headed, and we very much appreciate his willingness to prepare the Foreword.

Larry Gamm, professor of health policy and management, Texas A&M University Health Science Center, School of Rural Health Policy, was a reviewer of the manuscript of this book. John Koster, M.D., was, in addition to an interviewee, a reviewer of the final manuscript. Both Larry and John challenged us with many questions, offered numerous insights, and encouraged us as we made improvements to the final version of this book.

Don Arnwine, former chief executive officer of VHA Inc., who is currently affiliated with McManis Consulting, helped us crystallize our thinking in regard to strategies for hospitals and multihospital systems and in regard to the health system and hospital governance issues covered in Chapter Fourteen.

F. Kenneth Ackerman, vice president of McManis Associates and former executive director of the Geisinger System in Danville, Pennsylvania, worked with us in preparing a number of case studies of large integrated systems. We appreciate Ken's input, especially in connection with the chapters on governance, management, and the strategies of integrated systems.

Laura Wareham, also a vice president at McManis Associates, prepared the section on strategies for children's hospitals in Chapter Nine. Laura has consulted with a number of children's hospitals around the country and is an expert on the special issues facing these kinds of organizations.

Jim Vogel, former associate at the Denver office of McManis Associates and now director, Beansprout Pediatric Newtwork in Boston, conducted the research and prepared initial drafts for portions of Chapter Two that deal with quality of care.

Lowell Palmquist, associate in the Denver office of McManis Associates and former hospital chief executive officer, reviewed drafts of all chapters and was especially helpful in preparing Chapter Eight.

Colleagues

We also wish to thank the following colleagues at St. Paul Companies and McManis Associates:

Michelle Cooney, former vice president, knowledge network, St. Paul Companies, who supported our research efforts during the preparation of this book

Rhonda Wyn, Denver office of McManis Associates, who has assisted us with three previous books and whose expert word-processing and administrative support were invaluable in preparing the manuscript of this book for publication

Karen "Pete" Drury, Denver office of McManis Associates, who arranged for many of our interviews and performed a variety of tasks that enabled us to get the manuscript of this book into its final form

Other Contributors

We wish to thank the following individuals at MGMA, the Healthcare Financial Management Association (HFMA), and Jossey-Bass Publishers:

Cynthia Kiyotake, director, library resource center, MGMA, who helped with our review of the literature

Richard L. Clarke, president of HFMA, a coauthor of *Beyond Managed Care,* who reviewed the manuscript of this book and made numerous suggestions

Andy Pasternack, senior editor, Jossey-Bass Publishers, whose vision and encouragement merit our particular gratitude

Gigi Mark, production editor, Jossey-Bass Publishers, who was primarily responsible for ushering this book through the publication and printing process

Samya Sattar, assistant marketing manager, Jossey-Bass Publishers, whose marketing efforts on our behalf we also greatly appreciate

The Authors

DEAN C. CODDINGTON is associated with McManis Consulting. After more than a decade as a research economist with the University of Denver's Research Institute, Coddington cofounded BBC Research & Consulting in 1970, where he served as a managing director for twenty-seven years before leaving to help form Moore Fischer Coddington, LLC. He received his bachelor's degree in civil engineering from South Dakota State University and his master of business administration degree from Harvard Business School. He has supervised over one hundred health care assignments for hospitals, medical groups, integrated systems, and health plans in all parts of the United States. He has coauthored six books on health care, including *Beyond Managed Care,* and has written numerous articles on a range of subjects, including integrated health care, factors driving health care costs, and health care strategies. Coddington is former chairman of the board of trustees of the 328-bed Swedish Medical Center in the Denver area and has served on the board of directors of the Colorado Neurological Institute.

ELIZABETH A. FISCHER, also with McManis Consulting, was a founder of Moore Fischer Coddington, LLC, and before that a managing director of BBC Research & Consulting. Fischer holds a bachelor's degree in American studies and economics from Mount Holyoke College and a master's degree in city and regional planning from Harvard University. Fischer's work includes formation of hospital-affiliated group practices, product development for health plans, community needs assessment, and creation of health care networks. She also has extensive experience in rural health care and long-term care. Along with Dean C. Coddington and Keith D. Moore, she has coauthored three previous books, including *Beyond Managed Care.* She has completed more than one hundred assignments for health care organizations. She is a frequent speaker at professional meetings of various health care industry groups and coauthor of numerous articles and papers.

KEITH D. MOORE is chairman and chief executive officer of McManis Consulting. He previously served as chairman of the board and chief executive officer of Moore Fischer Coddington, LLC, and for fifteen years as a managing director of BBC Research & Consulting. He received his bachelor's degree in economics from the University of Texas and his master's degree in city planning from Harvard University. Moore's consulting assignments have included strategic planning, mergers of medical groups, and development of productive working relationships between physicians and hospitals. He has published several articles on health care and is coauthor of six books on health care, including *Beyond Managed Care*. Early in his career, Moore was a senior consultant with a Denver-based consulting firm, a teaching assistant at Harvard University, and a U.S. Marine platoon leader in Vietnam. He headed the Industrial Economics and Management Division of the University of Denver's Research Institute, where he was responsible for research into technology transfer, research and development management, corporate planning, energy and resource economics, and governmental management strategies. He is a former board member of Spalding Rehabilitation Hospital in Denver.

Strategies for the New Health Care Marketplace

Part One

Understanding the Health Care Marketplace

Let's get over the idea that health care is purchased based solely on price. There are many ways health care organizations can differentiate themselves and create value for their customers. This is not a commodity business.

BENEFITS CONSULTANT, MIDWEST, September 2000

Part One begins by summarizing the health care marketplace and environment of the future. Our previous research (Coddington, Fischer, Moore, and Clarke, 2000) indicates that the new health care marketplace will be radically different from what we have seen over the past two decades. The fundamental market and environmental shifts we foresee are covered in Chapter One, which outlines our thinking on the new health care marketplace and describes the factors likely to shape health care during the first half of the twenty-first century.

In Part One we also devote four chapters to explaining the values important to health care consumers. These chapters examine what consumers want now, what they will want in the years ahead, and what they value most. Based on our background in research and management consulting and the experience of a number of health care organizations, we believe that most consumers are interested in a combination of nine value-added characteristics. These characteristics are shown in Figure P.1.

Quality of Care, Clinical Outcomes, and Medical Information

We discuss quality of care, clinical outcomes measurement and reporting, patient education, and medical information in Chapter Two.

Quality of Care and Clinical Outcomes

In the past, most consumers have often been unable to differentiate between high-quality and mediocre medical care. In fact, when discussing quality, consumers often confuse quality of care with service. Also, consumers usually assume they will receive high-quality care from their physician and local hospital.

Figure P.1. Adding Value for Health Care Consumers.

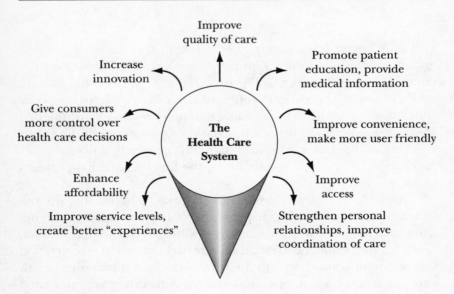

This is likely to begin to change over the first five years of the new millennium. In the future there will be more and better comparative information available about clinical outcomes, patient satisfaction, and other indicators of quality. These types of data will be available on hospitals, physicians, and medical groups, for use by health plans, business coalitions, and consumer purchasing alliances.

Evidence of inconsistent quality of care continued throughout the 1990s. For example, the comparative studies of John Wennberg, M.D., and his colleagues at Dartmouth continue to show substantial clinical variations among neighboring communities with comparable demographic characteristics (Dartmouth Medical School, 1996). There is general agreement that at least 20 percent of all health care spending (some would argue the percentage is much higher) is inappropriate and unnecessary.

One of the major strategies of most of the advanced health care systems in the United States is reducing clinical variation through the development and application of clinical process improvements, better electronic databases, and outcomes measurement. We believe that these sorts of efforts will begin to attract the interest of consumers.

Medical Information

Patients have access to vast new sources of medical information and are arriving at their physicians' offices much better prepared (at least in the consumers' view—physicians often disagree). Regardless of what physicians think or the extra work created for them, there is no doubt that consumers will seek out and use more health care information, including data on complementary and alternative medicine (CAM).

Another trend that promises to become important is consumers' access to their own medical records. Will this lead to improvement in quality of care? Some physicians are horrified at the thought, but we believe that consumers' access to their own medical records will lead to quality improvement. A growing number of physician leaders agree, and the experiments taking place around the country are likely to demonstrate that consumers' control over their medical records will lead to better quality.

Service, Convenience, and Access

Three value-added factors—service, convenience, and access—are intertwined; they are discussed together in Chapter Three. Consumers are demanding dramatically improved access and the convenience of obtaining health care services when they want them, not when providers find it convenient to offer these services. We also see increased evidence that consumers want a greater role in the choice of physicians and other providers.

Service

Chris Binkley, regional president of Kaiser Permanente in Denver, told us that his top priority for the next five years is to improve service to customers. "We have been trying to improve service," he said, "but we are nowhere close to the levels of service we are going to have to offer to remain competitive and maintain our market position" (interview, July 1999). If this is the perception of a leader from one of the top-rated health plans in the country, there are significant opportunities for service improvement in other health systems.

The leaders of nearly all of the health care systems we interviewed echoed Binkley's comment. There is general recognition that consumers, especially baby boomers, are more skilled than their parents at differentiating health care organizations based on level of service and that baby boomers will no longer tolerate inferior service.

What does our definition of good service include? Here are just a few examples:

- Friendly staff
- Prompt appointments with physicians
- Uncomplicated billing procedures
- Clear and concise statements of services rendered
- Good physician-patient communication
- Sufficient time spent by physicians with their patients
- Efficient systems of medical record keeping
- Timely reminders for routine checkups

The list could go on and on.

Convenience

The physician leader of a large health care system in the Midwest told us, "Consumers will put up with inconvenience when members of their family are facing a serious health care crisis. Under these circumstances they will gladly come to the main campus of a large multispecialty clinic to get access to the top specialists. But, for the routine, day-to-day health problems that come up in any family, consumers want convenience. They want a physician close by and want to get in to see their physician quickly."

There are at least three aspects to convenience: location close to home or work, office hours that make it possible to schedule an appointment at a convenient time, and the ability to see a physician or health professional on a timely basis. In order to satisfy the first criterion, location, many large health care systems have developed primary care networks covering a metropolitan area or region. The Mayo Health System is one example. It includes five hundred physicians, comprises several hospitals, and serves the region within 120 miles of Rochester, Minnesota. Hours of service have been extended in many communities, and the future promises even longer hours. Almost every large health care organization is taking steps to improve the availability of its physicians and health professionals, either in person or through electronic media.

Access

Access to the health care system means having a payment source that covers most or all of the types of medical services that consumers will need or desire, including drugs and advanced medical technology. Obviously, the uninsured and those on Medicaid do not have the same level of access as those with health plan coverage provided by their employer or individually purchased insurance.

Those on Medicare are concerned about whether they will continue to have access to the physicians and hospitals they want to use. With Medicare payment rates lagging, and the "hassle factor" and complexity increasing, an increasing number of physicians are closing their practices to new Medicare patients, and more are threatening to do so.

Affordability, Consumer Choice, and Personal Relationships with Physicians

Chapter Four deals with strategies for making health care more affordable and making consumers more accountable for their purchasing decisions. The chapter also addresses the growing importance of personal relationships between patients and providers.

Affordability

When we consider value added from the viewpoint of employers and payers, unit costs and quantity of services (utilization) are important. From a consumer perspective, however, the main financial consideration is affordability. Affordability depends on such variables as the types of health plan coverage available to an individual or family, the amount of total premium costs paid by consumers, the level of copayments and deductibles, and the extent of coverage of drugs, medical devices like hearing aids, and certain high-tech procedures. As the U.S. health care system increasingly focuses on consumers, there is growing concern about the share of health care costs borne directly by individuals.

Another aspect of affordability involves the increasing proportion of all health care procedures and products that can be characterized as improving quality of life and that are being paid for by consumers out of their pockets. Where will consumers get the discretionary income to be able to look better, have brighter teeth, grow hair on previously bald pates, and see better without glasses or contacts? To a large extent this depends on economic conditions, including the state of public equity markets.

Consumer Choice

One of the overall trends developing today is consumers' desire for more control over their health care. At the same time, consumers are becoming more willing to take personal responsibility for their own health and that of their families.

The more we analyze health care spending patterns and examine what consumers want out of their medical system, the more we are convinced that health care is evolving toward a focus on quality of life and away from a concentration on medical necessity. The shift toward medical services, drugs, and other products that basically improve quality of life—which is what consumers will be seeking—is noteworthy. Quality of life can be enhanced both in the process of obtaining health care (through friendliness, better service, greater convenience, and a better overall experience) and by the results of health care (seeing, hearing, looking, or feeling better). But what about consumers' responsibility to pay for improvements in their quality of life? We believe that in the new health care marketplace, consumers will take more responsibility for paying for their own health care.

Consumers' desire for freedom of choice and control is evident in the ongoing shift toward open-access health plans—preferred provider organizations (PPOs) and point-of-service (POS) health maintenance organizations (HMOs). Traditional HMOs with a primary care gatekeeper have lost market share and generally fallen out of favor. There is also substantial research on consumers indicating that when they have a choice of health plans, and thus a choice of physicians and hospitals, the level of their satisfaction with managed care increases significantly. However, this freedom of choice usually comes at a higher price.

Personal Relationships with Physicians

In most businesses personal relationships between providers of goods or services and the customers with whom they interact on a day-to-day basis are important. How much more important are personal relationships in health care?

There is no doubt that one of the by-products of managed care, particularly HMOs, has been the shattering of long-standing relationships between patients and their personal physicians. When large numbers of consumers were moving to HMOs during the 1980s and through the late 1990s, we concluded that personal relationships were not as important as we had once assumed. Many physicians are shocked by the number of loyal patients who have deserted them, mainly because of health plan restrictions and small differences in premium payments paid directly by employees.

However, we believe that personal relationships between consumers and their health care providers are making a strong comeback. If physicians and their staff take the time to develop relationships with patients and treat patients well, physicians will once again be rewarded with long-standing relationships.

Innovation and Entrepreneurship

Chapter Five, the final chapter in Part One, deals with innovation and entrepreneurship in health care. This chapter analyzes what has influenced innovation over the past twenty years and suggests what organizations can do to become more innovative in ways that will benefit consumers in the future.

Many in health care talk about the exciting innovations of the past two decades, but we think health care has become dull and predictable. Fortunately, the health care system will not be short on innovation during the first five years of the new century. We believe this is the way consumers want it; they want the benefits of new health-related products and services. Consumers can look forward to tremendous innovation in health care over the next five years.

Chapter One

An Environmental Assessment of Today's Health Care Marketplace

Health care is going to change more in the next five years than it has in the past two decades.
PHYSICIAN LEADER OF A MULTISPECIALTY GROUP ON THE
WEST COAST, September 2000

The purpose of this chapter is to describe the changing health care marketplace and present several scenarios for the initial years of the twenty-first century. Much of the discussion of the future of health care presented here is based on research and analysis conducted in connection with our previous book *Beyond Managed Care* (Coddington, Fischer, Moore, and Clarke, 2000).

The major market and environmental factors discussed in this chapter include the following:

- Growth and change in the overall health care market from 2000 to 2005 and the factors influencing the spending that will drive that growth
- Changes in the payer mix in the health care market and changes in the distribution of dollars among hospitals, physicians, and other providers
- Growth in the role consumers play in the health care market
- Impact of the Internet and other information technology (IT) on the health care market

- Implications of advances in genetic research, drug development, and medical technology for the future of the health
  care market
- Shifts in federal and state health care policy likely to affect the
  way health care is delivered and who is insured
- Patterns of consolidation among health plans, physicians, and
  hospitals and the ramifications of these trends
- Changes in the way health care is likely to be financed, such as
  through defined contributions, medical savings accounts
  (MSAs), vouchers, and individual insurance

Based on our analysis of these marketplace and environmental factors, we conclude this chapter by identifying and summarizing four possible scenarios for the future. A common theme among
the scenarios is the growing importance of consumerism and technology.

Growth and Change in the Health Care Market

The health care market of the future will grow much more rapidly
than at any time in the 1990s.

Growth in Health Care Spending

Total health care spending, $1.3 trillion in 2000, is expected to
grow at a rate of $100 billion per year, reaching $1.8 trillion in
2005. The rate of increase will be from 6 to 7 percent a year. Figure 1.1 depicts the increase in national health care spending between 1995 and 2005, showing total expenditures for 1995, 2000,
and 2005.

Factors Driving Increases in Health Care Spending

Among more than twenty identifiable factors driving health care
spending over the next five years, these five factors will be the most
important:

- *Aging of the population.* The aging of Americans, including the
  longer life spans of the frail elderly, continues to be an important driver of health care spending.

Figure 1.1. National Health Care Spending, 1995, 2000, 2005.

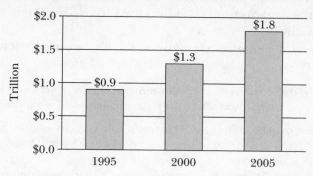

Sources: Health Care Financing Administration, 1999; authors' estimates for 2000 and 2005.

- *Growth in administrative expenses.* Given the growing complexity of the fragmented U.S. health care system, the overhead associated with health care financing and delivery represents a large and growing share of all health care costs.
- *Increase in consumer expectations.* Spurred by widespread use of the Internet and drug company advertising, the already high and growing expectations of consumers are bound to be a major factor driving up health care spending.
- *Proliferation of new drugs.* This has to be near the top of any list of factors pushing up health care expenditures, and there is no letup in sight.
- *Application of technology.* The availability and application of medical technology and IT will become even more important than in the past. In some industries the application of technology leads to lower costs, but this is unlikely to be the result in health care.

International Market Development

Part of the growth in health care spending will be attributable to international market development by U.S. physicians, hospitals, biomedical and drug companies, and producers of medical products.

Using telemedicine via the Internet and offering the most advanced medical technology and drugs in the world, a number of regional and national organizations will find ways to expand their services internationally.

A *Wall Street Journal* article spoke of health care as the new American export:

> In Sicily, there is an old joke about medical care. Question: What's the best Sicilian hospital? Answer: An airplane—to someplace else.
>
> Now that may be changing. This traffic-choked city of 750,000 [Palermo], where life has long been darkened by the dominance of the Mafia, boasts a new transplant center run by, of all places, the University of Pittsburgh. Financed by the Italian government, the center represents a new frontier for American high-tech exports.
>
> "If we learn to do this successfully," says Jeffrey Romoff, president of the University of Pittsburgh Medical Center Health System, "we will have developed a technology—running a major, high-quality facility overseas—that's eminently exportable to Egypt and Turkey and other countries" [McGinley, 2000, p. A1].

Citizens from Mexico and some countries in South and Central America, Europe, Asia, the Middle East, and the Pacific Rim, would have the disposable income to come to the United States for high-tech diagnostic and surgical procedures or to pay to have these services delivered in their home countries. The most prestigious health care organizations will have as much foreign business as they can handle.

Changes in Payer Mix and Spending Patterns

We anticipate major changes in the sources of health care dollars and the way they are spent.

Changes in Sources of Funds

Medicare and Medicaid will grow slightly in relative importance. Consumer spending, after twenty years of decline as a percentage of total health care expenditures, will hold its own in percentage terms and increase in actual dollars. The distribution of health care spending in 2000 and 2005 is shown in Figure 1.2.

Figure 1.2. Distribution of National Health Care Expenditures by Funding Source, 2000 and 2005.

2000

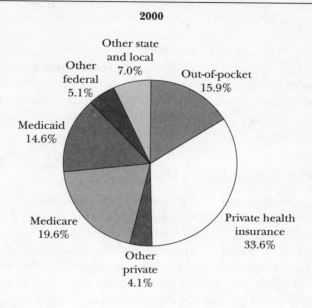

2005

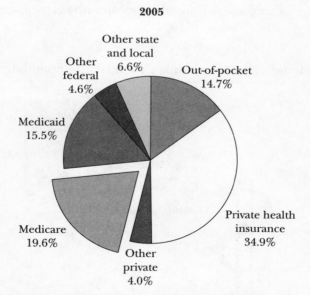

Sources: Health Care Financing Administration, 1999; authors' estimates.

Growth in Discretionary Spending

Figure 1.3 shows examples of several health care products and services that are largely or totally paid for by consumers out of their pockets.

Although we do not know the total proportion of health care spending that falls into the quality-of-life (or discretionary) category, we do know spending in this category is increasing rapidly. It will continue to be a major source of new health care market potential for physicians, hospitals, other health care providers, and product and service firms.

Stabilization of Spending on Managed Care

In 2000 managed care had 85 percent of the commercial market and, other than the potential for Medicare+Choice plans, could no longer be considered a growth industry. In fact, managed care is a mature industry in terms of market penetration. The historical growth of managed care, along with projections to 2005, is shown in Figure 1.4. As this figure shows, the rate of growth between 2000 and 2005 is expected to level off.

Along with the maturation of managed care, capitated payment (a fixed amount per member per month) is expected to con-

Figure 1.3. Discretionary Health Care Spending.

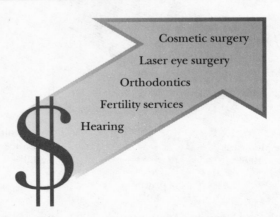

Cosmetic surgery

Laser eye surgery

Orthodontics

Fertility services

Hearing

tinue its decline, which first became evident during the period from 1998 through 2000. An increasing number of medical groups and hospitals, even those in advanced managed care markets, are refusing to take financial risk and are turning their backs on capitation. For example, Stan Pappelbaum, M.D., former CEO of Scripps Health, told us that following an evaluation of capitation that began in 1998, Scripps Health cancelled 120 health plans and other payer contracts as of mid-1999 and renegotiated nearly all of them by the end of the year. The result: the proportion of capitated dollars flowing to Scripps Health dropped from 28 percent in 1997 to 3 to 4 percent (interview, May 2000).

Decrease in Providers' Share of Spending

Hospitals will provide more intensive care and generate more revenues, but the long-term trend of hospitals' declining share of total health care spending is expected to continue. Hospitals' share of

Figure 1.4. Growth in Managed Care in the United States, 1980–2005.

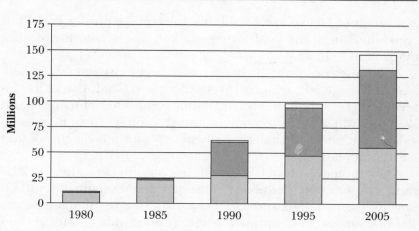

Note: As of January 1 of each year.

Sources: InterStudy, 1997, pp. v–viii; authors' estimates.

health care dollars declined from 41.5 percent in 1980 to 32.5 percent in 2000. By 2005 hospitals' share of health care spending is projected to drop to 29.7 percent. Figure 1.5 shows estimated percentages of national health care spending on various services for 2000 and 2005.

Physicians and medical groups can expect to maintain their share of the health care market—roughly 20 percent. Likewise, dental and vision services as a proportion of total health care spending are unlikely to change much. However, drugs, medical equipment, long-term care, rehabilitation, home health, disease management, and other personal and medical services will increase in relative importance.

We expect growth of at least 10 percent a year in the purchase and use of CAM and increased inclusion of CAM benefits in health plans. Physicians will increasingly accept these alternative "non-scientific" approaches, incorporate them into their medical practices, and work with consumers to meet their overall health care needs. CAM spending was estimated to be in excess of $50 billion in 1999 (Hofgard and Zipin, 1999)—this spending is *in addition to* total national health care expenditures as reported by the Health Care Financing Administration and other federal sources.

A Larger Role for Consumers

A number of factors are combining to create explosive growth in consumerism in the health care market. These factors are summarized in Exhibit 1.1.

With the consumer in charge, we expect more interest in wellness, self-diagnosis, self-care, prevention, and CAM. Use of the Internet will be at high levels, and a limited number of name brand Web sites will achieve acceptance and credibility. To an increasing extent, patients will challenge physicians on their diagnoses and treatment plans.

As a direct result of the growth in consumerism, there will be more emphasis on identifying consumer market segments and on developing products and services for specific segments (such as seniors, women of childbearing age, and individuals with certain types of chronic diseases). Figure 1.6 shows the key factors that define market segments in health care.

Figure 1.5. Distribution of National Health Care Spending on Various Services, 2000 and 2005.

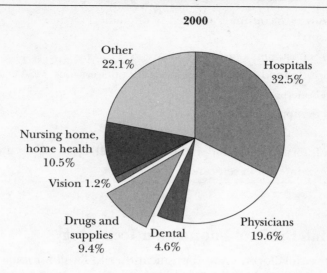

2000

Other
22.1%

Hospitals
32.5%

Nursing home,
home health
10.5%

Vision 1.2%

Drugs and
supplies
9.4%

Dental
4.6%

Physicians
19.6%

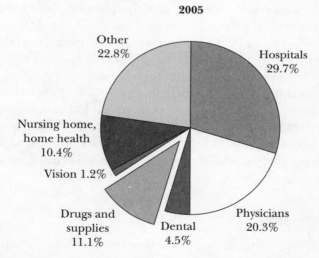

2005

Other
22.8%

Hospitals
29.7%

Nursing home,
home health
10.4%

Vision 1.2%

Drugs and
supplies
11.1%

Dental
4.5%

Physicians
20.3%

Sources: Health Care Financing Administration, 1999; authors' estimates.

Exhibit 1.1. Trends Converging to Create Consumer-Driven Health Care.

- Growth in direct-to-consumer marketing of medical technology, drugs, and services
- Rejection by consumers of loss of choice
- Trend toward defined-contribution models, vouchers, and MSAs
- Growth of CAM
- Changes in demographics
- Growth in discretionary spending
- Increase in Internet access and in the use of health-related Web sites
- Resurgence of interest in self-care

Use of the Internet and Information Technology

In our view the development and application of IT will far exceed the general expectations of the late 1990s. Bill Gates (1999, p. xxii) predicted that "successful companies of the [first] decade [of the twenty-first century] will be the ones that use digital tools to reinvent the way they work. These companies will make decisions quickly, act efficiently, and directly touch their customers in positive ways." We believe Gates's prediction will come to pass.

For the first time, health care organizations are likely to invest more than 2 to 3 percent of net revenues in IT. The admonitions of health care futurists to spend more on these kinds of systems and on research and development will finally be heeded. Of course, the payoff from these investments will become more substantial by, and continue well beyond, 2005.

Expected Developments in Information Technology

Here is a sampling of possible future developments in the application of IT:

- *Internet.* By 2005 nearly every home will have Internet access via high-speed transmission. Although the number of health-related Web sites will increase, a handful of highly credible

Figure 1.6. Key Factors That Define Market Segments in Health Care.

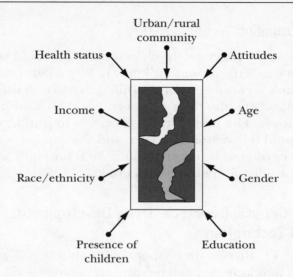

sites will dominate. Most medical groups of five or more physicians will have their own Web sites and will be linked to other clinical Web sites. Consumer e-mail communication with physicians will be routine.

- *Telehealth.* The potential for telehealth dreamed about in the late 1990s will become a reality by 2005. Remote monitoring of patients in their homes will be routine, reducing the need for home health visits.
- *Information systems.* The development of clinical and enterprise-wide information systems will accelerate. At least half of all hospitals and most large medical groups will have fully developed electronic medical records. At the same time, many consumers will assume ownership of their medical records, and new ventures offering medical record services directly to consumers will be common.

By 2005 many integrated systems, major hospitals, and large medical groups will be far along in developing a "digital nervous system" that provides real-time information for both clinical and management decision making.

Impact of Information Technology

The net effect of the expected developments in IT would be radical changes in medicine as we now know it. Physicians unable to invest in the new technologies or unwilling to learn to use them and incorporate them into their practices would be hard pressed to stay in business. The pressures on hospitals to purchase new technology would be greater than ever, and the gap between the kinds of services offered by inner-city and rural hospitals and tertiary care and academic centers would grow.

Advances in Genetic Research, Drug Development, and Medical Technology

In addition to IT, three other aspects of technology—genetic research, drug development, and medical technology—will have a major impact on the new health care marketplace.

Genetic Research

With the Human Genome Project completed ahead of schedule and several private ventures moving ahead rapidly, the results are likely to surprise the skeptics. "Personalized" medicine—the ability to target treatments and drugs to the needs of the individual—will become commonplace.

Drug Development

The rate at which new drugs are put on the market will be two to three times greater than in the late 1990s. Furthermore, claims by drug companies that these new therapies will reduce the need for many types of surgical interventions and cut the number of inpatient days in hospitals will prove to be correct. Advances in medications will reduce the need for some types of surgery (for example, coronary bypass surgery).

Drug company advertising directed at consumers will reach all-time highs. At the same time, we expect consumers to be pleased with the results they can achieve with these new drugs, especially in connection with the treatment of chronic illnesses and the substitution of drug therapies for some surgeries.

Spurred by the strong worldwide economy and their success in influencing consumers to insist on their name brand drugs, pharmaceutical companies will increase their spending on research and development. Better clinical information systems can be expected to reduce the incidence of errors in prescriptions, and patient compliance will improve.

Medical Technology

The growth of medical technology is accelerating and will continue to grow rapidly in the early part of the new millennium. Consumers will demand it and expect its benefits. We believe there will be at least two major breakthroughs as revolutionary as laparoscopic surgery or magnetic resonance imaging and hundreds—some say thousands—of smaller advances affecting every medical specialty. All of this will drive health care spending, and consumers will face the need to pay for access to the technology.

Who will decide which technology will be accessible to consumers and which will be restricted? In countries with national health care systems, it will be a public policy decision. We believe that in the United States these kinds of decisions will increasingly be made by consumers, based on the kinds of health plans they purchase and their willingness and ability to pay for the new technology out of their pockets. We do not believe any system of rationing access to demonstrably beneficial technology will be acceptable in the United States.

Shifts in Federal and State Policy

We expect Congress and the executive branch of the federal government to continue to provide limited financial relief to hospitals by continuing to relax some of the more onerous provisions of the Balanced Budget Act of 1997 (BBA). However, it is unlikely that

Medicare payments to physicians and hospitals will return to the levels of their heyday of 1990 to 1997, although reimbursement levels should be better than in 2000. In order to boost Medicare+ Choice, the Health Care Financing Administration is also likely to find ways to make payment to managed care organizations more attractive.

Passage of a patient's bill of rights mandating more benefits and of other legislation requiring certain HMO practices (such as longer lengths of stay for maternity cases) will have been accomplished by 2005. However, these new rules and regulations will be accompanied by added costs to employers and consumers; therefore, HMOs will be less competitive with PPOs. Of course, HMOs will continue to fight back with expanded information on clinical outcomes and other measures of the health status of members. There will be a continuing battle between those with quantitative data on health status, patient satisfaction, and clinical outcomes and those relying on anecdotal evidence.

We anticipate that medical groups and physician networks, including physician-hospital organizations and independent practice associations, will face continuing challenges regarding their pricing of services and other practices perceived as anticompetitive. In other words, the Federal Trade Commission and Justice Department will be actively seeking out physicians and medical groups that are colluding in pricing their services.

We do not anticipate universal coverage. However, given a continuing strong economy, the success of incremental reforms like the Children's Health Insurance Program (CHIPs) for children, increasing use of MSAs and individual insurance, and changes in eligibility allowing those between the ages of fifty-five and sixty-four to purchase Medicare coverage, the number of the uninsured is likely to drop to the range of thirty to thirty-five million by 2005. This is still high but a substantial improvement over forty-five million, the number of the uninsured in 2000.

Consolidation of Health Plans, Physicians, and Hospitals

The most noticeable consolidation will be among health plans. Start-up HMOs will find it even more difficult to succeed than in the 1990s, and many will either go out of business or be acquired.

But, contrary to conventional wisdom, we do not expect the total disappearance of provider-owned health plans that focus on local markets.

Physicians will continue to consolidate into larger groups, but the process will be slow and steady, not fast and spectacular. We do not anticipate a resurgence of physician practice management companies and their efforts to consolidate medical groups. Nevertheless, medical groups that are aggressive, long-term investors need capital, and they will combine with other medical groups, hospitals, or large integrated systems for that reason.

Hospital consolidation is likely to continue, but at a moderate pace. Because we do not expect the BBA to be as limiting as it was in its 1999–2000 form, we do not anticipate wholesale closure of hospitals, even in inner-city or rural areas.

Consumers will favor health care systems that already have regional or national brand name recognition or that develop a reputation for quality and cost-effectiveness. More emphasis will be placed on measuring and reporting clinical quality, which is more readily accomplished by larger groups of physicians; this will motivate physicians to consolidate. By contrast, gaining market clout with health plans will be a less important reason to consolidate than it has been in the past.

Changes in Payment Mechanisms

One of the key factors to watch over the next few years is how payment models change. Will employers continue their strong commitment to providing health benefits for employees and their families? Or, as many expect, will we move more toward a defined-contribution approach—paying a fixed amount per month to each employee and letting employees be responsible for purchasing their own health care benefits? What part will MSAs and vouchers play in health care financing? And will widespread use of individual insurance—an even more radical change—come to dominate? Figure 1.7 compares the degree of legislative change required against the level of consumer empowerment in the various payment models. A fully consumer-empowered future with individually purchased insurance would require the most substantial legislative change.

Figure 1.7. Continuum of Payment System Models.

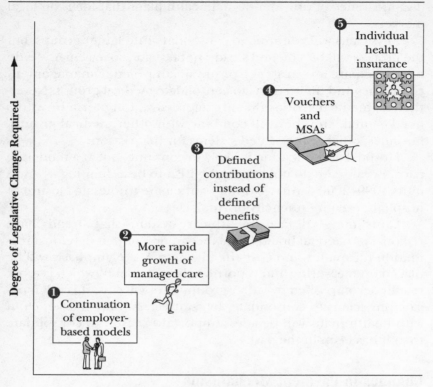

Degree of Individual Control and Responsibility ⟶

Four Health Care Scenarios

In our previous book *Beyond Managed Care* (Coddington, Fischer, Moore, and Clarke, 2000), we proposed four scenarios for the future: incremental change, constrained resources, technology dominant, and consumerism and technology (retail). Figure 1.8 lists the financial and marketplace factors used to define the four scenarios. Table 1.1 summarizes the characteristics of each scenario.

We believe that a combination of scenario 3 (technology dominant) and scenario 4 (retail) most accurately represents the likely

Figure 1.8. Four Scenarios for the Future.

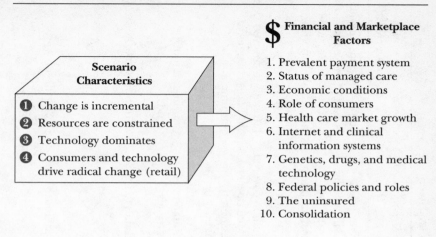

**$ Financial and Marketplace
Factors**

1. Prevalent payment system
2. Status of managed care
3. Economic conditions
4. Role of consumers
5. Health care market growth
6. Internet and clinical
   information systems
7. Genetics, drugs, and medical
   technology
8. Federal policies and roles
9. The uninsured
10. Consolidation

**Scenario
Characteristics**

❶ Change is incremental
❷ Resources are constrained
❸ Technology dominates
❹ Consumers and technology
    drive radical change (retail)

future of the new health care marketplace. Although most of the
rest of this book is based on the combination of these two scenarios, we do interject the implications of the other scenarios with regard to certain strategies.

Summary

Over the first five years of the new century, the health care market will grow more rapidly than at any time during the decade of
the 1990s and will reach $1.8 trillion by 2005. The ability of man-
aged care (as structured in the late 1990s) to slow the growth of
health care spending is suspect—the factors driving cost increases
are too powerful.

Major changes in the health care environment include five
aspects of technology: the Internet, clinical information system development, genetic research, new drugs, and advances in medical
technology. Other major changes include the aging of the population and the resulting growth in demand for medical products
and services (many of which relate to quality of life), continued
consolidation among medical groups, hospitals, and health plans,
and changes in the way consumers pay for their health care.

Table 1.1. Summary of the Four Scenarios.

Financial and Marketplace Factors	Scenario 1: Incremental Change	Scenario 2: Constrained Resources	Scenario 3: Technology Dominant	Scenario 4: Consumerism and Technology (Retail)
1. Prevalent payment system	Employer-based managed care with some increase in defined contribution	Defined contribution more prevalent; private pay shrinks	Wide variety of payment systems; Medicare pays full cost; private pay explodes	Employers phasing out as payers; move toward vouchers, MSAs, and individual insurance models
2. Status of managed care	100 million covered lives (one-third of population)	120 million covered lives; shift to HMOs and away from PPOs	110 million covered lives; Medicare moves aggressively to managed care	110 million covered lives; emphasis changes to consumers
3. Economic conditions	Continuation of 1990s trends	Recession; drop in equity markets	Continuation of 1990s trends	Continuation of 1990s trends
4. Role of consumers	Continues to grow	More emphasis on self-care; less discretionary spending on health care	Continues to grow	Consumers take control
5. Health care market growth	$1.8 trillion	$1.6 trillion	$1.9 trillion	$1.85 trillion

6. Internet and clinical information systems	Continuing investment in IT; growing use of Internet	Investment in IT slows; Internet use increases	Increased investment in IT; explosion in use of Internet	Pressures to show benefits from investment in IT; Internet use high
7. Genetics, drugs, and medical technology	Continuing progress; many new drugs	Slowdown in drug sales	Boom in gene therapy; new drugs and medical technology; rapid adoption	More selectivity by consumers in purchase of drugs and use of technology
8. Federal policies	Slight relaxing of BBA; focus on compliance; strong antitrust enforcement	No relaxation of BBA; added emphasis on corporate compliance	Significant relaxation of BBA to improve payment to hospitals	Medicare shifts to vouchers and premium support
9. The uninsured	55 million (18%)	60 to 65 million (20+%)	30 to 35 million (10+%)	20 to 25 million (less than 10%)
10. Consolidation	Trends of late 1990s slow accelerates	Physician and hospital consolidation accelerates	Health plan consolidation	Physician and hospital consolidation continues

In our judgment the potential changes in store for the U.S. health care system in the early years of the new millennium represent a fundamental market shift. Many of the old strategies and ways of managing will be outmoded, and successful health care organizations will undergo major transformations as they position themselves for the future.

Finally, consumers will increasingly take control of health care. The next four chapters in Part One, which discuss the value-added factors important to consumers, set the stage for the discussion of strategies in Part Two.

Chapter Two

Quality of Care and the Informed Consumer

*One thing we have found over the years is that consumers
don't really care about quality of care. They assume
quality and give more weight to services. Is this going
to change in the new health care marketplace?*
PHYSICIAN LEADER OF A LARGE INTEGRATED
HEALTH CARE SYSTEM

This chapter addresses two of the most important elements of
added value for consumers: the quality of the medical care they receive and the increasing flow of health-related information. We consider both present and future trends in these areas. A number of
forces are driving the public's growing interest in quality of care
and clinical information. In addition to the new wave of health
care information delivered by the Internet, HMOs have fueled consumers' concerns about health care quality. As Kassirer and Angell
(1997, preface) point out, "The spread of managed care, with its financial pressure to reduce costs, has caused widespread concern
that such pressure will lead physicians to skimp on care. Anecdotes
about patients who have received inadequate care in managed-care
settings fuel concern about this development."

We believe five basic questions will shape the national discussion over quality and determine essential health care strategies:

• What is quality, and how is it defined by different groups,
including consumers, employers, and physicians?

- How high is the quality of health care in the United States?
- What are some of the more advanced health care organizations doing to reduce clinical variation and improve quality of care?
- What are the existing barriers to improving quality of care?
- What role will consumers, who are becoming more demanding, play in improving quality of care, and what strategies must health care organizations adopt to serve these empowered consumers?

How Is Health Care Quality Defined?

The Institute of Medicine (IOM) defines *quality of care* as the "degree to which health services for individuals and populations increase the likelihood of desired health outcomes and are consistent with current professional knowledge" (Blumenthal, 1996, p. 892). We find this broad definition useful in understanding the multiple facets of quality, including population health and the involvement of the patient in decision making. By contrast, a discussion of the *quality of clinical care* might include the following definition: "The technical quality of care is thought to have two dimensions: the appropriateness of the services provided and the skill with which appropriate care is performed" (Blumenthal, 1996, p. 892).

Experts have struggled for years with alternative definitions of quality. A good deal of this challenge is attributable to the diverse stakeholders in the health care system. Perhaps the revised maxim "Quality is in the eye of the beholder" is most relevant today. As the health care environment continues to change, what does quality mean to the various stakeholders?

Physicians' Perspective

It is always interesting to ask physicians which of their colleagues in the community deliver the highest-quality medical care. They can almost always identify who, in their minds, are the best physicians.

How do physicians arrive at their conclusions? Discussions with nurses, anesthesiologists, and radiologists, their own observations, and feedback from patients shape their opinions. The credentials of physicians, including board certification, as well as their demeanor and how they conduct themselves at the hospital or in physician meetings, also factor into the evaluation.

Physicians have long understood that the "current professional knowledge" referenced in the IOM definition is a moving target—one that continues to change with the rapid advancement of medical science. Although universal agreement on the "state of the art" exists in some clinical fields, there are many areas where practitioners are far from unanimous. As such, variation in clinical practice is often considered part of the essential "art" of medicine.

When presented with data on variation at the local level, however, physicians often find the situation unsettling. Why are there local differences in areas of medicine where consensus has long been established? Why are there ongoing variations in training at medical schools and in residency programs? Frequently, comparative data are unavailable or simply ignored by physicians facing the time pressures of today's medical practice. Of greater concern is the defensive reflex of some physicians, who deny the need to change—often objecting that their "professionalism" is under attack from managed care.

Employers' Perspective

Employers look at quality differently. When American industry rushed to embrace quality tools to fend off foreign competition in the 1980s, many employers insisted that their suppliers—including health plans and provider groups—do the same. This was one of the driving forces behind many health care organizations' quality efforts in the late 1980s and early 1990s. Total quality management, continuous quality improvement (CQI), and quality teams proliferated in health systems at this time.

Meanwhile, employers such as Motorola employed advanced statistical process control tools, targeting six-sigma defect rates (or roughly three defects in ten thousand). From this perspective it is understandable that some employers were frustrated by the inability of health care to measure and demonstrate levels of quality approaching what had been achieved in industrial processes.

We believe that, in the final analysis, what most sophisticated employers are concerned about is ensuring their health care partners are applying systematic process improvement techniques. This process emphasis has had a beneficial effect on health care systems. Rather than trying to impress payers with their "excellent clinical outcomes," health care systems have viewed outcomes measurement as the critical feedback mechanism for clinical improvement.

The efforts of a few sophisticated employers and purchasing groups notwithstanding, the current focus among mainstream employers is on service levels and employee complaints. When asked about clinical outcomes in a focus group setting, the human resources manager of a two-thousand-employee firm told us, "When I think of quality of care, I think of the reports that we get from our HMO on utilization. Quite frankly, these reports aren't very understandable or helpful. I monitor the number of complaints we receive from employees about their treatment at certain hospitals and by certain medical groups. Even more important—how they were treated by the health plans we selected."

We believe the large employer purchasing coalitions will continue to contribute to advancements in quality measurement. However, the urgency of these endeavors will be less than before as employers shift more responsibility to employees through defined-contribution health benefits.

Consumers' Perspective

How do consumers evaluate health care quality? The anecdotal feedback from physicians and health care administrators has been nearly unanimous: most consumers assume a high level of clinical quality of care.

Our research with consumers of all ages from numerous focus groups and interviews confirms this relative disregard for clinical quality. Consumers tend to focus on access, convenience, service, staff friendliness, reputations, and cutting-edge technology rather than on clinical quality. The recent backlash against managed care, however, may be raising the importance of clinical quality in the public consciousness. Recent national news reports covering health care quality problems appear to be attracting attention to this issue. And consumers are reading published ratings of health plans and hospitals with greater attention.

In late 1999 the National Council on Quality Assurance announced the results of a study of health plan quality (Moore, 1999).

The report, based on results from its Health Plan Employer Data and Information Set (HEDIS) quality survey, reported for the first time a link between clinical quality and customer satisfaction. Although it is far from clear that one should assume causality from this finding, the results do raise interesting questions.

It is clear that in the future the quality of both nonclinical and clinical interactions will matter to health care consumers. But how and at what levels? We address potential responses to these new expectations later in this chapter. First, we examine the central question: How good is the quality of care Americans receive?

How High Is the Quality of Care in the United States?

John Wennberg, M.D., and his colleagues at Dartmouth Medical School continue to find significant regional variations in the health care delivery patterns of physicians and hospitals (The Center for the Evaluative Clinical Sciences, 1999). Variation exists in the incidence of common medical procedures, such as C-sections and prostate surgery. These variations occur from one community to another in towns of comparable size and demographic composition located in the same general region.

What is most disconcerting is that variation is often correlated with the number of physicians in a particular medical specialty practicing in these comparative communities or with the presence of hospitals that have various specialty areas and high-tech equipment. As an example, if one community has twice as many obstetrician gynecologists as another, the number of hysterectomies per thousand women could be as much as twice as high in the community with more obstetrician gynecologists.

Unexplained Clinical Variation

Unexplained clinical variation is the norm. Widespread clinical variation is present in procedures where there are generally accepted standards of care, including mammography screening, children's vaccinations, and post–heart attack medication. Experts believe many of these variations are attributable to differences in training among physicians, financial incentives (capitation versus fee-for-service payment), and the existence or lack of reminder systems in physicians' offices.

Report of the Institute of Medicine

The IOM report *To Err Is Human: Building a Safer Health System* (Kohn, Corrigan, and Donaldson, 2000) attributed forty-four thousand to ninety-eight thousand deaths per year in the United States to needless medical errors. Not surprisingly, the report created a furor and was front-page news.

This study brought quality of care to the forefront more than anything since the Clinton health care reform debates. It is clear that reduction of unexplained variation in clinical practice, and dismantling of the systems that support it, will be an ongoing focus of health care provider organizations, managed care plans, employers, the Health Care Financing Administration, and consumer groups. Here is an excerpt from a typical news story following the IOM study:

> Spurred by an Institute of Medicine report last month, big employers, healthcare organizations, state regulators and the federal government are stepping up pressure to revamp a healthcare system that calls itself the best in the world, yet hides and ignores mistakes that kill tens of thousands of patients a year.
>
> Executives of several large corporations, including General Motors and General Electric, formed an organization called "The Leapfrog Group." The group intends to encourage all employers to make safe medicine a top priority, and to steer workers to hospitals where the fewest mistakes occur [Kilborn, 1999].

The Leapfrog Group also includes two leading employer purchasing coalitions, the Pacific Business Group on Health and the Buyer's Health Care Action Group (BHCAG). The Leapfrog Group has set as its specific objectives the channeling of its employees to high-volume specialty centers for selected tertiary services (assuming higher volumes yield higher quality) and mandating of computerized order entry systems among providers to counter medication errors.

Dennis O'Leary (2000), president of the Joint Commission on Accreditation of Healthcare Organizations (JCAHO), characterized the issues of medical errors this way: "The fundamental need is for knowledge as to why medical errors occur. That knowledge will come from in-depth analyses of medical errors, beginning with the most serious occurrences. . . . These analyses must engage and be performed by those directly involved in caregiving. But that won't happen unless the caregivers involved feel safe—from blame and punishment—in participating. And organizations must feel safe in encouraging such participation. None of this, or any of the desired results of the IOM study, will happen without protective federal legislation."

Quality of Care in the United States: Summary

How high is the quality of care in the United States? Most physicians and other health care professionals would agree that even though the quality of care in the United States is the best in the world, there is plenty of room for improvement. This is true in both aspects of quality—the appropriateness of the care and the skill with which it is delivered. Many would also argue that quality problems are systemic and not necessarily related to the abilities of individual practitioners, echoing a view that is consistent with the quality movement efforts of many health care organizations.

Different Approaches to Improving Quality and Measuring Results

The organizations we have studied approach the matter of quality improvement and measurement in a variety of ways and with different motivations. Following are brief case studies of what four of the largest health care organizations in the country are doing to identify, improve, and measure the quality of care. All of these organizations believe that quality of care will become an increasingly important issue for consumers.

The Mayo Clinic

There had been continuous discussion among physicians at the Mayo Clinic about what was referred to as "the Mayo model of care," but the elements of this model had never been formally defined. In 1997 the clinical practice committee, one of the most powerful in the Mayo structure, appointed a work group to define the core elements of the Mayo model of care.

The work group interviewed ninety-two physicians and others at Mayo, and it conducted an extensive literature search. As a result of this research, the work group identified and prioritized the core elements, or attributes, that defined the Mayo model of care. Attributes of the Mayo model of care are shown in Exhibit 2.1 in two parts—patient care and the Mayo environment (or culture).

The Mayo model of care represents a comprehensive list of what consumers want from their health care provider in terms of quality. The track record of Mayo in providing this kind of quality—and the fact that Mayo cannot keep up with demand for its services—is further evidence that many consumers do in fact recognize and value quality.

In addition, Mayo has developed a number of clinical guidelines. There is also a strong cultural belief in evidence-based medicine. One physician leader told us, "This is where the real savings in health care will come. There is still tremendous variability in medicine, and we need to stay after it."

Dartmouth-Hitchcock Medical Center

The prestigious Dartmouth-Hitchcock Medical Center, based in Lebanon, New Hampshire, includes Dartmouth Medical School, Dartmouth-Hitchcock Clinic (comprising over six hundred physicians), and the 372-bed Mary Hitchcock Memorial Hospital. Dartmouth-Hitchcock is the site of significant research and educational programs aimed at improving quality and the delivery of health care.

The Center for the Evaluative Clinical Sciences (CECS), part of the Dartmouth Medical School, conducts cutting-edge research on critical medical and health issues with the goal of measuring, organizing, and improving the health care system. CECS offers a one-year master's degree program and had fifty-five students enrolled in early 2000. A focus of CECS is learning about the improvement of care. Paul Batalden, M.D., a national expert on health care process improvement, told us, "The basic idea is to dig deep into smaller systems to find out how processes can be improved." He said that within Dartmouth-Hitchcock, there are at least two hundred microsystems of care (interview, Jan. 2000).

Exhibit 2.1. The Mayo Model of Care.

The Mayo model of care is defined by high-quality, compassionate medical care delivered in a multispecialty, integrated academic institution. The primary focus, meeting the needs of the patient, is accomplished by embracing the following core elements (attributes) as the practice continues to evolve.

Patient Care

- Collegial, cooperative staff teamwork with multispecialty integration. A team of specialists is available and appropriately used.
- An unhurried examination, with time to listen to the patient.
- Physicians who take personal responsibility for directing patient care over time in partnership with local physicians.
- Highest-quality patient care provided with compassion and trust.
- Respect for the patient, family, and the patient's local physician.
- Comprehensive evaluation with timely, efficient assessment and treatment.
- Availability of the most advanced, innovative diagnostic and therapeutic technology and techniques.

The Mayo Environment

- Highest-quality staff, mentored in the culture of Mayo and valued for their contributions.
- Valued professional allied health staff with a strong work ethic, special expertise, and devotion to Mayo.
- A scholarly environment of research and education.
- Physician leadership.
- Integrated medical records with common support services for all outpatients and inpatients.
- Professional compensation that allows a focus on quality, not quantity.
- Unique professional dress, decorum, and facilities.

Source: Provided to authors by Mayo Clinic in December 1999.

MeritCare Health System

MeritCare Health System, formed by the merger of the Fargo Clinic and St. Luke's Hospital in 1993, reorganized in 1997 to improve its coordination and integration of care. A major benefit of this reorganization was improved quality.

Breaking Down "Silos"

According to Roger L. Gilbertson, M.D., president and CEO of Merit-Care, a number of problems with the governance and management structure flowed from the 1993 merger. "It was cumbersome," Gilbertson said, "and it created silos rather than clinical integration. It did not promote partnership and accountability between physicians and administrators. I became convinced of the need for more collaboration and standardization across departmental boundaries" (interview, Jan. 2000). The result was the creation of a matrix model that includes ten service lines, or "clinical aggregates" as they are called at MeritCare, each headed by a physician-administrator partnership.

Looking back on the reorganization, Gilbertson said, "We wanted to improve communications, better allocate resources, integrate physicians into accountable roles, speed up the decision-making process, and improve quality of care. There was too much of a 'we and they' attitude rather than 'us.'" One of the results of the new organizational structure has been a 25 percent reduction in the cost of heart services in just over two years. "Furthermore," Gilbertson added, "the quality went up, and mortality rates dropped. It was unbelievable" (interview, Jan. 2000).

Improving Care Through Clinical Guidelines and Disease Management

At MeritCare the emphasis on improving quality through better care processes, clinical guidelines, and outcomes measurement was linked with the development of disease management programs, especially in diabetes and congestive heart failure. Comprehensive guidelines for disease management were drawn up for depression, adult diabetes, cancer follow-up, carotid artery stenosis, congestive heart failure, upper gastrointestinal bleeding, tissue plasminogen activator use in stroke, transfusions, subarachnoid hemorrhage, and outpatient detoxification.

Bruce Pitts, M.D., executive partner in system/clinic support at MeritCare, noted that "when physicians realize that they can learn collectively, not just individually, it makes a big difference in the acceptance of quality improvement initiatives, guidelines, and outcomes measures." According to Pitts, outcomes measurement is an important area of emphasis at MeritCare. "It is better to benchmark against our own expectations than using outside standards," he affirmed. "We aren't doing this to impress people; we are seeking outcomes information in order to improve our practices here at MeritCare" (interview, Jan. 2000).

Park Nicollet Health Services

Park Nicollet Health Services, the result of a 1994 merger of the four-hundred-physician Park Nicollet Clinic and 426-bed Methodist Hospital in Minneapolis, has forty to fifty clinical guidelines, mostly relating to ambulatory procedures.

The average length of stay at Methodist Hospital has decreased from 4.4 days to 4.0 days over the past few years, and the readmission rate has been flat. Thomas Schmidt, M.D., associate medical director for quality/managed care, said, "We are focusing on the top twenty DRGs [diagnostic-related groups] on a physician-by-physician basis to see if we can improve quality and cut costs" (interview, Jan. 2000).

At Park Nicollet Health Services, what was called "CQI" in the mid-1990s is now referred to as "rapid cycle improvement." Examples of rapid cycle improvements include instituting hand-washing procedures, reducing adverse drug reactions, and increasing patient access to care.

Common Themes in the War on Clinical Variation

Despite considerable effort by many health care systems, the development and implementation of clinical guidelines has not achieved the expectations of five years ago. A number of systems have shifted their emphasis from big-ticket guidelines (such as those for open-heart surgery) to a limited number of guidelines that deal primarily with chronic illnesses like diabetes and congestive heart failure. These systems are merging the guidelines into the implementation of disease management programs.

Although the approaches to clinical process improvement vary widely among the four large systems just discussed, it is encouraging to find strong continuing interest in improving quality. These efforts to improve quality are occurring in the face of unsupportive physician and hospital reimbursement systems—fee-for-service payments that reward providers for providing more services. Nevertheless, these organizations are continuing to find ways to improve quality because they believe that patients do care and that it is the right thing to do.

Barriers to Improving Quality of Care

There are several barriers standing in the way of efforts to improve quality and implement systems of quality measurement.

The Assumption That Quality Is High

One of the reasons that efforts to measure and improve quality have lagged is that, as we discussed earlier, many consumers assume the quality of care is high. It is only when reports detailing the number of deaths due to medical and drug errors, like the one published by the IOM, come out that public confidence is shaken. Many physicians also assume that the quality of care they and their colleagues deliver is high, and for the most part it is. However, even error rates in the 2 to 3 percent range may no longer be acceptable.

Mixed Financial Incentives

Current systems of provider reimbursement represent another barrier to quality efforts. Capitated payment was a spur to the development of clinical process improvement, including clinical guidelines and their feedback mechanism, outcomes measurement. As capitation has stalled, the traditional fee-for-service payment system has not provided financial incentives for improving quality and reducing costs. One of the challenges for health care is to replace capitated payment with other financial incentives—incentives other than the fear of medical malpractice—in order to drive quality initiatives.

Differences in Training

The head of quality of a large integrated system in the southwestern United States told us that the three hundred physicians in the system were trained in over 150 different medical schools and graduate programs, including several in foreign countries. "They all come here with different ways of doing things," this director of quality assurance told us, "and this is understandable. However, by creating our own in-house university, we hope to introduce and sustain more consistency in the way we practice. We also have the opportunity to provide physicians with more evidence-based medical practice guidelines for many different chronic diseases and other common medical procedures."

Fragmentation of Physicians' Practices

Although there continues to be substantial consolidation among physicians and small group practices, many physicians are still in solo practices and small single-specialty groups. In many parts of the country, especially rural areas, this is the only feasible way for physicians to be organized. It is generally agreed, however, that for many medical procedures, quantity and quality go together. Therefore the low-volume heart programs (fewer than 150 coronary bypass surgeries a year) in some hospitals do not produce the same high-quality outcomes as the larger programs. Other medical specialties, such as orthopedics, neurosciences, and oncology, also appear to produce better quality when physicians are organized in larger single-specialty or multispecialty groups.

In a future where the ability to produce studies of clinical outcomes and measurements of patient satisfaction will be more important, larger groups are more likely to have the numbers of patients and the infrastructure to produce the necessary data. This should lead to more satisfied consumers and competitive advantage.

Resistance to Change

Physicians are no different from any other professionals when it comes to resisting new approaches. To date, efforts at developing and implementing clinical guidelines have achieved mixed results, and many large organizations have backed off.

Allan Kortz, a recently retired surgeon who writes about quality of care, identified several reasons for physicians' resistance to clinical guidelines and other efforts to change practice patterns. "We physicians have tended to be reluctant to accept the concept of practice guidelines," Kortz explained. "Perhaps this reluctance relates to our personal prejudice in favor of the therapeutic methods in which we have confidence. Furthermore, practice guidelines are often developed elsewhere and are imposed upon physicians, who understandably balk at acceptance. Lastly, guidelines may be misinterpreted as standards, either by those promulgating the guidelines or by those who are asked to accept them" (interview, Mar. 2000).

How do you overcome resistance to clinical guidelines or other efforts to change practice patterns? Many physician leaders tell us that the secret is to show physicians—with hard data—that certain surgical techniques or drugs yield better results. One physician told us, "Physicians will pay attention when they are presented data in a nonthreatening way. Most doctors don't want to be outliers. We can see immediate improvements in terms of reducing clinical variation just from collecting, analyzing, and distributing data."

High Cost of Quality Improvement

Many health systems have evaluated the costs of support staff and data collection, concluding that they cannot afford to continue intensive quality improvement and measurement efforts. At the same time, as we noted earlier, physicians paid on a fee-for-service basis have lacked financial incentives to make quality improvement initiatives a high priority.

In the early 1990s one prominent physician-led health system in the Southwest invested heavily in quality resources (thirty full-time-equivalent employees, including biostatistics, information systems expertise, and quality process facilitators). The system achieved significant quality breakthroughs—dramatic reductions in clinical variation in the areas of obstetrics, neonatology, and the treatment of heart disease, for example—only to divest itself of these resources when the system began losing money.

Quality pioneer W. Edwards Deming once commented that "quality is free," illustrating that reductions in unintended variation lead to less waste and enhance customer loyalty. In other words, when viewed in a broader perspective, the economic benefits of quality efforts—gaining patient loyalty and learning how to better use resources, including physicians' time—generally exceed the costs. But the financial payback is not immediate; investments must be made. And these investments are difficult to justify in times of belt tightening.

Lack of Accessible Data

The high cost and relatively slow pace of development of the electronic medical record (EMR) and central data repositories present barriers to the reduction of clinical variation. The cost of pulling data from conventional medical records is prohibitive, and the database that can be assembled from paper records is often of questionable accuracy.

One of the results of the lack of data at the medical practice or hospital level is the reliance on information provided by health plans. Although these databases are useful for some types of population-based measures of quality (such as inpatient admissions per thousand enrollees), they do not provide the kinds of information that physicians need to reduce clinical variation among physicians in a single practice or from practice to practice.

We believe that consumers will increasingly demand that their medical records be stored and available in digital form and will steer their business (and that of their aging parents) to those organizations that offer an EMR. Consumers in major metropolitan areas are unlikely to do business with medical groups or hospitals that do not have comprehensive EMR systems in operation.

Barriers to Quality Improvement: Summary

We believe that many of these barriers are coming down. For example, the continuing consolidation of physicians into larger single-specialty and multispecialty groups will encourage quality efforts. We also believe that despite the slow pace of IT adoption in the 1990s, we will see acceleration in the development of the EMR and central databases over the first five years of the new century. And, also important, much has been learned about quality and process improvement over the last two decades. We believe that given an increasingly informed and demanding public (described in the section that follows), these barriers will yield to progress at innovative health systems.

The Role of Consumers in Improving Quality

Health care leadership may be tempted to dismiss quality as they consider investment priorities. Some health systems were discouraged when early, unfocused quality investments produced few tangible payoffs. However, we believe that, in light of growing consumer awareness, health systems that ignore quality do so at their own peril.

A recent study cast light on this growing public awareness. According to a news poll conducted by the Kaiser Family Foundation and the Harvard School of Public Health, 51 percent of the American public followed the IOM report on medical errors. That compares with 56 percent who followed the World Trade Organization riots in Seattle in November 1999 (Moore, 2000).

If managed care–induced patient's rights legislation sparked public awareness, the medical errors issue only added fuel to the fire. It only takes one publicized medical error (most always attributable to undefined or uncontrolled processes) to create a public relations crisis.

Quality Report Cards and New Channels of Health Quality Information

The HEDIS measurement tool has become the industry standard for reporting health care quality to purchasers. Included in this "report card" are more than fifty indicators, primarily related to health plan providers' rate of screening and prevention practices. The criticisms of this tool are similar to those of other report card–type approaches.

Robert Kuttner (1998), writing in the *New England Journal of Medicine,* expresses the concern that HEDIS indicators have focused on *processes*—most notably prevention and diagnostic screens—rather than on *outcomes.* "Although the system as a whole needs to stress prevention," Kuttner says, "what consumers most need to know about a health plan is how it will perform if they become seriously ill" (p. 1562).

A number of employer purchaser groups became interested in quality report cards in the early 1990s, rating providers to influence health care purchasing. These ratings usually relied on publicly available outcomes data and existing indicators, such as those contained in HEDIS. The impact of these report cards has been mixed—primarily for two reasons. First, with health care inflation exceeding double digits, employers have been far more interested in costs than in quality. Only 11 percent of fifteen hundred employers surveyed in a recent study relied on quality data in selecting health plans. Second, ratings systems have had limited impact because of the limited role of employee choice. An estimated 47 percent of employees in large companies, and 80 percent in small firms, have no choice among health plans (Bodenheimer, 1999a).

Other report card experiments were those initiated by state health departments in the early 1990s, which studied outcomes of selected specialty procedures. A project begun in 1992, Pennsylvania's *Guide to Coronary Artery Bypass* (Pennsylvania Health Care Cost Containment Council, 1992), documented risk-adjusted mortality rates for all hospitals and surgeons with open-heart surgery programs. The result was that market share remained unchanged. Likewise, the New York Department of Health found that the publication of similar cardiac surgery data resulted in no market share movement among consumers toward programs with lower mortality rates (Schneider and Epstein, 1996; Chassin, Hannan, and De-Buono, 1996).

Despite the mixed results of the past, we believe consumer attention to quality information is now increasing. In Minneapolis–Saint Paul employees have begun to pay attention to the ratings of various care systems as provided by BHCAG. Although the number of employees engaged in the BHCAG experiment is limited, early evidence indicates quality seems to be influencing provider selection.

A handful of health care systems are publishing their own report cards to advertise their quality improvement efforts. Memorial Health Services, a five-hospital system in Los Angeles and Orange Counties, has begun publishing mortality rates for prenatal, maternity, and neonatal care, as well as survival rates for heart attack victims and long-term cancer patients (Weber, 1997).

The for-profit sector is now trying to tap growing public interest in comparative quality data. HealthGrades.com, sponsored by the publicly traded Specialty Care Network, rates all U.S. hospitals' performance by product line. Using mortality data reported annually by hospitals to Medicare, HealthGrades.com rates providers on a five-star scale for cardiac surgery, cardiology, orthopedic surgery, back and neck surgery, pulmonary and respiratory treatment, vascular surgery, and obstetrics. The site also hopes to include dentistry, ambulatory surgery, long-term care, and home health (Morrissey, 1999).

We believe that choice-empowered employees will be reading quality report cards with increasing attention and that these tools will establish a minimum "price of entry" for health systems. However, we believe the real value consumers are looking for goes far beyond the reporting indicators included in quality report cards to more fundamental quality efforts.

Impact of the Informed Consumer

The widespread availability of health care information has resulted in an increasingly informed consumer. This is manifesting itself in new demands on physicians. One physician in Minneapolis–Saint Paul told us about his eleven-year-old son who needed surgery to repair a hernia: "On his own, he went on the Internet and studied up on hernias. My son had me ask the surgeon in our health plan how many similar surgeries he had performed. Believe me, both my son and the surgeon were well prepared. If the surgeon hadn't given the right answers, my son would have insisted that we look elsewhere."

Robert Parker, M.D., former CEO of the Carle Clinic in Urbana, Illinois, told us that health care is entering what he refers to as a "knowledge-rich environment." He said, "In this type of environment, the gaps in knowledge between physicians and patients are tremendously reduced compared with what they have been in the past." He illustrated his point by referring to a telephone call from a patient concerning potential heart problems associated with a prescription drug:

> This patient called me at home about 7:30 P.M. Monday night after I had spent most of the day seeing patients. She asked me if I had seen the evening news that mentioned a new study that showed the possible link between the prescription she was on and heart dis-

ease. She also mentioned that there was an article in the local paper. Without hanging up, I asked my wife to find me the newspaper article. After reading through the article quickly, I told the patient I would call her back.

I got on the Internet and found that the latest research on the impacts of this drug took place in late 1999, and the results showed no side effects. I also found out that the manufacturer of the drug was mailing out a notice to physicians that same day, but I hadn't received my copy.

I called the patient back and told her that based on what I had found, I couldn't see any problems, but I would get back to her after I received the drug company information. I received the drug company letter on Thursday, and it indicated that there were no side effects. I called the patient again to reassure her [interview, Feb. 2000].

Parker's point in recounting this story was that he spent one and a half hours on this matter and received no reimbursement. "She was right in being concerned and to call," he said. "I would have done the same thing. This is what I mean by learning to work in a knowledge-rich environment. We have only seen the tip of the iceberg" (interview, Feb. 2000).

Donald Berwick, M.D., president of the Institute for Healthcare Improvement, sees great opportunity for quality improvement in this new environment through enhanced customer relationships. This new type of relationship—or "total relationship," as he calls it—is based on the flow of health care information to collaborate with and ultimately empower the consumer. This information, which flows both to and from the consumer, allows for greater consumer control through education and self-care, enabling consumers to fulfill in their health care the same need for control and self-mastery that they have in other aspects of their lives (Berwick, 1997).

How will this approach affect quality? Larry Staker, an internist practicing at Intermountain Health Care's LDS Hospital in Salt Lake City, is teaching diabetic patients how to keep statistical control charts of their blood sugar levels and how to adjust their insulin on their own. Results are positive: patients have achieved better control than when physicians were involved (Berwick, 1997).

Berwick also sees the opportunity for health care providers to shape the demand for services—not only through managing costs but also through managing quality. As consumers grapple with the glut of health care information available to them (some helpful but much of it bad), providers can cut through the misinformation to influence consumer behavior. For example, research has shown excessive use of fetal monitoring can raise the C-section rate unnecessarily. Realizing the payoffs of quality improvement, however, will require deliberate campaigns to influence consumer and physician behavior. And most health systems have yet to begin this important work (Berwick, 1997).

We believe tomorrow's successful health systems will be in direct dialogue with the consumer—including an ongoing exchange of information—to create lasting relationships. This new information flow to and from patients, in combination with enhanced information exchange among providers, will define new levels of quality.

New Issues for Physicians and Payers

The fast-changing role of medical information in the hands of consumers creates many new issues for physicians. For example, how will physicians be paid for the extra time it takes to read and absorb thirty or forty pages of material on a specific disease and discuss their conclusions with patients?

Physicians at Kaiser Permanente, Sutter Medical Group, and other health systems are addressing some of these issues through group visits for patients with common medical conditions. Some health systems are using "drop-in group medical appointments." These sessions include up to fifteen patients with chronic medical conditions. The ninety-minute sessions, where a physician, a nurse, and often a health behavioralist are present, begin with socializing among patients, which creates a valuable support network. Later in the session, providers have ample time to discuss treatment alternatives and answer questions posed by the group—much more time than available in individual appointments (Thompson, 2000). This format is just one example of an innovation that will enhance the quality of interaction with patients.

Impact of Consumers on Health Care Quality: Summary

We believe consumers, more than any other force, will speed up quality improvement in health care. Those physicians who do not like having their diagnoses and decisions challenged by managed care plans have not seen anything yet. Health care providers will need to be prepared for the new breed of informed patients, who will insist on being involved in decisions affecting their medical care. Although some physicians are disturbed by this prospect, one very senior surgeon sees this as an opportunity. He says, "I like working with patients who have taken the time to become informed and are interested in working with me as a partner in solving their medical problems. I never did like the fact that many patients placed me on a pedestal; I don't think that builds a healthy physician-patient relationship."

Quality of Care and Clinical Information as Measures of Value for Consumers: Conclusions

We conclude that there is plenty of room for improvement in the quality of care. Although the United States arguably has the highest quality of medical care in the world, it cannot be denied that despite the growth of clinical guidelines and process improvement, a tremendous amount of unexplained clinical variation persists. We suspect that among the biggest barriers to quality improvement are the ongoing absence of an EMR and the slow development of databases for outcomes analysis. In addition, continuing fragmentation of the medical community will make it difficult to gather systematic information, analyze clinical processes, and measure improvement.

Progress will be slowed by shifting financial incentives, such as the movement away from capitation and toward fee-for-service payment. At the same time, increasingly informed consumers will continue to reshape the way health care is delivered. Changes over the next five years will be dramatic. These changes will lead to a reevaluation of the way physicians are paid for the time spent with patients.

Successful health systems will learn how to manage these fundamental changes and to enhance quality. Those who build on quality principles to create more meaningful customer relationships—through enhanced information access, increased patient control, and improved consumer understanding—will achieve positions of market leadership.

Chapter Three

Service, Convenience, and Access

The Baby Boomers are coming, and they want change. If we don't partner with them, they will run over us. RUSSELL RICCI, M.D., GENERAL MANAGER, GLOBAL HEALTHCARE, IBM, Symposium on E-Healthcare Strategies for Physicians, Hospitals & Integrated Systems, February 2000

It is safe to say that over the next five years consumers will demand that their health care system be substantially more responsive to their needs than it is today. This includes convenience, access, and dramatically improved service. A physician leader of a large health care system in a southwestern state agrees. "Physicians need to come to grips with the fact that they are no longer the center of the universe," this physician leader said. "Patients are becoming more knowledgeable, and physicians need to become more service oriented. We find that patients are accessing the Internet for information on the quality of various medical groups and health plans, and they are especially interested in the results of patient satisfaction surveys."

A study by the Institute for the Future (1998) documented what we all know: consumers rate health care services poorly. For example, other than pharmaceutical companies and alternative medicine providers, health care generally received a rating of 2 out of 10 points. "But," the study says, "change is happening fast—by 2001 that score will climb to 5, and by 2005 to 7. Big improvements will be seen in the consumer-friendliness of services to the chronically ill, routine care and long-term care." We agree with this conclusion.

Changing Consumer Expectations of Their Health Care Providers

The CEO of a university-based health system told us that he believes service is becoming more important to patients than quality as they attempt to differentiate among various hospitals and medical groups. The CEO explained:

> People are at the point where they view the quality of health care as a commodity. When they visit a physician or come into a hospital, they expect to be healed. It is like going on a commercial flight—they expect the pilot to be competent and the plane to be in excellent condition. Travelers are not surprised or amazed when they make their destination. . . . By way of contrast, consumers are amazed at excellent service in health care. They are amazed when they don't have to wait to see a physician. They will be amazed when they have access to their medical record. The opportunities for impressing consumers with superior service are infinite.

Kurt Miller, a health services partner at Anderson Consulting, notes that health care will be subject to the same consumer pressures experienced by other industries. "Most executives will tell you," Miller (1999, p. 7) says, "that responsiveness to consumer demand is vital to success in their industries. Professional conferences, articles, and advertisements for services from healthcare plans to auto tune-ups proclaim the consumer as king. But down on the ground, as end-users find their expectations at significant variance from their experience, consumer demand is growing stronger and more strident." Miller goes on to note that this is particularly true for health care, "an industry in which consumers are emerging as extremely powerful customers. They want more from their providers, they are demanding and getting more choice in terms of plans and options, and they are making more informed choices" (p. 7).

Mary Hassett and Michael Rybarski, two professional marketers serving the health care industry, note that the parents of baby boomers tend "to respect medical authority and tolerate the inconveniences of the health care status quo (although this is beginning to change)" (Hassett and Rybarski, 1999, p. 2). However, as Hassett and Rybarski also explain, the baby boomers themselves are the future catalysts of change: "Enter boomer caregivers: predominantly well-educated, informed, working women, sandwiched between the stressful demands of their children and their parents—while already spread thin by the unrelenting expectations of their own self-actualizing generation. These assertive boomer caregivers will shake the system by their sheer size and the seismographic shock of their emerging dissatisfaction with their parents' healthcare experiences" (p. 2).

These baby boomers are looking ahead to their own potential health care needs. As they consider the future, they "expect healthcare to change to accommodate them. And why wouldn't they? Everything they have ever touched has changed to meet their needs. Boomers expect to live well longer and will demand a health system that supports their perspectives and preferences" (Hassett and Rybarski, 1999, p. 2).

We agree with these health care industry observers. Consumers are increasingly calling the shots in health care, and in the next few years their demands will lead to unprecedented change. The new consumers will not accept inconvenience in location or hours, and they will demand service that exceeds anything now offered by even the most patient-friendly health care systems.

What Do We Mean by Convenience, Service, and Access?

It is important to define in some detail, at the outset, what we mean by *convenience, access,* and *service* in health care.

Convenience

Convenience includes the availability of parking and the hours a physician's office is open for patients. It takes into account whether patients can receive services on the weekend or late in the evening. It also relates to patients' ability to receive health care services when they are traveling, even overseas. It is likely to include access to physicians via e-mail. For working women the inconvenience of taking half a day of work off to bring a child in for a routine appointment is a serious matter. One observer points out that "Americans really do crave convenience—yet the healthcare system just doesn't seem to get it. After all, an industry that labels its consumers 'patients' is clearly off to a bad start in factoring in convenience as a prime attribute of its services" (Herzlinger, 1997, p. 16).

Physician Bonding

One of the traditional physician-bonding strategies has been to build medical office buildings adjacent to the hospital in order to attract and retain physicians. The conventional wisdom of the 1980s went something like this: "Physicians are our best customers, and we need to make it convenient for them. They can make or break us." However, physician bonding works against *consumer* convenience.

The focus on physicians as customers is probably one of the most difficult impediments to overcome. As long as this attitude prevails, it is almost impossible to shift the focus to consumers and their best interests. As one hospital administrator told us, "You can say what you want about the growing importance of consumers, but the lifeblood of this hospital is its medical staff. If they don't want to work here, we might as well hang it up because we won't make it. So if I want to keep my job and the hospital is going to survive, I have to focus on physicians as my number one priority."

In a fee-for-service environment with solo practitioners and small medical groups, it is difficult to argue against the views of this hospital administrator. However, the trends of physician consolidation and medical group expansion are continuing. Physicians are being forced to look at the market, and this often means new locations.

Hours of Service

We remember well the hospital that lamented poor use of its mammography unit. "We have been disappointed in the number of women who have come in. The number of patients is falling well below our projections," said the associate administrator in charge of women's services. The unit was open from 9:00 A.M. to 4:30 P.M. Monday through Friday.

Several of the women who participated in a focus group on the mammography issue had a different perspective. One forty-three-year-old working mother said, "I know I need to go in for a mammogram periodically, but I hate to take off half a day of work just to have this test. I have to take time off fairly often for the kids, and that's my top priority." Others in the group echoed these sentiments with questions such as, "Can't the mammography center find a way to be more convenient?" The response of the associate administrator of the hospital was, "It is hard to find staff who are willing to work odd hours." So the impasse continued.

Service

We have noted over the years that when human resources (HR) executives or CEOs of major employers talk about health care quality, they almost always discuss service deficiencies. We hear comments such as "The reports we receive from our health plan almost always contain errors" or "We can't figure out what we paid for in terms of medical services for one of our employees who had open-heart surgery."

HR officers are often the ones who talk to employees when there is a problem with the health care system. One HR executive told us, "Most of the complaints from a visit to a physician's office relate to the way the employee or family member was treated or the long delays associated with a routine visit."

Given this background, it is not surprising that of the various measures of quality and service, patient satisfaction surveys tend to carry the most weight. This shocks and disappoints many physicians, particularly those who pride themselves on the clinical quality of care they believe they deliver to their patients. Yet, at the Henry Ford Health System in Detroit and BHCAG in Minneapolis–Saint Paul, for instance, patient satisfaction surveys are generating highly useful results in terms of consumer decision making and in terms of working with physicians and their staffs to improve service. Figure 3.1 gives a few examples of the kinds of health care service improvements that consumers desire.

Access

By *access* we mean primarily the ability to obtain medical services on a timely basis. When we discuss patient access in this context, we are not referring to a payment source for the uninsured. Coverage for

**Figure 3.1. Kinds of Service Improvements
That Consumers Desire.**

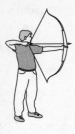

- Readily available appointments
- Fast turnaround of tests
- User-friendly systems
- Short waiting times
- Expanded choice
- Respectful treatment
- Personal service
- Telephone or Internet contact rather than personal visits
- Easy access to their personal physician
- Minimized paperwork

the uninsured is a critically important public policy issue that we analyzed in *Beyond Managed Care* (Coddington, Fischer, Moore, and Clarke, 2000).

Access is an especially important problem in rural areas where there are shortages of physicians. Whereas in most rural areas it is common to wait several days for an appointment, for patients of MeritCare in North Dakota and northwestern Minnesota, this is changing. MeritCare is implementing a program that guarantees patients access to primary care physicians on the same day they seek services. This means that patients in a predominantly rural area will have almost immediate access to primary care physicians.

Many large multispecialty clinics and integrated systems, especially those operating in more advanced managed care environments, provide walk-in clinics or after-hours care. From what we have seen, these types of clinics are extremely busy. Consumers, especially men, appreciate the convenience of being able to drop in without an appointment.

Marshfield Clinic: A Case Study in Access and Convenience

When we visited Marshfield Clinic in central Wisconsin, we were struck by something unusual: the best parking places near the entrance to the clinic were reserved for patients. Discussing this with us, Fritz Wenzel, executive director at the time, explained, "Physicians park in the remote lots. There is a shuttle bus, or they can walk." When asked who made this decision, Wenzel responded, "The doctors. They run this place, and they thought it was not only the right thing to do but also good business. It sends a signal that we care about our patients" (interview, Apr. 1993).

Regional Network of Care Centers

Marshfield Clinic is a multispecialty clinic with over five hundred physicians, located in the town of Marshfield (population twenty thousand, about thirty minutes southwest of Wausau). Marshfield also has thirty-nine regional centers, located within a two-hour driving distance. (In 1993, by comparison, Marshfield had twenty-two regional centers.) Most of these centers are in small communities and are staffed by family practice and other primary care physicians. Some of the larger centers have specialists. Figure 3.2 shows the location of Marshfield Clinic and its regional centers.

Marshfield is not unique among large integrated systems. Many other clinics and hospital-led integrated systems have impressive primary care networks. For example, Geisinger has sixty-nine care sites in its seventeen-county service area in Pennsylvania. MeritCare has thirty-four sites in North Dakota and Minnesota. Scott & White has twenty locations, many in smaller communities in central Texas.

Regional Outreach by Specialists

Marshfield has made a conscious effort over the past few years to send its specialists out to care for patients at the regional centers. In some cases a cardiologist might spend one day a month visiting a regional center. Consumers highly value this outreach.

Other Examples of Physician and Hospital Outreach

Marshfield is not the only example of a health care system that has regional primary care centers and that sends specialists to remote locations on a regular basis. We have observed numerous examples of effective outreach networks in many parts of the United States— from Hays, Kansas, to northern Maine. Physicians based in Hays, for example, regularly provide medical services to twenty small communities, some as many as 125 miles from Hays.

Figure 3.2. Marshfield Clinic and Regional Centers, 2000.

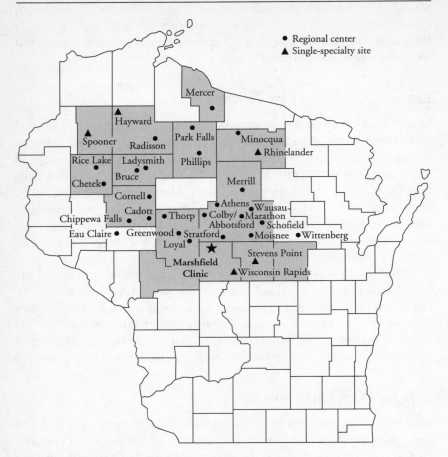

Source: Marshfield Clinic, February 2000.

Fort Kent

While visiting Fort Kent on the northern tip of Maine, right on the Saint John River and within a stone's throw of New Brunswick, we were pleasantly surprised to find that the local hospital hosts a number of specialists (in orthopedics and oncology, for example) from Presque Isle and other medical centers. People living in the Fort Kent area, especially those who are retired or work in the woods, appreciate the convenience of these kinds of medical services—particularly in the winter.

One resident of Fort Kent told us, "If we didn't have an unusually broad array of health care services for a community of our size, many of the senior citizens who live in the area would have to move somewhere else." Because retirees are a key element of the economy of Fort Kent, a community that struggles to maintain its economic base, the availability of specialty medical services is especially important and much appreciated.

Outreach: A Valued Consumer Benefit

Many of those critical of the U.S. health care system fail to appreciate the kinds of outreach efforts that exist in places like Hays and Fort Kent. Some of the motivation for providing outreach clinics in smaller communities is financial—it can help build a practice and fill a physician's schedule. But many of the physicians who provide these services do so because of the positive feedback they receive in smaller communities, especially from their older patients.

Resistance to Outreach: "Let the Customer Come to Me"

At the same time, we are aware of many other situations where physicians claim to be too busy to offer outreach services. One orthopedic surgeon told us, "I can make more money by staying in the office or working at the local hospital. The travel time to these small communities is not only a strain, but it cuts into my income." We know of numerous specialists who worked in outreach clinics when they were establishing their practices but who stopped their outreach efforts once they reached what they considered an adequate volume of patients (and revenue). Comments such as "I'm too busy to do it; it's not a good use of my time" are common.

Kaiser Permanente in Colorado

Kaiser Permanente (KP) in Colorado routinely rates high as one of the best HMOs in the country. Although, by the admission of its leaders, KP has a tremendous amount of room for improvement in the level of its services, this system is implementing several pioneering initiatives.

Improved Access Through an Enlarged Primary Care Network

In the mid-1980s KP planned to build its own hospital to serve its members in the Denver area. At about the time the ground breaking was scheduled, a Colorado Department of Health study showed that hospital bed capacity in the Denver area was in excess of any reasonable projection of future demand. The new $80 million hospital only would have added to the developing glut of inpatient beds.

As an alternative, KP entered into a long-term contract with the five-hundred-bed Saint Joseph Hospital and invested the funds that would have been used to build a hospital in building five new primary care offices instead. These were in addition to the four primary care offices KP already had. By 1999 KP had seventeen care sites in the Denver area; no subscriber lived more than a fifteen-minute drive from one of these clinics.

Improved Customer Service

Although some independent physicians and many others refer to KP as offering "military" or "production line" medicine, the organization has taken numerous steps to improve service. For example, KP guarantees that members can see a primary care physician the same day they call for an appointment.

Like many large systems, KP rigorously surveys patients after their visits to monitor their satisfaction. All physicians in the Permanente Medical Group receive a quarterly report evaluating their service from the patient's perspective. These reports contain suggestions for improvement.

Implementation of the Electronic Medical Record

KP of Colorado made a $160 million investment in developing an EMR. This is significant for members in that when they check in to any of the KP offices or call an advice nurse, their medical history is immediately available. Patients are also able to avoid the annoying pattern of having to respond to the same questions over and over, which patients in many health care settings are still asked to do—sometimes four or five times in a single day. A recent patient of the KP system described his experience this way: "I came in to see a rheumatologist. When he learned that I had recently had surgery, he pulled up and scanned [into a computer] the clinical notes and tests on the spot. Then he e-mailed the surgeon, asking for future lab results. I decided I was in very good hands!"

The EMR was operational in early 1999. KP is now one of a relatively small number of health care systems that are paperless. Kate Paul, a former KP executive, noted, "It has taken some time, but most physicians are very happy with the paperless system and have come to depend on its convenience. More important, we have had excellent feedback from our members."

Advice and Appointments

In its quest to provide ready access and service to its members and to be cost effective, KP has learned some hard lessons. KP's experience with centralizing one of its services, described here, is an example of one such lesson:

> The Colorado region centralized its advice and appointment system so members could call a single number day or night for advice and scheduling appointments. Prior to this change, members called their individual medical office for advice and another number for appointments.

> What KP found, however, was that telephone wait times increased, advice nurses were removed from the medical offices into a central facility, and they did not have direct contact with physicians and physician's assistants. An advice nurse could no longer walk down the hall to consult with a physician about a patient's case.

> After several months, physicians and administrators agreed that despite extensive investment in infrastructure and training, the system didn't work—it did not serve the members as well as the previous model.

As a consequence, KP moved advice nurses back to the medical offices, in close proximity to physicians. Members still call one number, but it is routed to their medical office for advice. Members might have to wait for a callback from their physician, but they are assured of getting that call within a prescribed time period.

Kaiser Permanente Online

Already in place in California, Kaiser Permanente Online (KP Online) is being rolled out in other markets. This system enables members to renew prescriptions electronically, communicate via e-mail with their personal physician and advice nurses, and make appointments on-line. KP plans to expand its range of on-line services to include consumer health information and educational materials. Ultimately, KP Online will allow patients to view portions of their medical record.

Beyond Service—to "Experience"

In their book *The Experience Economy*, B. Joseph Pine II and James H. Gilmore (1999) argue that the U.S. economy is moving beyond the provision of high-quality services to offering "experiences" to consumers. Here is the way they introduce the importance of experience:

> Consider Las Vegas, the experience capital of America (although Orlando, Los Angeles, Manhattan, and even Branson, Missouri, would win their share of votes in any poll). Virtually everything about Vegas is a designed experience, from the slot machines at the airport to the gambling casinos that line the Strip; from the themed hotels and restaurants to the singing, circus, and magic shows; and from the Forum Shops mall that recreates ancient Rome to the amusement parks, thrill rides, video arcades, and carnival-style games that attract the twentysomethings and give older parents a reason to bring their kids in tow [p. xi].

Pine and Gilmore devote an entire book to this proposition, and their arguments are compelling.

What does this have to do with health care? Most consumers who are forced to use the health care system would probably characterize it as an unpleasant experience. But is that the way it has to be? Dental offices have made great strides in improving the experience of having teeth cleaned and checked. Medical offices for cosmetic surgery try to create a pleasant experience by providing tasteful decor, extremely friendly office staff, cookies and coffee, computer imaging, and easy payment methods.

It is interesting to see how KP handles its annual flu shot programs. For three consecutive Saturday mornings in the fall, all offices are closed for all medical services except flu shots. Thousands of people show up at each office over a three-hour period. You are likely to run into old friends. The line moves quickly, and the whole experience has a festive atmosphere. With all of this the shot is less painful. You are through the line and out of the office in half an hour.

A visit to the Mayo Clinic for a physical is also a comparatively pleasant experience. Even though there are long waits for tests and for receiving test results, the entire experience is over in two days. There are thousands of patients around doing the same thing, and the atmosphere is upbeat. The nearby hotels are excellent and convenient. The assigned internal medicine physicians, who spend several hours with each patient, do their best to make it a pleasant experience.

The January–February 2000 issue of *Health Forum Journal* asked this question: What experience are you selling? In that issue Joe Flower (2000) argues that if a health care organization competes on the basis of price alone, it is dead. "The entire healthcare environment—people, architecture, technology, sounds, rules—makes up the healthcare experience," Flower says. "And that experience—whether healing or horrifying, exasperating or fulfilling—is the product we provide. It is not just a package of technological fixes" (p. 14).

Flower cites East Jefferson General Hospital in Metairie, Louisiana, as an example of a health care organization that has adopted an approach that considers the hospital to be a "theater" and the employees to be "actors" and "actresses." "If all of this seems Disney-fied," Flower writes, "it's no coincidence. East Jefferson has been sending employees to learn customer service at Disney University in Orlando for seven years. Some 30 percent of Disney's students come from healthcare, but East Jefferson seems to have learned better than most. In February 1997, The Walt Disney Company honored East Jefferson with its guest relations award, the 'Mouscar' (an Academy Awards take-off)—the first time the award has been given outside the Disney empire" (p. 14).

Has this raised East Jefferson's costs? The hospital claims it has not. East Jefferson also reports that employee turnover has dropped from 18 percent to 11 percent a year. (With tight labor markets in many parts of the country, a change like this can be especially important.) Moreover, the hospital's market share increased from 33 percent in 1993 to 40 percent in 1999 (Flower, 2000).

Conclusions

The good news for health care consumers is that the next few years will bring unprecedented improvements in service, convenience, and access. In all fairness to physicians and hospitals, there have been numerous service improvements over the past decade. However, we expect the changes of the past decade to pale in comparison with the "experiences" we expect over the first few years of the new millennium.

Here are some of the changes that consumers will value:

- *Recognition as valued customers.* This will be reflected in the courtesy and friendliness of staff in medical offices and hospitals.
- *Dramatically reduced waiting times and easier scheduling.* The hospitalist movement is helping to facilitate this by keeping many physicians in their offices rather than encouraging them to make hospital calls. Many medical groups will allow patients to schedule their own appointments on a Web site.
- *Longer hours of operation for offices and organizations providing medical services.* The hours can be expected to match the needs of consumers and not be dictated by what is convenient for physicians and their employees.
- *Reduction in the paperwork necessary for checking in to a physician's office or hospital.* Largely because of more widespread use of EMRs, when consumers arrive at physicians' offices or hospitals, they will be pleased to learn that the staff is already familiar with their case and medical background—that the staff "knows them."
- *Better access to health care information.* This will include consumers' ability to view medical records, and to retrieve health care information on specific diseases and care protocols, via

the Internet. On-line advice services will be accessible anytime, day or night.

- *Increasingly sophisticated and more widely distributed patient satisfaction surveys.* This type of survey will provide valuable feedback for providers and have a major impact on them. Consumers will benefit from having these surveys as a basis for comparison of multiple health care systems.
- *Identification of top-rated physicians and medical groups.* We are already hearing about "gold" groups being identified by some health plans. BHCAG in Minneapolis–Saint Paul periodically publishes reports that compare patient ratings and costs. These sorts of initiatives will proliferate in the consumer-dominated health care marketplace of the future.
- *More extensive use of e-mail and other technologies.* This will improve communication among physicians, their staff, and their patients.

This list barely scratches the surface of potential service enhancements in health care. But we could not possibly anticipate all of the improvements in service, convenience, and access that are likely to emerge in such a large—and increasingly innovative—industry.

Chapter Four

Affordability, Choice, and Personal Relationships

The conflict between the potential of medical science and the reality of limited dollars is permanent.
THOMAS BODENHEIMER, M.D., "The American Health Care System: Physicians and the Changing Medical Marketplace," *New England Journal of Medicine*, 1999

This chapter deals with three additional value-added factors: affordability, choice, and personal relationships between patients and providers. We add another important element to this mix—consumer accountability. By *accountability* we mean consumers being more financially accountable for the choices they make concerning which health care products and services they use.

"The demand for health care is insatiable," a former hospital CEO has often told us. The growth in demand for quality-of-life services over the past five years, and consumer expectations for more such services in the future, make his words seem prophetic. We believe it is inevitable, in this environment of continuously growing demand for more and better health care products and services, that consumers will be asked to pay an ever greater share of the cost of their health care—which is as it should be. This shift in health care spending in the United States will bring order to what many consider a dysfunctional health care system, in which patients typically pay little or nothing out of their pockets for the medical services they receive.

Affordability of health care has several different connotations. For families without health insurance coverage, affordability depends on whether or not they can pay the entire cost of medical services when they need them. For individuals and families who have health plan coverage or who are on Medicare or Medicaid, affordability refers to how much they have to pay in premiums, co-payments, and deductibles. Affordability also relates to whether or not consumers are likely to have the financial resources to pay for the new drugs, medical devices, and health services that are only partially covered, or not covered at all, by health plans or other payers. For example, even with an outpatient prescription drug benefit added to Medicare coverage, out-of-pocket costs would be substantial.

The following are four questions about affordability introduced and discussed in this chapter:

- What progress will be made in extending health insurance coverage to segments of the uninsured population?
- Will consumers have the financial resources to spend more on health care, especially on discretionary or quality-of-life medical services?
- Assuming the earnings and financial condition of most consumers remain strong, will they be willing to spend significant additional dollars on health-related services?
- What can health care providers, drug manufacturers, and others in health care do to improve the affordability of their products and services?

Health Plan Coverage for the Uninsured

Despite sustained economic growth and low unemployment, the number of the uninsured continued to rise in the 1990s and into 2000. Under an incremental change scenario (scenario 1 as described in Chapter One), we expect the number of uninsured to continue to increase by about one million a year during the first five years of the new millennium. In that case a growing proportion of the U.S. population would lack the financial resources to help purchase health care services. (It should be noted, however, that half of the uninsured have at least one employed person in the household.) But assuming a strong economy and an incremental approach to providing coverage (as in scenario 4, for example, adding coverage for children and for those between ages fifty-five and sixty-five), the number of the uninsured should decrease. This would mean more people would have the ability to pay for basic health-related services.

The implications of changes in the number of the uninsured are especially important for inner-city, urban, and teaching hospitals and for primary care physicians, many of whom have offices in lower-income areas (where the proportion of uninsured residents is typically high). But the problem is not limited to these kinds of areas. For example, one-quarter of the population of the San Diego metropolitan area was uninsured in late 1999 (Pappelbaum, 2000). Other large and prosperous metropolitan areas continue to have a high proportion of uninsured residents.

In summary, we believe that in scenarios 3 and 4 it is reasonable to expect progress in reducing the number of the uninsured. We project that in 2005 the uninsured population will be smaller than it was in 2000, perhaps as low as thirty to thirty-five million. If we are correct, several million Americans—mostly children, self-employed individuals, and early retirees—will have greatly expanded access to health care services. This will mean an increase in the number of Americans who can afford health care.

Ability to Pay

In the four-year period between 1996 and 2000, the proportion of the U.S. population we classify as having sufficient financial resources to be able to afford to pay more for health care increased from 63 percent to 69 percent. Furthermore, the proportion of Americans with the financial ability to pay more for their health care should increase steadily in a future characterized by much stronger consumerism and more advances in technology. We discussed consumerism and technology in *Beyond Managed Care* (Coddington, Fischer, Moore, and Clarke, 2000, Chapters Six, Seven, Eight, and Nine).

This trend of growing ability to pay leads to the next question we consider: Even if consumers have the financial resources, will they be willing to spend more on health care?

Willingness to Spend More for Health Care

In our judgment consumers will be willing to spend significantly more than they do currently on health-related products and services. What evidence do we have to support this opinion?

The rapid growth of cosmetic surgery, eye surgery, ultrafast heart imaging and other diagnostic testing, hearing aids, teeth whiteners, and a host of other health-related products and services indicates that consumers are willing to spend a great deal of money for products and services they believe are valuable. Consumers may be upset about small increases in copayments for office visits or prescriptions, but that does not stop many of them from spending thousands of dollars for big-ticket items. In the following paragraphs we offer several examples.

Corrective Eye Surgery

In early 2000 the average cost of laser surgery for vision correction was about $2,100 per eye. Unlike cataract surgery, which is reimbursed by Medicare and some health plans, most refractive eye surgery requires out-of-pocket payment by consumers. Is the high direct cost an important barrier?

Successful practices are overcoming this objection (the cost) by using a very consumer-oriented practice—financing options. An examination of current advertising for laser vision correction shows that the "$99-a-month" approach is working quite well (Dewey, 1999, p. 48).

By making financing available, physicians offering refractive surgery have been able to appeal to a broad market of twenty-five- to forty-five-year-old patients, many of whom are in middle-income, blue-collar occupations. The rapid growth of refractive eye surgery provides compelling evidence that consumers will pay for something as valuable as improved vision.

Complementary and Alternative Medicine

One study showed that of the two-thirds of Americans who want CAM coverage in their health plans, half are willing to pay extra for it. Merlin Olson, a principal at Deloitte & Touche, says, "Still, that's a significant finding for HMO's, because if 50 percent of subscribers are willing to pay for CAM services, then it can be a financially feasible option" (Daily, 1999, p. S6). The landmark studies by David Eisenberg, M.D., published in the *Journal of the American Medical Association* in 1993 and 1998, found that three-quarters of the money spent on complementary therapies was paid out of pocket (Baldwin, 1998).

On-Demand Laboratory Services

An article in *USA Today* reported that in Jacksonville, Florida, there is a medical lab called HealthScreen America, where aging baby boomers can stop in for a quick checkup. "No symptoms or doctor's referral required," the article explained. "In fact, most customers won't even see a doctor. Cash, checks and credit accepted" (Appleby, 2000, p. 1B).

Robert Aycox, a customer of HealthScreen, said, "I love my doctor, don't get me wrong. I just don't think the details the doctor would give me are as extensive as what I'll get here." Aycox paid $1,100 for a package of tests, plus special high-speed CT scans of his heart and lungs. The recent death of a friend, plus a family history of heart problems, prompted him to get tested (Appleby, 2000, p. 2B).

Chris and Fred Fey, the founders of HealthScreen, say that their program is for the masses. "But," the *USA Today* article noted, "to capture the high-end market as well, their centers offer 'luxury getaway' testing weekends. For $2,650, customers can have 25 health tests and spend three days at a Florida resort" (Appleby, 2000, p. 2B).

Preventive CT Scans

The *Wall Street Journal* reported that his fortieth birthday "prompted California attorney Joseph S. Schuchert to ponder the question that that milestone begs: How many years remain? Instead of just wondering, Mr. Schuchert took action. He underwent a full-body [CT] scan at an out-of-pocket cost of $695" (Spurgeon and Burton, 2000, p. A1). The article went on to say that the CT scan, designed to diagnose illness, is being used more and more by people who feel fine.

"Never mind," the article pointed out, "that insurance doesn't cover it on a preventive basis. The number of [CT] scans—which reached 26 million in 1997, the most recent year for which figures are available—has been rising by about a million a year, and a big chunk of that growth is coming from seemingly healthy Americans willing to fork over hundreds of dollars of their own money for it" (Spurgeon and Burton, 2000, p. A1).

Avoidance of Unpleasant Procedures

There is also evidence that consumers will pay significant dollars out of their pockets in order to avoid an unpleasant or painful procedure. The *Wall Street Journal,* for example, reported on the following new technique that is meant to make a medical procedure less unpleasant: "One 3-D application that shows huge promise but isn't refined enough for routine use is the 'virtual colonoscopy.' Without using a scope, it takes a picture of the colon that allows doctors to check for signs of cancer" (Gentry, 2000, p. B4).

According to the vice chair of the department of radiology and the New York University School of Medicine, when patients first heard about virtual colonoscopy, they clamored for it. Following a television program reporting that New York University was working on the test, the hospital had four hundred calls in a single day. "The test hasn't been fully proven, let alone approved for insurance, but patients wanted to cover the $300 cost themselves" (Gentry, 2000, p. B4). In our view this is not an isolated incident. Patients will increasingly be willing to pay for tests that provide high-quality results and are less painful.

One of the continuing challenges for health care marketers will be to determine how much consumers are willing to spend for quality-of-life products and services and for less unpleasant procedures, such as three-dimensional imaging in place of a regular colonoscopy. An understanding of what motivates consumers to pay for certain health care products and services is part of the new skills base required for market segmentation.

What Manufacturers and Health Care Providers Can Do to Make Their Products and Services More Affordable

Most health care providers are paying attention to their costs and searching for ways to improve the operational performance of their organizations. This is an especially high priority for hospital

CEOs, group practice administrators, physician leaders, and leaders of all other types of health care organizations. This brings us face to face with a difficult question: How much "fat" remains in the health care system?

In our view many health care organizations—those that have invested in massive development and implementation of IT or in improvements leading to reductions in clinical variation—have already cut most excess spending out of their budgets; there is not much more "fat" to trim. Furthermore, given a continuing strong economy, the cost of labor—the single largest expense item in most health care organizations—is likely to increase dramatically. Therefore, in our judgment, any expectation of significant reductions in the cost of health care products and services is unrealistic. Perhaps the best we can hope for is moderation in the rate of increase in unit prices, but even in that regard the outlook is not promising.

Despite this discouraging prognosis about the ability of health care organizations to reduce their expenses or put a cap on annual increases, we believe most Americans will be able to afford most of the health care they want. This, of course, depends on a continuing strong economy and no major shocks to the equity markets.

It will be a beneficial change for health care organizations to begin to think in terms of the value of their services for consumers rather than negotiating rates with health plans. As this change occurs, health care will begin to resemble other segments of the U.S. economy. Individuals and households will balance the value received against the costs they pay, not against the cost to third parties, such as their employer or Medicare.

Affordability: Conclusions

Although we are concerned about the issue of affordability, we believe that the dollars to pay for health care will be available as long as health care providers and suppliers continue to develop and offer innovative products and services that meet real needs.

Consider other industries. The cost of new cars is also high. However, after much soul searching and comparison shopping, most potential car buyers who initially experience "sticker shock" still ultimately purchase the vehicle of their choice. The same is true in housing. In many large metropolitan areas and other communities, the price of housing appears to be outrageous—yet there are purchasers.

Carrying the automobile analogy a step further, we expect to see an increasing number of health care providers arranging financing for their customers. Many plastic surgeons now do this for their cosmetic surgery patients, and they make it relatively painless. Automobile dealers have been doing it for years. In fact, it is sometimes difficult to get salespeople to discuss the price of a car; all they want to talk about is the monthly payment. Is this a preview of what we will see in health care in the new millennium? We believe it is.

In summary, paying a higher proportion of the cost of health care products and services will come as a cultural and economic shock to many consumers. However, we believe that consumers will adjust as long as the value of the services is apparent. This poses a new challenge for health care providers: looking at themselves through the eyes of their customers.

Consumer Choice, Control, and Accountability

Consumers want more choice and control over which health care providers they use and when they use them. They also want more involvement in decisions affecting their health and that of their family.

More Choice for Consumers

There are significant differences in the attitudes of consumers toward their health plans when they have a choice. When they can choose among health plans, they tend to select PPOs and other open-access plans that give them a greater ability to choose the physician and hospital they want.

A central theme of our previous book *Beyond Managed Care* (Coddington, Fischer, Moore, and Clarke, 2000), and of this book as well, is that consumers are becoming more informed and demanding and that they have higher expectations for the health care they need or want. Part of the reason for this is the increasingly important role of baby boomers as direct consumers of health care and as members of the "sandwich" generation (which refers to their involvement in the health care of both their parents and their children).

Consumers' desire for choice practically eliminates the option of health plans' controlling costs by reinstituting small panels of physicians and primary care gatekeepers. Health plans will have to find other ways of controlling rapidly increasing demand for health care products and services, such as more thorough retrospective review and the development of much more advanced clinical information systems. We are not optimistic that health plans and government payers will be successful in implementing other alternatives for containing costs.

If we move toward defined contributions and greater use of individual insurance, consumers will truly have choice in terms of their health plan and provider options. This is one reason that we give this scenario more credence than do many health care industry observers who believe individual insurance is too radical a departure from the present employer-dominated system.

Consumer Control and Involvement

The growing desire of consumers to be in control of their own health care, including prevention and wellness, is a related factor. This desire is evidenced by, among many other things, consumers' increasingly frequent use of CAM. In the future, consumers will be more involved with physicians in understanding treatment options and in selecting the best course of treatment for themselves and their family members.

Although they are not sure whether or how they will be reimbursed for accommodating consumers' desire to be more involved in their health care decisions, many physicians welcome this idea. One physician said, "How can you be opposed to the idea that consumers might become more knowledgeable and more responsible for their own care?"

Consumers' Financial Stake in Treatment: "Bring Some Skin to the Game"

We hear physicians and health care executives using the phrase "Bring some skin to the game" more and more in referring to consumers' having a financial stake in their treatment options. This old saying about bringing skin to a game comes from golf and other sports; it refers either to placing a bet or to literally leaving some skin on the ground (as a result of diving for a loose ball in volleyball or basketball, for instance).

One physician leader told us, "In the exam room, a physician can't stand up against a patient unless there are some significant dollars coming out of the patient's pockets. With money being no object, as it is for most patients who have private insurance, patients want the brand name drugs and the most expensive tests and treatments. Things have to change, or our health care system will become even more dysfunctional."

The need for consumers to pay more out of their pockets is the downside of choice and control. However, we do not believe that Americans can have one without the other. Without a price tag attached to health care, the demand will become virtually infinite, as is already the case in many parts of the country.

Quality-of-Life Products and Services

The growing number of quality-of-life products and services complicates the issue. In the past, when there seemed to be general agreement on what constituted "medical necessity," it was less difficult to decide what health care benefits would be covered in employer or government health plans. But with quality-of-life products and services representing a growing share of health care spending, the issue of who should pay is increasingly muddled.

Because we do not have a clear definition of what health care services fall into the category of medical necessity and which fall into the category of quality of life, we cannot make a reasonable estimate of the relative proportion of the health care dollar spent on each. However, our strongly held opinion is that the number of dollars spent on improving the quality of life of consumers is increasing much more rapidly than the amount spent on medical necessities.

Why is this distinction important? Primarily, because it makes the determination of health care policy much more difficult—some might say impossible. We are not in favor of the federal government mandating certain procedures or products as medically necessary when it could be argued that these products lean toward improving quality of life. Policymakers could not do this anyway; the rapid and constant changes brought on by genetic research, new drugs, and advances in medical technology would make it unfeasible.

If health plans and public policymakers are not capable of clearly distinguishing between medically necessary and quality-of-life products and services, who is? We can see only one choice: the consumer. But in order to make that distinction, the consumer must have a financial incentive to weigh the costs of alternative treatment options and to consider forgoing a test, new drug, surgery, or other procedure. How else could it be in a rational health care system?

This discussion shows why we have combined affordability and consumer choice in this chapter: the two are intertwined.

Personal Relationships with Physicians

As the baby boomers age and join the more than forty million Americans already on Medicare, we expect renewed emphasis on long-term relationships with a personal physician. This is already happening: consumers are increasingly opting for open-access health plans, such as PPOs and POS HMOs, so they can maintain a relationship with their preferred physician and medical office. The movement of more medical groups and integrated systems into disease management will further lock patients in to a particular personal physician and group practice.

With the advent of managed care in the 1980s and early 1990s, it appeared as though patients did not place much value on a personal relationship with a physician or medical group. It was often noted by "experts" in health care that a $10 a month additional cost to consumers would make the difference between switching to a different physician and not doing so. This, of course, was a crushing psychological and economic blow to many physicians who had thought consumers valued the personal relationship.

It now appears that consumers were not quite as sanguine about their personal relationships with physicians as was first thought. Older Americans, in particular, place a special value on their own physician. In focus groups we often hear seniors talk about "where they do their doctoring," and it is evident that they are more loyal to their particular physicians than we may have believed a decade ago. For younger consumers, having a personal relationship with a physician is not as important. However, the many younger and middle-aged Americans serving as caregivers for elderly parents realize the importance of continuity of care.

Conclusions

Affordability is a concern, but we see substantial room for providers and manufacturers to push consumers further than they have been pushed in the past in terms of paying for what they want. Many consumers have been receiving basic health services and paying a smaller and smaller percentage of the cost. Small increases in the employees' share of premiums, copayments, or deductibles are greeted with loud complaints. In companies where employees are unionized, the cost of health care borne by employees is a hot issue, particularly in tight labor markets.

At the same time there is no denying that a growing proportion of Americans are paying $4,600 for digital hearing aids, $5,000 for facial surgery, $2,100 per eye for vision correction surgery, $500 for the "personal security" of knowing there is nothing wrong with their heart, and $300 for a quick fix to whiten their teeth. In vitro fertilization can cost $10,000 to $15,000. Assisted living, which is not covered by Medicaid, costs $1,800 to $2,500 a month. Parents cough up several thousand dollars over two or three years in order to have their kids' teeth straightened. Much of the $50 billion CAM industry is "cash and carry."

So people may complain about relatively small increases in the cost of health care services they are accustomed to receiving free, but the data show that they will pay relatively large amounts for products and services that are not covered by health plans or Medicare. As for "financial" access to health care, such access would be much improved in a future where consumerism and technology are key drivers. In this type of scenario the proportion of Americans without health insurance coverage would be two-thirds of what we might expect under an incremental change scenario.

The implications of the increased purchase of health care products and services by consumers with their own money and better access to these services are that many hospitals and medical groups must improve the way they operate. They will need to become more consumer friendly by offering such benefits as more convenient hours, easier scheduling, and better service.

Chapter Five

Innovation in Health Care
The Next Wave

The amount of change going on in every medical specialty is phenomenal. We haven't seen anything yet compared to what the future will bring.
NEUROLOGIST, DENVER, COLORADO, October 2000

Entrepreneurship and innovation are arguably at an all-time high in the United States. Most economists acknowledge that entrepreneurship and innovation have played a key role in driving the economic prosperity of the 1980s, 1990s, and the beginning of the twenty-first century, particularly in the high-tech, telecommunications, entertainment, retailing, and financial services industries.

After a flurry of innovation in the late 1980s and early 1990s—including the development of new businesses centered on integrated delivery systems, physician practice management companies (PPMs), and health care information systems—hospitals have become almost dormant in comparison with other sectors of the economy. The conventional wisdom is for hospital executives to "hunker down," cut costs, and implement existing business plans. "Getting back to the basics" is a popular theme in the hospital sector. Most recent innovation has been taking place among the multitude of product- and service-oriented health care companies. Internet companies serving health care are a prime example.

If hospitals, medical groups, physician networks, health systems, and health plans are to prosper in the new millennium, they must adopt a new spirit of innovation. The next wave of change is taking shape now, driven by the increasing power of consumers, the expanded capabilities and use of the Internet, health care systems' investment in IT, genetic research, new drugs, advances in medical technology, and related innovations in marketing and management. *Opportunities for innovation and entrepreneurship in health care during the first five years of the new century will exceed anything we have seen in the past two decades.*

This chapter addresses the following issues related to entrepreneurship and innovation in health care:

- The relationship between entrepreneurship and innovation
- The conditions that make the health care industry ripe for a new wave of entrepreneurship and innovation
- The likely shape of the next wave of innovation
- Strategies for increasing the chances of success in innovation

Entrepreneurship and Innovation

What do we mean by *entrepreneurship*? How does it differ from *innovation*? And how do the two interrelate?

Entrepreneurship

"The entrepreneur," said the French economist J. B. Say around 1800, "shifts economic resources out of an area of lower and into an area of higher productivity and greater yield" (quoted in Drucker, 1993, p. 21). In other words, an entrepreneur devotes his or her efforts to making organizations (business and others), and the economy in general, function more efficiently.

Merriam-Webster's Collegiate Dictionary defines an entrepreneur as "one who organizes, manages, and assumes the risks of a business or enterprise" (the assumption usually being that the entrepreneur does so for the sake of profit). This is the way most people think of entrepreneurship.

Others view entrepreneurship as something more than just starting a new venture. For example, according to management guru Peter Drucker (1993, p. 22), "In order to be entrepreneurial, an enterprise has to have special characteristics over and above being new and small. Indeed, entrepreneurs are a minority among small businesses. They create something new, something different; they change or transmute values."

Using the economist's definition, an entrepreneur redeploys resources—products, services, people, money, markets, facilities—in an innovative manner in order to add new value for customers. This definition includes those who establish new businesses or other entities (including not-for-profits) as well as those who work to lead established organizations in fundamentally new directions (often referred to as "intrapreneurs").

Innovation

Many in business think of innovation in terms of new products. The cellular phone and the personal computer were innovations, as were magnetic resonance imaging and laser eye surgery. But innovation can also come from changing the way things are organized. PhyCor represented an innovative approach to consolidating medical practices that spearheaded the PPM industry. The efforts of many hospitals to find new ways to work with the physicians on their staff have produced innovation.

Innovation is not a hit-or-miss proposition. It is not usually based on brainstorming sessions, although focus groups with customers can be important. And true innovation is a far cry from mere improvisation (the same could be said for entrepreneurship).

How Does Entrepreneurship Create Innovation?

Some innovations spring forth as fully formed, significant changes in and of themselves—the airplane and the Internet would be examples. However, these are few and far between. Most innovations, and the entrepreneurial activities that bring them about, are more prosaic. Rather than creating something entirely new, entrepreneurs exploit the changes taking place around them in order to produce innovation. In other words, although entrepreneurs are in the business of causing change, most successful entrepreneurs begin with and feed on changes already occurring around them.

Most entrepreneurship consists of exploiting one or more of the seven generic sources of opportunity (Drucker, 1993):

1. New knowledge
2. Changes in customers' perception, mood, and meaning
3. Changes in industry or market structure
4. Changes in demographics
5. Needs for process improvement
6. Incongruities in the marketplace
7. Unexpected changes

The key is that change feeds on itself. Each change produces opportunities for entrepreneurial initiatives, which in turn produce changes and still more opportunities.

Opportunities for Entrepreneurship and Innovation

The implications for health care of each of the seven forms of opportunity are discussed below. Examples of expected opportunities are summarized in Exhibit 5.1.

New Knowledge

Drucker (1993) says that knowledge-based innovation is the superstar of entrepreneurship: "It gets the publicity. It gets the money. It is what people normally mean when they talk of innovation" (p. 107). It is difficult to imagine an industry where new knowledge is as pervasive as in health care. For example, the findings from genetic research and the subsequent development of new drugs require vastly greater knowledge than in the past. What lies ahead in the area of knowledge-based change and entrepreneurial opportunity? By most accounts, we can expect a whirlwind of further technological innovation, including rapid progress in genetic manipulation, pharmaceuticals, bioengineering, and IT.

One of the challenges for entrepreneurs is to figure out how consumers will be able to afford the new drugs and advances in medical technology. In other words, we expect the technology to develop more rapidly than the market can finance it. At the same time, consumers will demand access to the new wonder drugs and latest medical advances. *Tremendous opportunities for innovation and entrepreneurship now exist in the marketing, financial, and business aspects of medical technology.*

Exhibit 5.1. The Seven Common Sources of Innovation: Examples in Today's Health Care Marketplace.

1. *New knowledge*
   - Genetic research
   - Pharmacology
   - Biomedical engineering
   - Information technology
2. *Changes in customers' perception, mood, and meaning*
   - Growing discontent with the first generation of managed care
   - Increasing customer participation in health care decision making
   - Continuing customer segmentation (by age, income, lifestyle, health needs, and approaches to information and problem solving)
3. *Changes in industry or market structure*
   - Shifts in federal reimbursement away from a fee-for-service approach and toward care management
   - Withdrawal of employers from decision making and risk taking in health care
   - Shifts in health plan roles and positioning
   - Changes driven by technology
4. *Changes in demographics*
   - Aging of the population
   - Growth in consumers' income and net worth
   - Increase in importance of international payers to U.S. providers
5. *Needs for process improvement*
   - Disease management
   - Integrative management (involving physicians and other process managers)
6. *Incongruities in the marketplace*
   - Declining health care payments versus growing and inelastic demand
7. *Unexpected changes*

Sources: Drucker, 1993, p. 31; authors' projections.

Changes in Customers' Perception, Mood, and Meaning

Survey after survey has shown that Americans dislike the health care system, particularly managed care, but are pleased with their physicians. In many communities the local hospital is a highly regarded institution. At the same time, consumers complain vociferously about their health care costs and, increasingly, their health plans.

The growing role of consumers—consonant with their demand for greater freedom of choice and more involvement in their own health and that of their families—is part of a change in perception. The fact that a growing number of consumers consider freedom to choose their own health plan, physician, and hospital important is another example of a change in perception. Just a few years ago it was widely believed that virtually all consumers would change health plans (and physicians) for a $10 reduction in their share of the monthly health plan premium.

The explosive growth in cosmetic surgery represents one of the best examples of innovation and entrepreneurship designed to meet the changing needs of Americans. Performed by board-certified plastic surgeons, otolaryngologists, dermatologists, general surgeons, and other specialists, cosmetic surgery is a rapidly growing field. It is not unusual for a cosmetic surgery center to offer computer imaging ("before" and "after" pictures), a surgery suite, and specialized financing. A consumer might be told, "If you are worried about what this face-lift will cost, just fill out this card, and we will have your credit approved within five minutes." This is the way it is done in many parts of the country, and consumers are delighted with it.

Consumer research is an area where health care can borrow heavily from other industries. Other industries devote significant resources to segmenting the consumer market and then tailoring products and services to the needs of specific segments. As discussed in Chapter Fifteen, we expect to see more refined market segmentation based on consumers' age, lifestyle, health care needs, and preferred approaches to obtaining information and making decisions.

Changes in Industry or Market Structure

Actual and projected changes in the health care industry and market structure have driven the strategies of most health care provider organizations for the past two decades. How will the health care industry structure change in the future? The retreat of employers away from key roles in health care financing and decision making threatens to become a stampede. If increasing numbers of employers decide to stop providing health insurance benefits or to begin offering plans with a defined contribution, significant structural changes will ensue. Meanwhile, the same trend is occurring in Medicare. The expectation is that, one way or another, the consumer is about to pay more but also be more in control of the choice of providers and other aspects of care.

Changes in Demographics

The biggest demographic change affecting health care has been the growth in the number of persons sixty-five or more years of age and on Medicare. The aging of the population, particularly the increase in the number of those over eighty-five years old, has had a dramatic impact on hospitals, home health, and long-term care organizations (such as independent living, congregate care, and assisted living facilities and nursing homes). What are the implications of these demographic shifts for innovation and entrepreneurship? It is difficult to imagine a more significant area of opportunity.

Here, in brief, is the story of how one entrepreneur approached this market opportunity: "A former hospital and health plan executive, Michael Schonbrun, has moved from being a healthcare manager to an entrepreneur by forming Balfour Senior Care with an emphasis on a continuum of services for one segment of the elderly. In approaching this segment, Schonbrun has gathered a group of business advisers from across the country—including the executive VP of a biotech firm, a psychologist and a former administrator of HCFA [the Health Care Financing Administration]" (Austin, 1999b).

The new company opened Balfour Retirement Community of Boulder County, Colorado. Reminiscent of a country estate, the upscale development offers everything from Internet access and waist-level outdoor gardens to a cocktail lounge and hair salon. But what really sets Balfour Retirement Community apart from other developments of its kind, said Schonbrun, is that once residents make the move to Balfour, they do not ever have to move again.

Balfour took an innovative approach to health care staff retention: "To attract and retain quality nursing staff, one of the problems in long-term care, Balfour offers employees stock options. While in the Silicon Valley, Schonbrun says that, 'I saw the power of people that had stock in their company'" (Austin, 1999b). It is also interesting that Schonbrun and his colleagues recognized early on that one size does not fit all in retirement communities and designed a facility that appeals to one market segment: seniors with high income and significant accumulated wealth.

Needs for Process Improvement

Almost everyone acknowledges that health care needs to invest in process improvement or automation. For example, the need for hospitals to streamline admissions processes is obvious to patients, physicians, employees, and volunteers.

In the next wave of process-oriented change, we expect to see more intentional pursuit of multiple goals. For example, one of our recent consulting assignments was intended to produce simultaneous improvements in a hospital department's clinical activities, regulatory compliance, and financial performance. We also expect to see more efforts to improve the effectiveness of departments and organizations in working together. Although the goal of becoming a fully integrated health care delivery system is no longer shared by many provider organizations, the goal of providing organized and coordinated clinical services to customers remains critical.

Incongruities in the Marketplace

Entrepreneurs are adept at finding and exploiting incongruities in the marketplace, such as mismatches between reality and perception or between the willingness to pay for a service and the cost of delivering it. New ventures crop up to remove incongruities in much the same way that nature fills a vacuum.

POS HMOs were born to respond to an incongruity. On one hand, consumer research indicated that people were resisting HMOs that limited their choice. On the other hand, research also revealed that, given a choice to go outside of the network for a small fee, consumers almost never exercised the option to do so. This afforded an opportunity to design POS plans that were financially viable and that at the same time garnered a substantial market share.

For health plans and employers there will be a need to find ways of holding down utilization without relying totally on financial incentives to providers (such as capitation or withholding). There is a tremendous need to find new types of health plans that motivate more cost-effective behavior by consumers.

Another incongruity is that, even as payers try to wring costs out of the health care system, many consumers are willing to pay significantly more for what they regard as better coverage and more user-friendly care. The next wave of health care change may well include "premium priced packages"—offerings of very comprehensive coverage (after high deductibles) matched with accessible and attentive customer service and high-quality providers.

Unexpected Changes

There is one final category of innovation: those opportunities to come from unexpected changes. By definition, we do not know what the next round of unexpected changes leading to entrepreneurial ventures will be. However, from past experience, we know that many successful innovations will come without being planned or anticipated.

The Marshfield Clinic's development of its primary care network (discussed in Chapter Three) is one example of an unexpected change that led to a substantial innovation. In the early 1970s Marshfield was a traditional multispecialty clinic, in a single location, without family practice or most other primary care specialties. At that time a physician in Stratford (ten miles north of Marshfield) died, and a Marshfield Clinic doctor began serving people in the area on a part-time basis. In the mid-1970s the town of Mosinee (twenty-five miles northeast of Marshfield) came to the clinic after their physician left. By coincidence, a physician came to the clinic looking for a practice in a small town, and the clinic recruited him to fill the spot in Mosinee. This small start led to a network of thirty-nine medical offices.

Innovation in the Future

What do we expect in the next wave of entrepreneurship and innovation in health care, and how would we describe the context in which we believe it will occur?

Key Trends

Several general trends appear likely, especially in a future dominated by consumerism and technology.

The market will become less predictable. Despite the feeling of many in health care that the industry is dynamic and has been changing at a rapid pace over the past few years, we take a contrary view. We believe that many aspects of health care have become predictable and somewhat dull. For example, managed care has achieved maturity in many markets, and with 85 percent commercial market penetration nationally, it has already nearly reached its maximum growth potential. Similarly, the trend toward consolidation of hospitals, health plans, and medical groups has slowed. However, the factors likely to induce innovation that have already been discussed will accelerate the pace of change in health care. Changes in one innovation factor (such as use of the Internet) will produce additional rounds of changes in other factors (such as process improvements and industry structure).

Cost containment pressures will coexist with growth pressures. With medical spending reaching $1.3 trillion in 2000 and growing at the rate of $100 billion a year, there is renewed concern about an escalation in health care costs. The promising results of genetic research, drug development, and advances in medical technology are putting increased upward pressure on health care spending. Concurrently, the ability of Medicare, Medicaid, and commercial managed care (the three largest payment sources, accounting for about three-quarters of all health care dollars) to keep health care spending in check is suspect. With nearly forty-five million uninsured Americans and the coming impact of the baby boomers on Medicare spending, health care is facing unprecedented challenges. (Keep in mind that most of the baby boomers will not turn sixty-five until after 2010!)

Consumers will pay more but gain in self-determination. We see deepening cracks in the foundation of the employer-based health benefits system, parallel and still deeper cracks in the foundation of Medicare and other public sector reimbursement programs, and increasing interest among consumers in taking more control of their health care. We believe the U.S. health care system is headed for profound changes. Consumers will drive these changes through greatly expanded use of the Internet, a desire for freedom of choice, greater use of CAM, and increased sophistication leading to intensified demand for better quality, access, and service.

The Internet, telehealth, and new clinical information technology will begin to drive strategy and market structure. Although it takes many years to realize the benefits of investment in health care IT, the continuing high levels of investment in this area are likely to affect health care in significant ways over the next five years. There will be more and more talk of "e-health."

Genetic research, new drugs, and medical technology will cause acceleration in both innovation and costs. Largely because of genetic research, the number of new drugs will grow rapidly; they will be effective, highly sought after by consumers, and expensive. We have already seen evidence of the impact of new technology in such inventions as laparoscopic surgery and laser eye surgery, and dozens of technological advances are in the pipeline.

Consumers will become better informed and more demanding. The shift toward consumerism is being accompanied by demands for higher-quality care, better access, and substantial improvements in service—and we have only seen the tip of the iceberg. More and more consumers will have "done their homework" (via the Internet, through review of direct marketing materials, or through consumer buying groups) before they see their health care providers.

The Next Generation of Entrepreneurs

Where will the next generation of health care entrepreneurs come from? One traditional source has been physicians. And why not? Many physicians are smart, have access to start-up capital, and are intimately involved with the technology and the workings of current products and services. Experience suggests, however, that only a select group of physicians should consider playing the role of entrepreneur.

For years, we have found it useful to divide physicians into four attitudinal groups:

- *Early adapters.* These are physicians who cannot wait to try the newest device, business model, or staffing or marketing approach. These physicians can tolerate the frustration of being on the leading edge of innovation. They are inherently optimistic. Ask them how their practice will be five years from now, and most will say it will be the same or better than it is now.

- *Defensive adapters.* These are physicians who aggressively make changes but who do so as a defensive strategy. This group continues to merge and affiliate with others, add products and services, and otherwise adjust their practice. They take these steps in order to minimize their risk. Ask them how their practice will be five years from now, and most will say it will be much worse than it is today.

- *Traditionalists.* These physicians believe that medicine has, in too many ways, gone downhill. They refuse to submit to most changes and bitterly chafe at those they do have to accommodate.

- *Pure practitioners.* These physicians say they never intended to have to deal with the business aspects of their practice. They would like to be removed from business considerations and just left alone to practice good medicine.

Successful physician entrepreneurs come almost exclusively from the first two groups. In addition, they have a business idea and feel passionately about it. Finally, they are relatively stubborn and are not put off by the possibility of failure.

A second source of entrepreneurs is certainly the executives already in the industry. Some, like Michael Schonbrun, the former health care executive who started Balfour Senior Care, will organize their own companies. Many others will be intrapreneurs, leading significant innovations within their existing organizations.

Some believe that health care executives, particularly hospital managers, are unlikely to lead innovation and entrepreneurial efforts. Some of the attempts by hospitals to build physician-hospital organizations and integrated systems may support this theory. However, there are also numerous success stories regarding innovation from the hospital sector, and we expect many more.

A third source of entrepreneurs will be successful executives from other industries. It is important that potential entrepreneurs from within the health care industry anticipate the involvement, and never discount the potential, of successful innovators and investors from other sectors of the economy.

Best Practices

What can we learn from past successes and failures? As in any industry, in health care there will always be failures in efforts to innovate. The willingness to face the possibility of failure is part of the very essence of entrepreneurship. This is the way it should be. There are lessons to be learned from past entrepreneurial efforts in health care—including the unsuccessful efforts—that may make the process less painful and more rewarding, both financially and professionally. Based on the experiences of those who have gone before, we can make several suggestions.

Begin with a strongly held concept. All of the entrepreneurs we have ever met and worked with have had a unique idea, vision, or concept of a product or service that they believed would fit with one of the seven sources of innovation discussed earlier. An entrepreneur with a strongly held concept who is mentioned in *Capitalizing Medical Groups* (Coddington, Moore, and Clarke, 1998, p. 209) is a good illustration: "Joe Hutts, the founder of PhyCor, told us that his feelings about forming an organization to work with physicians grew over a long period of time until it became 'compelling.' He added, 'I have always been impressed with multispecialty clinics, especially those with a large primary care base. These are the types of organizations that have the greatest potential to impact the way health care is delivered.'"

Pursue the concept with enthusiasm and energy. This is another characteristic of any entrepreneur we have met. For example, Richard Ruben, M.D., founder of Women's Health Connecticut, was the key person in putting together a statewide organization of obstetrician gynecologists. Here is how Ruben describes his efforts:

> I went back to my group and said we need to measure quality and costs. We asked each physician to "tithe 10 percent of revenue" to spend on research and development. We hired consultants and looked carefully at what we were doing. Within eighteen months we were able to increase the income of each doctor by over $100,000 by merely doing things differently.

One of the attorneys who worked with this group during the formation of Women's Health Connecticut referred to Dr. Ruben as "Noah." The attorney said, "We call him by that name because he not only saw the impending flood of changes in healthcare, but he took the lead in building the ark" [Coddington, Moore, and Clarke, 1998, pp. 262–263].

Focus on creating value. Most PPMs added value to the medical groups they acquired, but not enough to continue to impress physicians and to offset the management fees they charged. In many cases there was too much emphasis on external expansion (adding new physicians and smaller groups) and not enough on fostering "same-store" growth, improving back-office operations, and developing medical management (including quality, service, and cost-effectiveness).

Conduct a careful analysis of the market or need. A limited amount of market research and analysis, coupled with a feasibility assessment, pays big dividends relative to its cost. In reviewing start-up plans, we are often shocked that financial models contain tremendous detail on expenses but make broad assumptions about the market or need for the innovation. Often these plans "put the cart before the horse," focusing on expenses and neglecting what should receive most of the emphasis in the analytical stage—the market or the need for the innovation.

Be realistic in matching capital sources to opportunities. In our view most medical groups need a capital partner. They need access to clinical and management information systems and more clout in negotiating with managed care. They need increased ability to perform medical management. They need to offer senior physicians an exit strategy. Most PPMs were designed to serve all of these needs. So what went wrong?

Many physicians and entrepreneurs, particularly in PPMs, have learned the hard way that it is impossible to meet Wall Street's growth and earnings expectations. The ability to generate 20 to 35 percent annual increases in revenues and profits in order to satisfy investors' earnings expectations is simply not possible for most medical enterprises involving physicians. Entrepreneurs in different settings have learned a related lesson the hard way: never, ever start a venture that is undercapitalized.

Minimize risks. Most definitions of an entrepreneur would include wording about accepting the responsibility and taking the financial risks (as well as accepting the rewards) associated with an innovation. However, Drucker (1993) claims this is nonsense—entrepreneurs are not risk takers. He quotes a successful entrepreneur who says, "The successful [entrepreneurs] I know all have one thing—and only one thing—in common: they are not 'risk-takers.' They try to define the risks they have to take and to minimize them as much as possible. Otherwise none of us could have succeeded. As for myself, if I had wanted to be a risk-taker, I would have gone into real estate or commodity trading, or I would have become the professional painter my mother wanted me to be" (p. 139).

This is consistent with our experience. The successful entrepreneurs we have worked with over the years have been analytical and careful in committing resources—money, people, or energy—to an innovation. They are not afraid to abandon an idea if they have serious questions about whether or not it will succeed. Not only do successful entrepreneurs take the necessary steps to discontinue those initiatives that do not work, but they also carefully avoid being trapped in activities that are only marginally successful.

Conclusions

Some are still getting accustomed to living with or working in a market-driven health care industry. This is understandable—it has been less than two decades since Medicare initiated the move away from "usual and customary" fees. Part of getting used to the new health care industry is learning to live with change and uncertainty. The first major wave of entrepreneurship and innovation brought many successes and numerous failures. The next wave promises to be more broad based and sustained.

In the future, innovation will come not from a single source (such as, in the past, the introduction of DRGs) but from multiple sources, including the growing role of consumers and technology. From the entrepreneur's perspective, things could not be better—the greater the number and extent of changes, the more attractive the opportunities. Consumers, for their part, will be pleased with the results.

Health Care Delivery and Financing Systems

Developing Strategies in Anticipation of Fundamental Change

> *Given your views on how health care will change in the future—more emphasis on consumerism and technology— what are we supposed to do about it? How will these changes impact our investment decisions? Our strategies and business planning?*
> PHYSICIAN LEADER OF A LARGE MULTISPECIALTY CLINIC IN THE MIDWEST, July 2000

The seven chapters in Part Two focus on strategies for most of the major players in health care: physicians, medical groups, physician networks, hospitals, multihospital systems, academic medical centers, specialty hospitals, integrated health care systems, other types of health care services, and health plans. If technology dominates and consumers take charge, many health care leaders and their organizations will be compelled—if they are to survive and prosper— to make quick changes to keep pace with the dynamic, ever changing health care marketplace of the future.

Physicians and Medical Groups

We believe that physicians and medical groups will have tremendous opportunities in a health care future dominated by consumerism and technology. Chapter Six reviews strategies for physicians with an emphasis on those in single-specialty groups.

Physician Networks

There are hundreds of physician networks, including independent practice associations (IPAs), "clinics without walls," physician-hospital organizations (PHOs), management services organizations (MSOs), PPMs, and single-specialty physician networks, that will be affected in different ways by the four scenarios for the future. Chapter Seven discusses strategies for the various types of physician networks.

Hospitals and Multihospital Systems

Chapter Eight identifies a dozen major strategies for hospitals and multihospital systems and analyzes how these strategies might change depending on perspectives of the future. One hospital CEO told us, "I don't really see the core strategies of this organization changing. It is more a matter of the intensity of management effort and resources that will be applied." We agree with this assessment, which is reflected throughout Chapter Eight.

Academic Medical Centers and Specialty Hospitals

Chapter Nine features a case study of a university medical center that is moving from its old location in a congested area of Denver to a large campus in the eastern suburbs, on the site of the old Fitzsimons Army Hospital. In the course of the move, the new facility will be positioning itself to be a true research and educational center for the future, including innovative approaches to accessing the Internet and conducting clinical trials. In Chapter Nine we also highlight strategies for children's hospitals and rehabilitation facilities.

Integrated Health Care Systems

Are integrated systems relics of the mid-1990s, when "single-signature contracting" was the way many organizations were positioning themselves for the future? What value do integrated systems bring to the new health care marketplace? Chapter Ten discusses two broad types of integrated systems—those established by multi-specialty clinics and those initiated by hospitals or multihospital systems. In most cases they are different types of entities, and although their strategies for the future have similarities, there are differences in emphasis.

Other Types of Health Care Services

What about the strategies for other types of health care services, many of which are growing in relative importance? These include long-term care, home health care, dental care, vision care, disease management, and CAM. Chapter Eleven summarizes the major strategies for these players and explains how consumerism and technology are likely to affect them.

Health Plans

With the shift toward vouchers, defined-contribution benefit plans, MSAs, and individual insurance, the role of health plans will change dramatically. Instead of working primarily with employers, health plans are more likely to market directly to consumer purchasing alliances and individuals. These and other issues related to health plans are the subject of Chapter Twelve.

Chapter Six

Strategies for Physicians and Medical Groups

Strategy is needed; the future is mainly unpredictable.
ROBERT H. WATERMAN JR., *The Renewal Factor: How the Best Get and Keep the Competitive Edge,* Bantam Books, 1987

Physicians are accustomed to making decisions under conditions of uncertainty, and they usually make these decisions fast. By contrast, scenario planning may be frustratingly slow and complex for many physicians and medical groups. One physician told us, "Just give me your best estimate of what you think will happen, and we can plan around that." But uncertainty, or lack of predictability, is not the enemy. As an article in *Business Week* (Coy and Gross, 1999, p. 82) points out, "English essayist Francis Bacon figured this out nearly 400 years ago. 'If a man will begin with certainties, he shall end in doubts. But if he will be content to begin with doubts he shall end in certainties.'"

Before we discuss strategies for physicians and medical groups, it may be useful to summarize what we have learned about physicians and their risk-taking behavior. Just as there are differences among individuals in their investment criteria—time perspective, acceptance of risk, income versus capital gains—there are differences among physicians and medical groups in their investment approach. When it comes to investing in the future of their practices, physician groups can be divided into at least four distinct types. Figure 6.1 highlights the characteristics of each type.

Throughout this chapter we devote a disproportionate amount of space to the first three types of physician investors. We expect physicians and medical groups of the fourth type, defensive investors, to follow prevailing trends and not spend much time strategizing about the future of their practices.

We have found that primary care and single-specialty medical groups typically use one or more of eleven general strategies:

1. Expanding the practice
2. Consolidating with other physicians and practices
3. Implementing IT, including the EMR
4. Enhancing quality of care
5. Improving service and access
6. Increasing cost-effectiveness
7. Generating ancillary income
8. Positioning the practice for managed care contracting, including the acceptance of risk contracts
9. Creating relationships with CAM providers
10. Gaining access to capital
11. Joining a union—a relatively new strategy

Other strategies might include disease management, coordination of care, and development of physician leadership.

As an illustration, Table 6.1 shows the strategies that might be used by a cautiously optimistic orthopedic group in each of the four scenarios we propose for the future of health care. (See Chapter One for an overview of the four scenarios.) The importance of each strategy in each scenario is ranked on a scale of 1 to 10, where 1 signifies that the strategy is unimportant and 10 represents the greatest financial and management commitment. Our purpose in including this example is to suggest that although strategies might be the same regardless of the future, the emphasis will change rather dramatically.

Expanding the Practice

There are a variety of reasons to expand a medical practice: to meet demand from patients that exceeds present capacity, to gain more

Figure 6.1. Investment Characteristics of Four Types of Medical Groups.

1. Aggressive long-term investors

    Anticipate change
    Invest proactively
    Defer present income for investing in the future
    Position themselves for the future

2. Aggressive short-term investors

    Seek to maximize revenues today
    Attempt to avoid risk

3. Cautiously optimistic investors

    Remain receptive to change but are not overly aggressive
    Endeavor to maintain past successes

4. Defensive investors

    Stay completely focused on maintaining
    what they have today

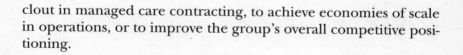

clout in managed care contracting, to achieve economies of scale in operations, or to improve the group's overall competitive positioning.

Satellite Offices

For both primary care and specialty physicians, there may be opportunities to open offices in generally attractive but underserved areas. This is a strategy that broadens the size of the market area and expands the number of physicians and support staff. In a future dominated more and more by consumerism and technology, medical groups—in particular those that are aggressive long-term investors—will be opening a number of additional satellite offices in attractive markets within or adjacent to their service area. The availability of higher-quality and more cost-effective telemedicine, increased use

Table 6.1. Changing Strategic Emphasis in the Four Scenarios, for a Cautiously Optimistic Orthopedic Group.

Strategy	Scenario 1: Incremental Change	Scenario 2: Constrained Resources	Scenario 3: Technology Dominant	Scenario 4: Consumerism and Technology (Retail)
1. Generating ancillary income	7	3	8	9
2. Contracting with managed care plans	8	4	5	5
3. Centralizing the business office	6	7	5	5
4. Expanding geographical coverage	6	5	8	9
5. Establishing outpatient surgery centers	6	3	7	9
6. Improving quality	7	4	8	9
7. Establishing a brand name	5	3	6	10
8. Improving governance and decision making	7	8	8	8
9. Improving relationships with primary care physicians	7	7	6	5

of videoconferencing, and new IT will facilitate this type of expansion. Many large integrated health care systems, especially those led by multispecialty clinics, are already expanding their regional networks (see Chapter Ten).

Outpatient Facilities and Services

It is becoming more common for physicians to invest in outpatient facilities and services. In many communities the growth in outpatient surgery and diagnostic centers represents one of the major changes of the past decade. Because the earnings potential for these kinds of facilities has been high, it has been relatively easy to attract outside investors in order to construct and equip ambulatory centers that are partially owned by physicians. We know of cases where hospitals have also been partners with physicians in such endeavors.

These kinds of opportunities may be diminished in an incremental change scenario or in a scenario where resources are constrained owing to poor economic conditions. However, we anticipate continued expansion of physician-owned (or physician-controlled) outpatient facilities and services in a future where consumerism and technology gain in importance. This is not good news for hospitals.

Disease Management

A surprising number of individuals we interviewed said that medical groups should consider getting into chronic disease management or establishing relationships with organizations that provide disease management services. Consumers, health plans, and Medicare will expect physicians and medical groups to provide these kinds of services. An internal medicine physician told us, "If I had a group of eight or ten physicians, the first thing I would do is either start a disease management program or find a partner for such a venture. This has to be of vital importance to our patients who have chronic illnesses. I don't want them going somewhere else for this service."

The increased availability of the Internet, e-mail, and telemedicine makes the management of chronic diseases more feasible. Furthermore, with the aging of the population, the number of Americans with one or more chronic conditions requiring some sort of monitoring and management is growing dramatically. A relationship with a person with a chronic condition is a potentially important factor determining referrals to physicians and hospitals. Disease management services offer an opportunity for medical groups to expand the size of their service area and to generate new revenues, and the initial evidence about the cost-effectiveness of disease management is promising.

Physician Recruitment

We expect many types of practices, especially those that are aggressive long-term investors, to continue to seek out physician associates in order to expand. This should be possible in most markets, given that newly trained physicians often prefer to work in established practices. However, we anticipate that physicians hired as associates will not be guaranteed the same types of compensation packages as in the 1990s. We expect employment contracts to contain more incentive compensation clauses and few guarantees. The lessons of the 1990s will not be lost on physician leaders of medical groups that are expanding.

Local Outreach Clinics and Long-Distance Business Development

Having a specialist leave the office one day each month or week is a relatively low-risk strategy, and we foresee continued growth in outreach clinics. In the past many busy specialists have resisted this approach; taking time out of the office costs them money. However, this strategy has proved to be extremely popular with consumers. We anticipate that in the consumer-driven health care system of the future, more and more services will be available in smaller communities and in medical offices distant from the home office of the specialist. For certain large and prominent medical groups, especially those in clinical and surgical specialties, the future will present many new opportunities for major geographical expansion outside the normal service area—even overseas.

Improvements in technology will facilitate this approach to delivering health care. These technological advancements include increased use of e-mail, scheduling on Web sites (thus eliminating the need for a person in the local community to take time to schedule the visiting specialist), telemedicine, and other communication technologies. The bottom line is that consumers want specialists to visit their communities, and we expect this approach to delivering care to explode in popularity.

Consolidating with Other Physicians and Practices

One of the discernible long-term trends among physicians and medical groups is consolidation into larger groups.

Merging with Other Practices

Physician mergers will continue at the same rapid rate as in the past, especially with consumerism and technology playing more dominant roles. In several markets, such as Minneapolis–Saint Paul, the expansion of single-specialty medical groups in fields such as gastroenterology and cardiology is accelerating. The factors at work in the first strategy we discussed, market expansion, are the main reasons for merger and consolidation. Access to capital (or lack of it) will be a major consideration. In addition, the ability of larger groups to demonstrate higher quality of care and improved services will drive this long-term trend.

Selling to a Hospital

Considering the reported large losses of hospital-affiliated medical groups, this may seem far-fetched. It is not. In fact, surveys of hospital CEOs continue to show that many plan to acquire medical groups and establish ventures with single-specialty groups.

Given the failure of many PPMs and the sell-off of acquired medical groups, we expect a number of PPMs and medical groups to end up with hospitals as capital partners. It will be easier for a medical group to align financial incentives with a community hospital than with a publicly traded PPM.

Partnering with a Physician Practice Management Company

Until early 1998, partnering with a PPM was the consolidation strategy of choice among most medical groups. Although PPMs are far from extinct, the lack of capital caused by a failure to deliver on their promises limits the kinds of deals that PPMs are able to offer prospective partner medical groups. In other words, many PPMs are in much less favorable competitive positions to acquire medical groups than they were during most of the 1990s.

The nature of PPM agreements with medical groups has changed dramatically and can be expected to continue to change in the initial years of the new century. For example, up-front cash and stock payments to physicians have been reduced substantially (and in some cases totally eliminated). Management fees are also down from 15 to 20 percent of net revenues to half or two-thirds of this amount.

In a future where technology and consumerism reign, PPMs can be expected to regain some of their past glory. After all, medical groups that are aggressive long-term investors still need capital for expansion and IT, and PPMs have the potential to meet this need.

What Are the Positive and Negative Aspects of Consolidation?

We do not foresee a reversal of the trend of the 1990s toward significant consolidation among physicians and medical groups. The same forces that led to consolidation continue—the needs for capital, economies of scale, and market clout in dealing with managed care and the growth in the number of physicians who prefer practicing in larger groups. We expect physician practice consolidation to be rapid.

Implementing Information Technology

The continuing need to invest in IT is a challenge for most medical groups. They often lack the capital necessary to make the kinds of investments needed to position the practice for the future. One expert on medical groups told us, "Physicians are terrified about making a mistake on this. There are so many black boxes that companies are pushing, and the ability to make comparisons is often lacking. A mistake could be devastating." Despite these concerns over bad investments, physician groups must take advantage of the opportunities provided by today's and tomorrow's IT. The emerging opportunities for physician practices to deliver better patient care faster and more economically far outweigh the risks of bad investments in IT.

Investing in Web Sites

It is difficult to imagine a competitive medical group in the twenty-first century that does not have a Web site. Why a Web site? A carefully constructed Web site is a wonderful way for physicians to market their distinctive expertise. Résumés of each physician and physician's assistant can be included, along with references to articles written and papers presented. The good news is that the cost of establishing Web sites is dropping; they are not capital intensive.

Adding hyperlinks to other medical group Web sites in the community and around the world also makes sense. One physician leader told us, "I can see a medical group making cross-references to the Web sites of other reputable groups in the community and to some of the more prestigious large medical groups, like the Mayo Foundation and the M. D. Anderson Cancer Center in Houston." He went on to say that this will help to improve the uneven quality of information presently available on the Internet.

Moving Toward an Electronic Medical Record

For most medical groups, we recommend a cautious approach to selecting an EMR system. There are dozens of vendors offering EMRs. Of course, the explosion in the number of for-profit companies offering Internet-based medical record services directly to consumers has to be taken into account.

One company has developed an optical card that is a portable database. Jack Harper, president and CEO of the company that developed the card, said, "It's an extremely easy system to use. You go into the clinic to see the physician and all the updates to your medical record are changed within one or two minutes" (Austin, 1999a).

One former group practice administrator told us, "While it is true that patients own the information about their own health, physician practices must also have a medical record for their patients. Medical groups can transmit medical data to a centralized medical record firm if the patient instructs them to do so (and perhaps pays for this service), but this doesn't mean that the medical office doesn't have to continue to maintain its own records."

Communicating via E-Mail

Despite security issues and resistance from some physicians, most physicians will soon be communicating regularly with their peers and patients via e-mail. One physician told us that he expects the real opportunities in e-mail to be between physicians and their patients, between physicians, and between physicians and health plans. Looking to the future, he said, "If consumers can schedule their own airline tickets and vacations, there is no reason that they won't be able to make their own appointments with physicians. Also, physicians and the office will be able to communicate test results to patients."

For some large multispecialty clinics, communicating with patients via e-mail is likely to become absolutely essential. As one chief information officer of a large clinic told us, "We can't hire the people to answer the phones, transcribe dictation, and do all of the other basic jobs. Our volume of telephone calls exceeds several million a year, and we can't manage this without making use of new technology, including the Internet and e-mail."

Leveraging Information Technology to Manage Back-Office Operations

Whereas using IT to help with patient interactions will be important for some practices, leveraging IT to manage claims processing and other back-office functions will be essential for all practices. Cost savings are available now for physicians, hospitals, and payers who are willing to make small investments and behavioral changes. Electronic processing is already better, faster, and cheaper for accomplishing several administrative tasks:

- *Eligibility verification,* including verification of what a patient's insurance covers and what the relevant copayments are
- *Referrals management,* including receipt of referral authorizations from payers and tracking and management of referrals

- *Treatment certification and review,* including precare certifications, postcare reviews, and similar tasks
- *Claims processing,* including submission, adjudication, and payment of claims

Electronic processes for performing these functions are getting better every month. They are already good enough to reduce the need for physician support staff, cut down significantly on claims submission errors, improve response time to the patient, and speed up cash flow to the physician.

Managing the Costs and Benefits of Information Technology

Figure 6.2 illustrates a hierarchy of value added to physician practices by IT. Connectivity is at the lowest level in the diagram. Simply giving physicians and their office staff access to e-mail, lab results, and clinical notes entered at other locations provides some value. More important, electronic connectivity provides a foundation for other services. Basic information sharing also adds value. Physicians can use their Web site to refer patients to reliable health information and provide many other forms of useful background data.

Transactions processing is the next logical step. Physicians, hospitals, and payers can cut back significantly on their administrative overload by replacing processes that rely on a large quantity of staff and paper with electronic processes. A transaction processing revolution is coming in health care, and the potential cost savings and processing time improvements are large. We even expect to see an added dividend in the form of a reduced claims error rate.

As practices move further up the IT-leveraging pyramid, other added value will accrue, in several forms. Some practices will provide patient consultations via the Internet; some will also allow patients to schedule their own visits. In some cases patients will be able to submit and access their own lab results via a customized version of their physician's Web site. Physicians will have on-line conferences while each is viewing the same relevant clinical data.

Further up the pyramid lies a still bigger payoff: practices will be able to analyze their clinical and financial data by patient, by type of patient, by payee, and by many other criteria. Medical groups

Figure 6.2. Increasing Levels of Value Added to Physician Practices from Information Technology.

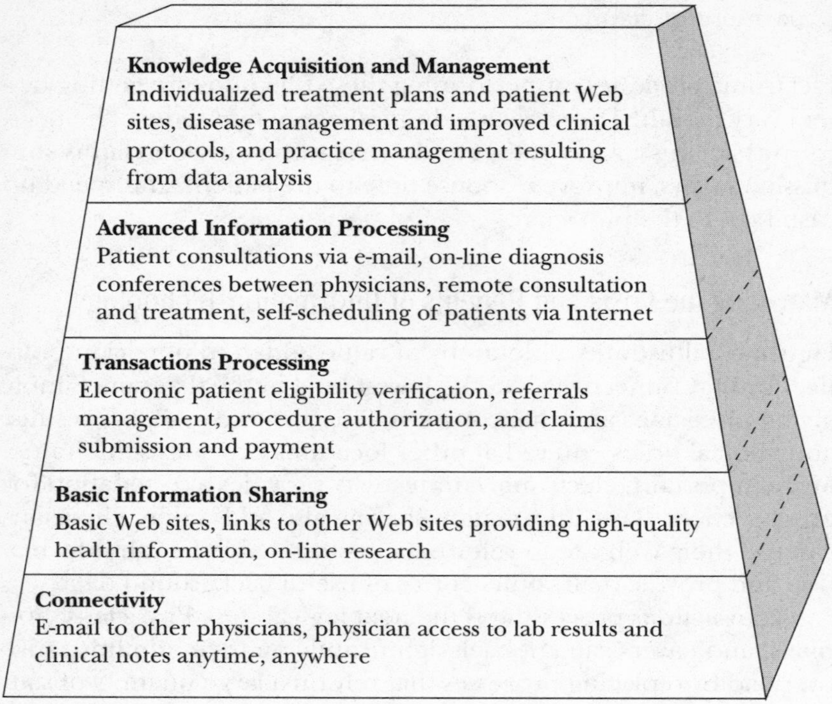

Knowledge Acquisition and Management
Individualized treatment plans and patient Web sites, disease management and improved clinical protocols, and practice management resulting from data analysis

Advanced Information Processing
Patient consultations via e-mail, on-line diagnosis conferences between physicians, remote consultation and treatment, self-scheduling of patients via Internet

Transactions Processing
Electronic patient eligibility verification, referrals management, procedure authorization, and claims submission and payment

Basic Information Sharing
Basic Web sites, links to other Web sites providing high-quality health information, on-line research

Connectivity
E-mail to other physicians, physician access to lab results and clinical notes anytime, anywhere

will be able to pool and compare their data with other practices and draw still more powerful conclusions. Physicians will be using the foundation of electronic information they have developed to acquire, manage, and leverage new knowledge.

Improving Quality of Care

We anticipate major advances in standardizing definitions of clinical quality of care and in presenting quality indicators to the public in terms that are understandable and meaningful. Physicians will be under increased scrutiny regarding the quality of the care they provide, and this information will be more broadly disseminated by a variety of sources (such as health plans, purchasing alliances, and government agencies). In the health system of the future, consumers will be more interested in what they can learn about the quality of care provided by various physicians and medical groups.

Using Patient Satisfaction Surveys

Patient satisfaction surveys are becoming common for all types of medical groups, and the survey instruments will continue to be designed to better differentiate clinical quality from service levels. Furthermore, the results of these surveys will become widely disseminated. In the future that we anticipate, where consumerism and technology dominate, we expect patient satisfaction surveys to be accomplished on a real-time basis using e-mail and other types of IT. This will offer medical groups the opportunity to make immediate adjustments to the way they interrelate with patients.

Reducing Clinical Variation

Process improvement and clinical guideline development accelerated during the last half of the 1990s, and these efforts continue to gain acceptance among physicians, hospitals, and health plans. Furthermore, payers, including Medicare and consumers, want to know whether guidelines are in use and will consider this information as part of their judgment about the quality of care provided by physicians and medical groups.

We expect there to be at least one scandal about the amount of unexplained clinical variation between communities during the first five years of the new millennium. The potential to embarrass physicians over clinical variation is substantial. (Consumers will take an increasing interest in the types of health care utilization data provided by Dartmouth Medical School.) Physicians in practices that leverage IT will be able to generate their own data to use in minimizing clinical variation.

How Will Quality of Care Change in the Future?

Concern over reducing clinical variation and improving quality of care will gain momentum, especially in a new era of consumerism. We expect consumers to take more interest in health care quality than the typical human resources manager of the 1990s did. (Corporate human resources managers will also develop a more sophisticated understanding of quality variations and what can be done about them.)

Improving Service and Access

Here is an e-mail message from the brother of one of the authors. The individual who sent this message lives in northern California and is on Medicare; he suffers from adult-onset diabetes.

> I filled out the forms today to switch from a medical group and HMO in Santa Rosa to Health Plan of the Redwoods. I haven't been able to get a physician assigned to me by the HMO; it has been over six months. When I try to call patient relations, I get an answering machine, and invariably miss their callbacks; they end up sending me a letter. I finally decided to go to a physician I visited before joining the HMO. The cost of filling prescriptions will be higher, but I can get them locally. If I can't see a physician, or find someone who cares about my medical history, what good are all the great capabilities of this HMO?

Unfortunately, this kind of experience with medical groups and health plans is not uncommon. However, consumers will not accept this sort of thing much longer. With the growth in consumer choice and power, improved service and access will be increasingly important regardless of which of the four scenarios for the future predominates.

As demonstrated in survey after survey, when making a decision about which physician or medical group to use, consumers are better at judging service and access than they are at evaluating clinical quality. Service and access are more important for physicians and medical groups, which are on the front lines of dealing with consumers, than for hospitals. Assuming greater consumer choice and a reduced role for health plans, demands for service and access will grow at a rapid rate, especially in a future where consumerism and technology are drivers of change.

Opportunities for Service Improvement

Most criticisms of physicians' offices and medical groups fall into one or more of eleven categories:

1. Unduly long waits
2. Unfriendly staff
3. Difficulty in making appointments
4. Poor communication with physicians and staff
5. Rushed visits with physicians
6. Uncomfortable surroundings
7. Delays in reporting diagnostic results
8. Inadequate emphasis on prevention
9. Inordinate amounts of paperwork
10. Lack of respect
11. Breach of confidentiality

Each of these eleven areas offers an opportunity for physicians and medical groups to improve their level of service.

Access Problems

Problems with access to physicians' offices relate to several issues, including the requirement of going through a primary care gate-keeper, long waits for appointments, inconvenient location of physicians' offices, and limited hours of operation. These problems tend to be more pronounced for baby boomers, most of whom are still working and pressed for time. Based on our experience, many seniors (other than the frail elderly) are not as upset about having to travel relatively long distances to see a physician.

Impact of the Four Scenarios on Service and Access

We anticipate that even if the health care system does not change as fast as we project, consumers' expectations for better service and improved access will be substantially higher in 2005 than in 2000. There will be some medical groups that will become national models of service and access, and their reputation will spread rapidly. Many of the old excuses—"We're too busy," "We can't get good help," "Managed care made us do it"—will no longer suffice. The verdict on primary care gatekeepers is already in: consumers do not like this model of delivering care.

We expect technology to assist many medical groups in improving their service levels. For example, the use of Web sites for scheduling appointments and e-mail for reporting lab and other test results to consumers will become commonplace. Filling prescriptions will be much easier for patients.

We also expect that demand for higher levels of service and more convenience will skyrocket. The use of twenty-four-hour minor emergency centers will grow (which will be to the advantage of larger medical groups and integrated systems). Medical groups will achieve substantial success in differentiating themselves from competitors by the services they provide. Levels of service will truly be the difference between the winners and the losers.

Improving the Cost-Effectiveness of Physician Practices

How much potential is there for improving the cost-effectiveness of most medical groups? Many physicians believe there is substantial room for improvement; in fact, a number of them turned to PPMs for this type of assistance, only to find that it was much more difficult to achieve significant cost savings than most physicians expected. In our analysis we take a broad perspective on improving cost-effectiveness, considering the payer mix, back-office operations, and benchmarking information.

A More Favorable Payer Mix

Most physicians will not admit that Medicare has been one of their best payers over the past decade. In fact, we continue to hear about medical groups that will not accept new Medicare patients. Managed care plans, especially those that are capitated, are generally not popular either. Where will physicians and medical groups turn next?

A number of different medical specialties are attempting to improve their payer mix by going directly to consumers. For example, over the past four years, board-certified plastic surgeons have shifted their mix of patients from 60 percent reconstructive surgery (almost all paid by Medicare, managed care, and worker's compensation) to 60 percent cosmetic surgery (all private pay). Ophthalmologists, who are still paid well for many procedures, are moving to the private-pay market with vision correction surgery. Other medical specialties moving toward private pay include orthopedics, dermatology, otolaryngology, urology, obstetrics and gynecology (with in vitro fertilization, for example), and cardiology (with ultrafast heart imaging, for example). We expect a future dominated by consumerism and technology to offer the best opportunities for physicians and medical groups to improve their payer mix.

More Efficient Back-Office Operations

Most physicians believe that their back offices are not operating at peak efficiency. For most primary care groups, administrative overhead can range from 55 to 65 percent of revenue. Overhead for specialists is typically lower—in the 30 to 40 percent range. Therefore, primary care physicians have more to gain by investing in efficiency improvements.

Improving the efficiency of medical groups is more difficult than it appears on the surface. This is a hard lesson many PPMs learned; most could not generate sufficient savings in back-office operations to come close to covering their management fee. Technology is a big part of the answer for improving the efficiency of medical groups. With a properly constructed Web site, for example, patients could do their own scheduling, thus reducing telephone traffic. Patients' taking control of their own medical records could reduce the workload for the practice. (As noted elsewhere, this does not eliminate the need for medical practices to maintain medical records on their patients.) Billing, collections, and accounting could be simplified with new information systems, and greater use of the Internet for communicating with health plans and other payers could help increase efficiency.

Improved Benchmarking

We have only begun to achieve what is possible with benchmarking practices to help regulate expenses, enhance physician productivity, customer service, and clinical outcomes, and introduce improvements in many other areas. We expect the sophistication of all types of benchmarking to improve dramatically over the next five years.

Cost-Effectiveness: Summary

Consumers will demand more than lower costs, and this may diminish the usefulness of the cost-effectiveness strategy somewhat. We expect the more advanced medical groups to ensure they have access to sufficient capital (discussed later in this chapter) to acquire the support systems necessary for providing better service in order to please consumers.

Generating Ancillary Income

Most physicians will tell you that they would like to find ways to make money while they are sleeping. The possibility of ancillary revenue from a variety of services, including laboratory, pharmacy, outpatient surgery, testing, imaging, and other services, is attractive to many doctors. One otolaryngologist we work with has expanded his practice to include allergy treatment, audiology, and cosmetic surgery. Some plastic surgeons, in addition to performing cosmetic surgery, sell different types of beauty products. Many vision centers, as well as employing optometrists, dispense contact lenses and glasses.

We expect that, in an incremental change scenario, physicians and medical groups will continue an aggressive pursuit of ventures that generate ancillary revenue. As the hospital sector continues its "back to basics" approach and moves away from partnerships with physicians in PHOs and integrated systems, hospitals are becoming especially vulnerable to competition from physicians. If we assume an economic downturn and constrained resources, we expect opportunities for investing in ancillary products and services to dwindle. However, we anticipate that as technology and consumerism become increasingly important, opportunities for physicians to invest in and manage outside ventures will exceed anything seen in the past.

Positioning the Practice for Managed Care Contracting

Medical groups have tried a variety of approaches to position themselves for managed care contracting, with mixed success. The PHO movement (discussed in more detail in Chapter Seven) has been a disappointment. Some IPAs have been successful in obtaining managed care contracts and in providing cost-effective, high-quality care for health plans, but the overall track record is mediocre to poor.

Assessing the Drawbacks of Accepting Risk

There are numerous reports of medical groups losing substantial sums in accepting risk (such as through capitated payment). In 1999 and 2000 there were frequent reports of medical groups declaring bankruptcy or being forced to merge with other organizations, largely because of losses attributable to managed care contracting. As discussed further on, medical groups in California have been hit especially hard.

Looking Back on Past Experience

For the most part, physician strategies of consolidating to increase their appeal and clout in the eyes of managed care plans have not worked as expected. In the case of single-specialty groups, such as neurology and neurosurgery, and others that represent a small share of per member per month costs, health plans have often exhibited disinterest.

A neurosurgeon who heads a network of specialists in the neurosciences told us that this has been one of his biggest sources of frustration with managed care. "We have the data demonstrating our quality, outcomes, and cost-effectiveness," he said, "but the health plans aren't interested. We are insignificant compared with primary care, some of the other medical specialties, hospitals, and drug costs." A group of orthopedic surgeons composed of six practices had a similar experience. Health plans were not interested in contracting with the large group, especially when there were a number of solo practitioners and smaller groups available. The orthopedic surgeon who heads this group told us, "We know that we are the highest-quality group in the metro area, and we are cost effective. The health plans are unimpressed. Even if we invested extensively in improving our measurement of clinical outcomes, I doubt that they would take us seriously. Besides, they would think our data is self-serving."

Avoiding Catastrophic Contracting Arrangements

At least two dozen California medical groups were expected to go out of business by the end of 1999. The California Medical Association reports that over one hundred organizations have declared bankruptcy since 1996. Reports from Texas, New York, Colorado, and other states indicate a similar problem: medical groups' lack of the financial resources and actuarial know-how to be successful with capitated contracts. Many health plans are refusing to contract with medical groups that are not financially strong. When it comes to capitated contracts, medical groups should proceed with great caution, if at all.

Planning for the Future: What Can Be Done?

As far as managed care contracting is concerned, primary care physicians have an advantage in most markets. Specialists, who tend to be in greater supply, face more difficult challenges and usually have no interest in capitated arrangements. We believe that health plans and consumers will become more discriminating and knowledgeable about medical specialists and will ensure that they have access to specialists of the highest quality who provide the best service. Therefore, as consumerism gains momentum, the bargaining position of many specialists may improve.

In summary, it is too early to give up on strategies to position medical groups for success in managed care contracting. However, the growing role of consumers will change the rules of the game. Health plans will increasingly contract with physicians and groups that consumers want and that can demonstrate cost-effectiveness, excellent service, and high quality. Furthermore, these contracts are more likely to be based on a discounted fee-for-service arrangement rather than on capitation.

Creating Relationships with Providers of Complementary and Alternative Medicine

We are already beginning to see traditional physicians and medical groups partnering with CAM providers, and we expect this trend to accelerate regardless of which of the four scenarios for the future prevails. However, opportunities to bring CAM (which is discussed in greater detail in Chapter Eleven) into medical groups will be especially attractive in a future dominated by consumerism. Rather than ignore or fight CAM practitioners, physicians will join with them, and in ever greater numbers. The situation will be analogous to the way ophthalmologists have worked with optometrists and opticians in eye centers.

The physician leader of a large multispecialty group in the Midwest told us that four orthopedic surgeons in the group had been trained in acupuncture and that they were adding a chiropractor. "Let's get real," this physician leader said. "This is what consumers in our area want, and if we don't give it to them, they will pass us by." A staff member of a medical group association had a similar opinion. "If the economics are favorable," he told us, "there is no doubt that many medical groups will bring CAM into the practice. I saw the same thing several years ago with physician assistants in teaching hospitals; at first there was resistance, but as pressures built to control costs, it soon became the norm." He added, "Give physicians credit for being extremely adaptive." A group practice administrator agreed, saying, "If physicians can see that they can make money and protect their markets by offering CAM products and services, they will do it. They aren't that proud."

Gaining Access to Capital

Two of the authors wrote an entire book on the subject of obtaining access to capital, *Capitalizing Medical Groups: Positioning Physicians for the Future* (Coddington, Moore, and Clarke, 1998), and the need for capital continues to be a critically important issue for most medical groups. With the failure of a number of PPMs and with many hospitals experiencing financial problems, the sources of capital for medical groups are more limited than in the latter half of the 1990s.

Capital Needs and the Lack of Ready Capital

Exhibit 6.1 shows the top ten reasons that physicians and medical groups need capital. Most groups do not require funding for all ten reasons; typically, they have two or three of the needs listed.

The key reason that access to capital is restricted is that well over 90 percent of all medical groups do not retain earnings. They operate on a cash basis and fully distribute annual earnings to the physicians who own the group. Despite increased criticism of this approach, it is still dominant (long-standing habits are hard to break).

Exhibit 6.1. Top Ten Reasons for Physicians' and Medical Groups' Capital Needs.

1. Expanding and optimizing the existing practice
2. Adding primary care physicians and sites
3. Investing in new profit centers
4. Adding next-generation facilities and equipment
5. Adding next-generation information systems
6. Developing single-specialty networks
7. Accepting and managing medical risk
8. Providing an exit strategy for retiring physicians
9. Covering cash flow shortages
10. Insulating against risk

Options for Obtaining and Financing Information Technology Support

A future where the application of IT accelerates is scary for most medical groups in that the capital requirements would be larger than many groups could meet from readily available sources. If the pressure on medical groups to invest in IT continues to grow, many more physician practices will be driven to join forces with hospitals, larger medical groups, or PPMs.

Fortunately, we foresee the development of new IT service provision and financing arrangements that will take some of the pressure off medical groups by allowing physicians, patients, and in some cases even health plans and others to adopt a "pay as you go" approach to IT. Companies that specialize in providing individual IT services (application service providers) or suites of IT services (e-health service companies) and groups of companies that allow customers to comparison shop as well as to mix and match IT solutions (e-health trading communities) will become common. Together, they may well offer many physician practices service and financing options that obviate the need for frequent capital investments.

With rampant consumerism, the need for capital will not go away. However, with the continuing strong growth in health care, the shift to more consumer choice, and an overall optimism about the future of health care, it is likely that new sources of capital will emerge. Will this be another wave of Wall Street financing of health care? It is possible.

Nevertheless, we see capital availability as the major limiting factor in physicians' efforts to position themselves for the future. Those groups that begin to retain earnings and give a high priority to developing a capital plan will be the ones that succeed. We have been encouraged to find medical groups that have five-year capital plans. We believe that an increasing number of medical groups will realize the necessity of planning for future capital needs.

Joining a Union

How many physicians will choose to join a union over the next five years? Why would they take this drastic step? John Koster, M.D., an executive at Sisters of Providence in Seattle, noted that physicians are increasingly turning to unionization as a way to stand up to health plans and organizations that employ physicians. "I don't really expect to see physicians giving much more ground to health plans," Koster said. "Most feel that they have already given more than enough."

A physician executive involved in a malpractice insurance company told us, "Physicians are doing this because they are mad, and this is a way of striking back at managed care, Medicare, Medicaid, and the health care system in general." Another physician, who served on the American Medical Association board in the late 1990s, explained that there is more to it than striking back at the system: "I was initially opposed to unionization as being unprofessional. However, because of the antitrust laws, other legal issues that stand in the way of physicians working together, and the growing power of health plans, I concluded that for many physicians, it makes sense. Unionization will make it easier for them to work together."

We expect membership in physician unions to increase slowly. Physicians generally should do well professionally and financially if the health care system develops as we expect it to. In addition, managed care will be much weaker if the country moves more toward individual insurance. Thus we anticipate that there will not be a pressing need for unionization.

Are Single-Specialty Groups Uniquely Positioned for the Future?

It appeared a few years ago that single-specialty groups (other than primary care) were in dire straits. However, single-specialty medical groups are making a comeback in many markets and could well become a dominant form of physician organization over the next five years. The strategies for single-specialty groups overlap with the more general medical group strategies discussed in the first part of this chapter. However, the focus here is on single-specialty groups in the surgical and diagnostic specialties.

"Focused Factories"

Regina Herzlinger (1997), Harvard Business School professor and author of *Market Driven Health Care,* endorses single-specialty groups. She calls these groups "focused factories"—medical practices that can focus on patients with certain needs and meet these needs in a cost-effective and high-quality manner. She provides numerous examples of physicians working in a single clinical area, such as hernia repair, orthopedic surgery, or heart surgery, who could offer superior service and a track record of satisfied patients.

In the Minneapolis–Saint Paul health care market, single-specialty groups are growing stronger and becoming a greater source of competition for multispecialty clinics and independent physicians. One physician told us, "They have some real advantages in recruiting physicians. Their overhead is low, and they aren't supporting primary care networks. They can measure and report their quality, and physicians in these groups tend to take home more dollars."

Most Medicare beneficiaries have the freedom to choose any physician or hospital, and this has boosted business for many single-specialty groups. Although administrators of many of these groups might disagree with us, we believe that, in general, medical specialists have been able to more than cover their costs with Medicare patients. In some specialties, such as ophthalmology, reimbursement levels have gone down but are still attractive.

Market Clout with Managed Care Companies and Other Payers

Many single-specialty groups were formed during the 1980s and mid-1990s partly as a defensive move in response to the threat of managed care and the perceived need to band together to stand up to large health plans. The hope was that market clout would ensure access to the health plans' provider panels and reduce discounts on billed charges.

This strategy worked when the single-specialty group had a virtual monopoly position in a market, leaving managed care plans no choice. We have seen this happen in several midsize markets (communities with fifty thousand to four hundred thousand residents). However, when the markets get larger, it is difficult for a single group to control a medical specialty, which gives managed care plans other alternatives. As the physician leader of a large orthopedic group told us, "There are always bottom feeders out there, and as long as managed care companies only care about price, these physicians will be selected to be in the health plans' panels."

In more recent years health plans, doing an "end run" around larger groups, have begun to enter into contracts with physicians in solo practices and very small group practices. This has caused a number of single-specialty groups, especially those that came together quickly and more out of necessity than desire, to reconsider their strategy and often disband.

Extended Geographical Reach

Many single-specialty groups require relatively large service areas to provide a sufficient number of referrals to keep their specialists busy. This is particularly true in cardiology, cardiovascular surgery, orthopedics, oncology, and the neurosciences.

We worked with a group of six cardiologists in a metropolitan area of seventy-five thousand and witnessed their aggressive marketing efforts to attract patients from as far away as three hundred miles. Leaving the office to make personal calls on primary care physicians was part of their strategy. Of course, providing high-quality care and exceptional service led to patient satisfaction, and the patients told others, including their primary care physicians.

One of the cardiologists said, "As a group of six cardiologists, we couldn't survive without attracting at least half of our patients from outside this metropolitan area. We want to keep our group together. It enhances the quality of care we can provide and reduces the call coverage we have. We also do better financially by keeping our volume up."

Other single-specialty groups extend the boundaries of their service area by operating outreach clinics in surrounding communities. Outreach clinics are especially common among surgeons, radiologists, otolaryngologists, urologists, and orthopedic surgeons. This is a valuable service for small hospitals, which benefit from the increase in local surgeries and patients. Patients, particularly the elderly, greatly appreciate having physicians come to them, obviating the necessity of traveling to a larger city to see a specialist. We have observed an increase in outreach clinics over the past five years and expect this trend to continue in all of the four scenarios we propose for the future of health care.

Measurable Improvements in Quality and Cost-Effectiveness

We know of many single-specialty groups that have been successful in establishing themselves as the premier medical group in their community or region. In fact, we have noticed that almost every community of fifty thousand to one hundred thousand residents has two or three single-specialty groups that have achieved substantial success in establishing strong reputations for quality and service. One of the benefits of a single-specialty group of reasonable size is that it can implement significant initiatives for clinical quality improvement and outcomes measurement and reporting. Furthermore, if the group is of sufficient size, the sheer volume of procedures increases the probability of above-average clinical outcomes.

Direct Marketing to Consumers

A cosmetic surgery group is an excellent example of a single-specialty group that can achieve success by marketing directly to consumers. Nearly all of this type of surgery is private pay, and patients usually come to cosmetic surgery centers on their own—they are usually not referred by another physician. Newspaper and television advertising to consumers is effective, as are more targeted approaches, such as direct mail aimed at individuals with the right demographic characteristics (for example, women between the ages of forty and sixty-five with above-average income in households with above-average net worth). One of the themes of this book is the need to become more sophisticated in market segmentation— definitely a key to success in cosmetic surgery.

Improved Service

For single-specialty groups, improving service is usually a high priority and easier to accomplish than for other types of medical groups. By definition, single-specialty groups are dealing with a more homogeneous group of customers, and service enhancements can be designed specifically around the needs of these individuals.

In comparison with primary care practices, single-specialty groups typically see a much smaller number of patients each day. Therefore, they can devote more attention to the needs of individuals and not be overwhelmed by the volume of patients waiting to be served. Moreover, many single-specialty groups have greater financial resources to devote to service enhancements than primary care practices do.

When it comes to service enhancements, cosmetic surgery centers again offer a good example. Many of these centers allow consumers to see the "results" of a planned surgery beforehand, using computer imaging to show a customer's appearance before and after surgery. In addition, most cosmetic surgery centers have prearranged credit to eliminate an important potential barrier for consumers.

Ancillary Services

Providing ancillary services is not a new strategy for specialists. The freestanding ambulatory surgery center is a prime example. Other examples include laboratory services, imaging, and diagnostic testing. These types of services are often the major profit producers for hospitals, so the strategy of generating ancillary revenues is often a source of conflict between single-specialty groups and their hospitals.

Given that referrals from specialists are among the top sources of hospital admissions, there usually is not much hospitals can do to defend against the loss of ancillary revenues to its "best customers." Of course, as we discuss in Part Four, we prefer to see hospitals and their best physicians (both primary care and specialist) find ways to work together to meet the needs of consumers and other customers. In our opinion, internal competition for ancillary revenues is usually not in the best interests of the community.

Greater Efficiency

By their very nature, single-specialty groups tend to have lower overhead than multispecialty groups, primary care physicians, and many independent specialists. And because they are devoted to a single specialty, they can design administrative processes that are less complex. They are more likely to have the financial resources to implement information systems and automate various procedures, such as scheduling appointments and sending reminders to patients when certain tests (mammograms or pap smears, for example) are due.

Looking ahead, we believe that single-specialty groups are more likely to develop an EMR for their patients and to have physicians trained in and enthusiastic about using new systems such as the EMR. A computerized medical record, in turn, will facilitate studies of clinical outcomes and help to identify prospects for clinical trials.

Competition with Multispecialty Clinics

Single-specialty clinics in some parts of the country are outperforming multispecialty clinics—attracting physicians and paying them more, demonstrating high-quality and cost-effective care, and providing high levels of service for consumers. Furthermore, the cost and complexity of developing an infrastructure, including such necessities as information systems, methods for clinical performance improvement, and means of outcomes measurement, are not as great an obstacle for single-specialty clinics as for multispecialty clinics.

In comparison with large multispecialty clinics, successful single-specialty groups can often offer physicians a better compensation package. Call coverage may also be better in single-specialty groups (a larger number of specialists means fewer evenings and weekends on call). As one physician told us, "This makes a big difference, particularly to younger physicians, who seem to place a higher value on their family and free time."

Conclusions

The initial years of the new millennium will be a challenging yet rewarding time for most physicians and for many medical groups. The strategic opportunities are almost infinite. When we consider the number of generic strategies for medical groups (refer back to Table 6.1), an obvious conclusion is that medical groups will exhibit more variation than other types of health care organizations in the way they position themselves with respect to the four scenarios for the future.

The strategies for primary care physicians and medical specialists do not differ as much as might be expected. Given the fact that they earn less, primary care physicians will have more difficulty in gaining access to capital. However, their capital requirements are usually not as high as those of multispecialty and single-specialty groups.

Of the four general types of investors among medical groups, the future is brightest for the aggressive long-term investor. Assuming this category of medical group can generate capital, it is difficult to imagine any player in health care with greater opportunities for the future.

Chapter Seven

Strategies for Physician Networks

*Physicians are consolidating their practices, but for the
most part, medicine is still a cottage industry. We attempt
to get organized to meet the challenges of managed care,
but most of these efforts have been ineffective.*
PHYSICIAN LEADER OF AN IPA, MIDWEST

Over the past twenty years there has been an explosion in various
types of physician organizations, primarily network models. Most
of the activity has been driven by managed care and by physicians'
response to what they perceived as pressures from health plans to
get organized and accept risk in the form of capitated payment. In
addition to forming or joining group practices, physicians and small
medical groups joined PPMs or networked with other physicians
in IPAs, "clinics without walls," MSOs, and PHOs in the hope that
they could gain market clout with health plans.

In preparing for a future dominated by consumerism and technology, physician networks face several issues:

- What will the economic drivers of physician networks be in the
  future? If managed care becomes less important and capitation declines, what pressures and opportunities will there be
  to maintain existing networks or form new ones?
- What types of network models—IPAs, "clinics without walls,"
  MSOs, PHOs, single-specialty networks, or a model not yet
  designed—are most likely to be successful?

- Do PPMs address a need and have a future? If so, what kind of future?
- What are the best networking strategies for independent physicians and small medical groups who are positioning themselves for the new health care marketplace?

These and other issues relevant to physician networks are the subject of this chapter. In Chapter Six, we assessed strategies available to larger and more formally organized medical practices, including single-specialty groups. In this chapter we consider physicians who have, at least for the past decade, relied on networks or other loosely knit relationships in order to participate in managed care contracting.

Types of Physician Networks and Their Development

The number of physician networks grew dramatically between 1980 and 1995—from around one hundred to nearly twenty-five hundred according to our estimates. The number of physician networks continued to grow in the late 1990s, but the rate of increase declined significantly compared with the early 1990s. Our research indicates that there were at least three hundred PPMs in various stages of formation in 1998 but that the number of PPMs declined to fewer than two hundred from late 1998 to 2000.

Independent Practice Associations

IPAs began to form in the 1970s, mainly as delivery systems for IPA-model HMOs. With the growth of managed care, there was a need for HMOs and PPOs to be able to contract with physicians on either a fee-for-service or capitated basis. IPAs are a legal way for physicians to join together for the purposes of managed care contracting. Many of the IPAs we have worked with or observed over the years have had a high percentage of medical specialists and a low proportion of primary care physicians. This, of course, has made IPAs less attractive to many health plans.

Hal Sadowy, who has worked with and studied IPAs, says, "What IPAs have in common is that they all serve as vehicles for private practice physicians to contract with managed care organizations

(MCOs). In short, IPAs are intermediary contracting organizations that provide a conduit for connecting private, self-employed, solo and small-group physicians to MCOs through a single contract between the IPA and the MCO" (1999, p. 3).

Sadowy reports that the percentage of physicians who participated in managed care contracts through IPAs increased from slightly under 20 percent in 1990 to well over 60 percent in 1998. "For the average physician with IPA contracts," Sadowy says, "these contracts represent about 22 percent of total revenue. The range extends from under 5 percent in markets with low managed care penetration to well over 85 percent in markets with high penetration" (1999, p. 2).

A common criticism of IPAs is that they have not made sufficient investment in the infrastructure needed to accept the financial risk involved in managed care contracts. However, not all IPAs fall into this category. We are familiar with several in California that have well-developed infrastructures (including, for example, the ability to pay claims, assess utilization, and develop financial and management reports) and that have successfully accepted capitated payment and the financial risks associated with this payment system.

The comments of Steve McDermott, executive director of Hill Physicians Medical Group based in San Ramon, California, at a symposium on e-health care strategies provide an overview of the way one IPA works. Hill Physicians, McDermott explained, "had almost 2,500 physician members—680 primary care doctors and 1,800 specialists. Enrollment in the health plans served by Hill increased from 50,000 in 1991 to 400,000 by the end of 1999." According to McDermott, Hill Physicians has focused on identifying best clinical practices, building interdependence among physicians, and introducing financial accountability. "The group has also learned a lot about how to manage populations as well as treating individuals," he added (McDermott, 2000).

In terms of the ability of Hill Physicians to serve patients, McDermott noted that in 1985 the standard number of patients a primary care physician could manage was two thousand. By 1995 this number had increased to three thousand patients per full-time-equivalent physician. "Before 1985 and the advent of capitated payment," McDermott said, "we used to think that 1,000 to 1,500 patients was a full practice" (McDermott, 2000).

Hill Physicians had invested in IT. An IDX basic platform was implemented in 1995, a Healtheon Web enabler was added in 1998, and electronic referrals and authorizations were being implemented in early 2000. As a result of investment in IT, the number of claims submitted by member physicians and processed electronically increased from fewer than ten thousand a month in December 1998 to seventy thousand in October 1999. The number of practices submitting claims electronically increased from 20 to 180 over the same ten-month period. "A key task," McDermott concluded, "is to create effective delivery systems. Although Hill Physicians has done well, most of the real work is ahead of us" (McDermott, 2000).

Physician-Hospital Organizations

PHOs are a more recent phenomenon and were popular in the late 1980s and early 1990s. The primary reasons for forming PHOs were the expected growth of managed care, the ability to offer "single-signature" contracting, and the expectation that the health care system of the future would be vertically integrated. However, with the consolidation of managed care and the willingness of managed care firms to separately contract with solo-practice physicians, small medical groups, and hospitals, the need for most PHOs has declined. As one expert on PHOs noted, "A significant number of the PHOs created over the past decade have either ceased to exist, or are essentially dormant organizations" (Hopkins, 1999, p. 8).

Our experience is consistent with Hopkins's findings—we do not hear much about PHOs anymore. There is little effort being put into forming new PHOs, and there are reports that a number of these organizations have ceased operations or have continued to function, but with greatly diminished force and significance. By and large, PHOs have failed to meet the expectations of their physician leaders and hospital administrators.

There have been success stories among PHOs, but these are few and far between. Thomas Gorey (1994), an attorney and health care consultant who has studied a number of physician organizations that are based on a network model, reports that among the eight PHOs he studied, the number of managed care contracts ranged from two to more than thirty. The number of covered lives was from fewer than five thousand to more than eighty thousand.

Gorey and others who have analyzed the performance of PHOs cite among the positive attributes of this type of organizational model the development of physician leadership and the unification of previously independent physicians. Gorey observes, "A key ingredient of whatever success has been achieved to date in the physician organizations and PHOs included in this study is the leadership role played by a handful of dedicated, respected physicians" (Gorey, 1994, p. 8).

Other PHO successes include adequate financing, an infrastructure (including clinical and management information systems), and an appropriate ratio of primary care physicians to specialists. Gorey found that the two most important issues for PHOs were the need to address the balance between primary care physicians and specialists and the need to provide a significant degree of primary care physician involvement in governance. But perhaps the most important factor in the success or failure of PHOs has been the level of their responsiveness to managed care and health care market needs. As Gorey points out, "A PHO will not be effective unless it is based on a keen understanding of the local market and is responsive to the needs of payers" (Gorey, 1994, p. 14).

Managed care plans and other payers have changed dramatically in the past five years, and more changes are ahead. For example, capitated payment has been declining, dramatically in some markets, and may be insignificant in most health care markets by 2005. In the future, consumers will play a much larger role in purchasing health care, and consumer purchasing coalitions may exist. Can PHOs play a role in this fundamentally new market? We think so. (We address this issue in greater detail later in this chapter.)

Clinics Without Walls

The most notable clinic without walls was the Sac Sierra Medical Group established in 1984 by physicians associated with the Sutter hospitals located near downtown Sacramento. According to one of the physicians who participated in forming Sac Sierra, the initial vision was that the organization would become a multispecialty clinic. "In addition," the physician explained, "we also wanted to impact the healthcare environment rather than reacting to it. We wanted to be in a position to engage in direct contracting. And we wanted to have leverage at the bargaining table with payors, the hospital, and others" (Coddington and Bendrick, 1994, p. 114).

Sac Sierra grew rapidly, from its initial 28 physicians in 1984 to 143 in 1992. Participating physicians retained their offices and staff. Sac Sierra had a central office that offered contracting help and pursued other business ventures aimed at generating ancillary revenue, such as a clinical lab, a cardiac diagnostic center, and a share of an endoscopy center. The central office also provided assistance in purchasing, personnel, payroll and benefits, accounts payable, patient billing, malpractice insurance, and financial reporting (Coddington and Bendrick, 1994).

In 1991, Sac Sierra leaders determined that to accomplish the objective of becoming a multispecialty clinic, the organization needed $20 million in capital. Sutter Health was selected as a partner. The following year Sutter and the physicians began to develop three medical foundations that would take the place of the seventy locations clustered around the two Sutter hospitals. These three medical foundations were strategically located in the Sacramento metropolitan area. In other words, the Sac Sierra Medical Group evolved into a foundation model (common in California) for the delivery of health care (Coddington and Bendrick, 1994).

Gary Susnara, a senior vice president of Sutter at the time, concluded, "The concept of a clinic without walls is flawed. This kind of organizational structure doesn't generate enough revenues to cover its costs. With around 70 practice sites, plus a corporate office, it was inefficient. There was no reduction in the number of employees and there were no economies of scale. And, this kind of group doesn't generate ancillary revenues to help subsidize its operations. If you started a clinic without walls from scratch today, you would get creamed" (Coddington and Bendrick, 1994, p. 124).

However, we continue to find clinics without walls functioning in New England and other locations. Here is one example. In 1997 Dartmouth-Hitchcock Medical Center in Lebanon signed a management agreement with forty independent physicians in Rutland, the second largest community in Vermont. Half of the physicians were in primary care and half in medical specialties; the group was known as the Vermont Physicians Clinic.

There is no managed care in the Rutland market. The purpose of the clinic without walls was for the physicians to preserve their independence from the local hospital, to be able to operate more efficiently, and to have a business relationship with Dartmouth-Hitchcock, the largest system in the two-state region. According to the administrator of the Dartmouth-Hitchcock/Vermont Physicians Clinic relationship, Rob Rosenbaum (interview, Jan. 2000), physicians appreciate the advice and assistance they have received on how to establish and operate a group practice, including administrative support to implement cost reduction and revenue enhancement initiatives and technical support for their information system.

Will clinics without walls emerge again in the new millennium? In certain situations, as in Rutland, clinics without walls may be a means for independent physicians to find a way to work together and gain support from large multihospital systems or integrated systems.

Management Services Organizations

What is an MSO, and how does it differ from other types of physician networks? There are a wide variety of MSOs, including physician-only organizations, physician-hospital MSOs, and those with private and public equity capital. We think of the latter group as PPMs, and they are discussed in the following section on PPMs.

The main difference between MSOs and clinics without walls is that MSOs usually purchase the assets of medical practices and employ all of the staff except physicians. In an MSO, physicians usually form a single professional corporation to function as the physician partner in the organization. In other words, an MSO is a tighter organizational mechanism than an IPA, PHO, or clinic without walls, but it falls short of a merger or outright employment of physicians by a hospital.

In the case of the type of MSO where physicians partner with a hospital, there is usually a corporation formed with representatives of both the physicians and the hospital on the governing board. In a sense, the hospital provides support services; it might also be the capital partner in the relationship.

St. Joseph Medical Center in Stockton, California, is an example of an MSO. In 1994 the medical center responded to a request from a number of independent primary care physicians. As Gary Spaugh, senior vice president for St. Joseph's Regional Health System, said, "They wanted to organize themselves for managed care contracting and to link with the hospital to do so." Spaugh further explained, "We settled on an MSO because it fit our philosophy of physicians leading clinical decisions and the hospital providing capital support and assistance on the business side" (Coddington, Moore, and Clarke, 1998, pp. 125, 126). Although physicians did not invest their own capital, they retained a 50 percent representation on the MSO's governing board.

The MSO grew and experienced success in managed care contracting. Spaugh cited these factors as leading to success: "First, we didn't let the hospital run the MSO. We hired an experienced practice administrator who serves the physicians' interest and facilitates physician decision-making" (Coddington, Moore, and Clarke, 1998, p. 127).

Although MSOs facilitate managed care contracting, and that has been a primary driver for the formation of many MSOs, they also serve other purposes. It appears that MSOs can add value through improving practice management (including information systems), enhancing professional administration, and attracting limited amounts of capital. By virtue of being a tighter organizational model than an IPA, a clinic without walls, or a PHO, the MSO provides physicians a greater opportunity to develop a strong culture that can ultimately lead to the formation of a group practice.

Physician Practice Management Companies

PPMs typically have many of the characteristics of MSOs. Some health care industry observers refer to PPMs as "MSOs with private capital." This describes most PPMs that have gone public or have been in the latter stages of going to the public equities market with an initial public offering (IPO).

PhyCor, established in January 1988, was generally considered the first PPM and, until recently, would have been considered the "blue chip" of the more than three hundred PPMs in various stages of development over the past few years. PhyCor partnered with multispecialty clinics and at its peak comprised over fifty clinics and thirty-eight hundred physicians (Coddington, Moore, and Clarke, 1998).

In the mid-1990s, PPMs were the darlings of Wall Street. With physicians and medical groups perceived as a "cottage industry," the opportunities for realizing economies of scale and market power through consolidation appeared to be enormous. By late 1997 there were approximately thirty publicly traded PPMs and at least as many more preparing for an IPO. During this time many PPMs traded at price-earnings multiples exceeding fifty times earnings.

In attending conferences on PPMs, we frequently heard investment bankers talk about the importance of meeting or exceeding Wall Street's earnings expectations. However, most PPMs did not meet those expectations. By mid-1998 a number of PPMs were in severe financial difficulty, and two highly publicized failures—MedPartners and FPA Medical Management—shocked the investment community and many physicians. In early 1998, following the failed merger of PhyCor and MedPartners, relationships with a number of PhyCor's clinics began to unravel. The period from late 1997 to early 1998, which corresponds with the aborted PhyCor-MedPartners merger, marked the beginning of a dramatic downturn in the fortunes of nearly every PPM.

Despite the dismal performance of many of what Wall Street considered the most solid PPMs, a few continue to do quite well and have an impact. MedCath, which builds specialized heart hospitals, is one example. U.S. Oncology, the result of a mid-1999 merger between American Oncology Resources and Physician Reliance Network, is another example. This PPM has 750 affiliated physicians and treats an estimated 13 percent of all new cancer cases in the United States. U.S. Oncology also runs the nation's largest network of outpatient cancer centers, with fifty-two sites in twenty-four states (Saphir, 1999).

We agree with a health care consultant who observed, "Because the physician needs that gave rise to the [PPM] industry have certainly not gone away, neither have [PPMs]. In response to market challenges, [PPMs] are experimenting with new business models to improve their economic viability" (Feorene, 1999, p. 10). In light of the anticipated fundamental market shift in health care toward consumerism and technology, several additional observations about the future of PPMs can be made:

- More than ever, physicians and medical groups need access to capital in order to develop and apply IT, purchase new medical technology, and meet consumer demands for better service.
- The need for expertise in medical management, one of the selling points of many PPMs, may not be as pervasive as when it appeared that health care was moving at full speed toward capitated payment. At the same time, most medical groups have a continuing need for improvements in processes, outcomes measurement, and patient safety; fulfilling this need requires expertise and funding.
- Even though most physicians have turned their backs on PPMs, medical groups—especially those that are taking a long-term view of the future—could benefit from creative efforts to develop new models to meet their financial needs. We expect new medical group financing models to emerge in the future.

In summary, we believe PPMs were a good idea and could, with a number of changes, represent a promising model for solving many problems of independent physicians, small groups, and even some large medical groups. PPM-like organizations appear to be especially promising for single-specialty groups, such as cardiology, oncology, high-risk obstetrics, and pediatrics groups.

Single-Specialty Physician Networks

Thomas Gorey (1997, p. v), who has studied a variety of physician network models, defines the single-specialty physician network (SSPN) as follows: "A business entity formed and owned by physicians in the same medical specialty in order to pursue managed care contracting opportunities and other cooperative ventures, either independently or in cooperation with a hospital or other entity." Gorey reports that SSPNs tend to be clustered in certain markets and are not represented in all geographical areas. "This situation is likely to persist," he says, "as physician and payer contracting strategies continue to evolve in a market-by-market fashion" (p. 26).

Examples of Single-Specialty Physician Networks

One example of an SSPN is Georgia Dermatology Network in Atlanta, which included 110 physicians and other providers and served over twenty counties. The organization had no staff and relied on the Dermatological Services Corporation, a three-employee organization originally established for administering health plan claims, to provide limited administrative services such as claims processing, contract negotiations, and publication of a network newsletter. In this network each practice had its own staff and computer system and handled its own billing and accounts receivable. This is an example of a very loosely knit, low-cost network.

Pediatric Subspecialty Network in Dallas is another example of an SSPN. This network of sixty pediatric subspecialists was established in 1995. "The network was created out of recognition that in the Dallas market, medical care is driven by managed care payers, and that there was an unfilled niche for pediatric subspecialty contracting because none of the area IPAs included a comprehensive grouping of pediatric subspecialists" (Gorey and Bannon, 1997, p. 55). One of the founding physicians of Pediatric Subspecialty Network said, "We didn't need to make this hard from day one. We didn't want an MSO on day one. All we needed to do was to agree to begin working together in providing services and to recognize that we could address the other issues eventually" (Gorey and Bannon, 1997, p. 56).

The Future of Single-Specialty Physician Networks

In SSPNs there is much discussion about the need to remain flexible, about being open to new opportunities, and about "moving to the next level." Gorey and Bannon view SSPNs as an interim step: "It is likely that many specialty networks will evolve into something else: fully-integrated specialty groups, MSOs, physician practice management companies, or other types of entities. A number of SSPN representatives recognized the strong possibility that specialty networks, as presently constituted, may be a transitional model with a short life expectancy" (1997, p. 26).

In our view it is impressive that in some parts of the United States specialty physicians have set aside competition, agreeing to take the first tentative steps toward working together. Although the motivation for many of these networks may be defensive—to establish a bargaining position with managed care companies—they appear to be a promising first step that could lead to more significant working relationships in the future.

We discuss the strategies of more formally organized single-specialty medical groups in Chapter Six; we are generally optimistic about their ability to succeed in a future where consumerism and technology are key elements of the health care marketplace. SSPNs may be the forerunners of larger single-specialty group practices that could be effective in a more consumer-driven health care environment.

Failed Physician Networks: Lessons Learned

The performance of physician networks is definitely mixed: some notable failures, a few successes, and an abundance of unimpressive results. This section describes one failure with an emphasis on trying to understand the underlying reasons for the problems that arose.

What began as an ambitious undertaking in Colorado in 1998 ended in failure a year later. Millennial was an association of IPAs and other physician organizations established for the purpose of contracting with PacifiCare and other health plans. At its peak the organization comprised seventeen hundred physicians in eight organizations, including several IPAs. Here is one report of what happened: "A vast Denver-area physician network voted to dissolve last week, a month after the state's largest health plan terminated capitation payments. PacifiCare of Colorado said the network, called Millennial, wasn't making timely payments to doctors. PacifiCare had delegated claims payment to Millennial under a three-year contract that started in January" (Jaklevic, 1999).

One physician in family practice who was involved in Millennial, John Kaicher, M.D., initially allied his practice with Aurora Associated Physicians (an IPA) and then with Millennial. Millennial told Kaicher he was spending too much on drugs for his capitated patients, and this led him to hand out more samples. According to Kaicher, he was forced to refer patients to specialists he did not know, surgeries were delayed when the IPA was low on funds, and he had to turn over hospitalized patients to a hospitalist. This last requirement, he said, cost him a quarter of his income and his patients' confidence (Hubler, 2000). "I think that when we first formed this IPA," Kaicher commented, "the whole idea was to have an organized group of physicians that could have some negotiating power, some clout in numbers to deal with the health plans, particularly PacifiCare, and I saw that they went from being the solution to actually being the problem" (Hubler, 2000, p. L8). Kaicher's solution was to close his practice and move to Springfield, Missouri, where there is less managed care. His partner also left, for Yakima, Washington.

What are some of the lessons learned from the experiences of Kaicher and Millennial? Perhaps the first is that physicians often have unrealistic expectations of what an IPA or group of IPAs can do in terms of negotiating with health plans, particularly in a marketplace characterized by a large surplus of physicians. We have observed this often over the years.

Second, although Kaicher's frustrations with capitation were not unusual, he may have given up too quickly. The use of capitation is declining in most parts of the country, including Colorado. In fact, many primary care physicians who serve PacifiCare patients have since been shifted to discounted fee-for-service payment.

Third, it is evident in reading Kaicher's story that he resisted changing some aspects of his practice (for example, he still wanted to visit patients in the hospital) and that he joined the IPA as a defensive strategy in order to maintain access to his patients and receive higher capitation rates. This approach to practicing medicine will fail even in markets where there is little managed care.

The growth of technology and consumerism is likely to place an entire set of new requirements on solo-practice physicians, such as e-mail communication with patients, patients arriving for their appointments armed with information from the Internet, a desire on the part of many patients to integrate CAM with traditional medical treatments, more intensive retrospective review by health plans, and restrictions on pharmaceuticals that can be prescribed. For many physicians these are likely to be disagreeable aspects of practicing medicine.

Preparation for the Future

Which organizational model is likely to be the most successful? What strategies will work best? And what changes will be required?

The Future of Independent Practice Associations

We believe that IPAs will continue to be popular with independent physicians and small groups. As managed care continues, for example, IPAs should be successful in providing a network for contracting with health plans. Payment will increasingly be on a discounted fee-for-service basis and will be acceptable to many independent physicians and their IPAs.

As health care moves more toward individual insurance, IPAs that do not invest in infrastructure (including, for example, information systems, medical management, greater physician accessibility, and patient satisfaction surveys) will be at a competitive disadvantage. There may also be opportunities for IPAs to develop the capability to be involved in disease management and in the measurement and reporting of clinical outcomes. Those IPAs that make an investment in infrastructure and enter the market as a unified, coordinated group of physicians are likely to be rewarded.

In several instances IPAs are becoming technology-based learning and purchasing mechanisms for their practices. For example, Hill Physicians Medical Group in California subscribes to Healtheon's services on behalf of its members. The Sand Hills IPA in North Carolina is contracting with Merallis for its transactions processing. We expect to see several IPAs serve as the vehicle through which practices link up with application service providers and e-health trading communities.

The Future of Physician-Hospital Organizations

It is generally believed that to be successful, PHOs must develop the capability to share risk. We think this viewpoint reflects the past, not the future. With combined physician and hospital capitation declining rapidly, how much need is there for entities that can share financial risk among physicians and a hospital?

Despite the characteristics that have been pointed out as shortcomings of PHOs, we believe that prospects are bright for the "PHO of the future"—a new type of PHO that can reorient itself away from the past focus on single-signature contracting toward our meeting consumer needs. In a future dominated by consumerism and technology, the winners will be physicians and hospitals that can collaborate as partners in developing innovative approaches to serving consumer markets.

If physicians and hospitals focus their efforts on consumers, and not on each other, they should be able to develop effective strategies for marketing, improving service, increasing convenience and access, and measuring outcomes and patient satisfaction. They should also be able to develop a common brand and achieve high levels of consumer recognition in their service area. Exhibit 7.1 compares the characteristics of the traditional PHO with those of the consumer-oriented PHO of the future.

The Future of Clinics Without Walls

We expect clinics without walls to continue, but on a limited scale. This network model tends to perpetuate the status quo—physicians do not have to change very much. However, physician practices that are not ready to respond to a future dominated by technology and consumerism are unlikely to be a significant factor in most markets.

The Future of Management Services Organizations

We believe that MSOs, particularly those that involve a local hospital or large integrated system, have a bright future. MSOs allow hospitals to maintain close relationships with their best physicians and yet avoid the financial liability of guaranteeing income as is the case when physicians are salaried employees of a hospital. There is financial risk in controlling overhead expenses, but this is more manageable than being at risk for physician productivity.

Furthermore, MSOs typically have a broader purpose than managed care contracting. Physicians who participate in an MSO remain at financial risk for their own productivity. At the same time, the administrative infrastructure, especially communications and information technology, can be more readily financed and developed through the cooperative effort of an MSO, particularly one with a hospital or integrated system as a partner. *We expect MSOs, or something similar, to largely replace the employment of primary care physicians by hospitals.*

We expect MSOs to follow the pattern of large multispecialty clinics and use partnership management models—a physician

Exhibit 7.1. The Traditional Physician-Hospital Organization Versus the Physician-Hospital Organization of the Future.

Traditional PHO	PHO of the Future
• Adopts a defensive strategy • Positions both physicians and hospitals for capitation • Makes no real change in physician practice patterns • Lacks an adequate infrastructure (for example, IT, financing)	• Creates a true partnership focusing on consumers • Constitutes a "learning and buying group"—learning how to optimize customer-based care, learning about and acquiring new forms of IT support • Emphasizes clinical process improvement • Works together to coordinate and improve service • Pursues joint marketing strategies • Develops information systems and Web-based technologies to communicate with consumers

leader and an administrator functioning as a team, for example. This should extend the scope of most MSOs to clinical process improvement, outcomes measurement, and, by a natural evolution, disease management. In addition, more advanced MSOs should do very well in an environment where consumers play a more important role.

The Future of Physician Practice Management Companies

Some of the PPMs that never got a good start in the hectic market leading up to the 1998 downturn were in the middle of developing new models involving different relationships with physicians. One PPM, for example, required physicians to buy in rather than the PPM purchasing the physicians' practices. It is clear that PPMs are unlikely to have access to significant amounts of capital. They will depend on their founders and physician participants to fund the needed infrastructure development and care management systems so lacking in the PPMs of the 1990s.

At the same time, access to capital remains one of the continuing needs of medical groups. This problem is not going to disappear; on the contrary, it is likely to grow in importance. PPMs represented a creative way to deal with this issue. Unfortunately, a number of large, popular PPMs failed to deliver on their promises, and this cast the entire industry in a bad light. As a result, access to Wall Street capital appears to be out of the question, at least in the foreseeable future. Therefore funding will have to come from other sources, including physicians themselves (in the form of retained earnings), suppliers of medical products and information systems, hospitals, commercial banks, and other types of financial institutions.

The Future of Single-Specialty Physician Networks

The loosely knit SSPN appears to be evolving into the more tightly knit MSO or the full-fledged medical group. (Strategies for single-specialty groups were discussed in Chapter Six.)

Conclusions

Although physician networks have a mixed record to date, we expect physicians to continue to participate in various types of networks, particularly IPAs, PHOs, and MSOs. Those IPAs and MSOs that develop their infrastructure—in such areas as information systems, medical management, consumer market research, patient satisfaction surveys, and outcomes measurement—could be long-term players. The Hill Physicians Medical Group described earlier in this chapter is an example of an IPA investing in technology and database development.

We are more optimistic about the future of MSOs than we are about clinics without walls and SSPNs. In our view MSOs offer the potential for significant infrastructure support for physicians and, if properly organized and governed, may also be a source of capital. Clinics without walls will continue, but because they tend to be a defensive strategy in the sense that they allow physicians and small group practices to continue to function as they have in the past, we do not see this model doing much to position physicians for the future.

Traditional PHOs are not providing significant benefits to payers or participating physicians and hospitals, and they are not well positioned for the future. PHOs are often viewed by both physicians and hospital administrators as a dead end. However, a change in the underlying purpose of PHOs along the lines of what we propose in Exhibit 7.1 could help renew PHOs. *PHOs that see themselves as true partnerships designed to better meet the needs of customers, mainly employers and consumers, have an excellent future.* This change in vision and culture could pay dividends for physicians and hospitals. A report sponsored by VHA Inc. comes to a similar conclusion: "Efforts at health system collaboration will continue to fall short of expectations and will prove unsustainable, unless both parties share core values and make a commitment to transforming the patient experience through better clinical outcomes and a renewed focus on the human element of care delivery" (VHA/Tiber Group, 1999, p. 1).

Despite their many failures, PPMs meet a need, and we expect entrepreneurs to continue to try to find creative ways to make the PPM model work. The purchase of physician practices, often involving large premiums, was a flawed strategy and is essentially dead. *However, new PPM models in which front-end capital requirements are significantly less are emerging.* Although it is popular to write off PPMs as an experiment that was a spectacular failure, there are lessons to be learned from the experiment that should be useful in the future.

Chapter Eight

Strategies for Hospitals and Multihospital Systems

With the financial pressures we are facing, how can we focus on positioning our hospital system for the future? If we don't figure out how to survive the BBA, there won't be a future for our organization!
CEO OF A THREE-HOSPITAL SYSTEM IN THE MIDWEST

Comments such as those of the CEO quoted at the beginning of this chapter were common in late 1999 and early 2000. In fact, these sentiments are typical of the majority of health care executives we have met in conducting research for this book and in our consulting practice. A typical remark might be, "Don't talk to me about technology and consumerism—tell me how to cut our costs so we can have a positive bottom line." We agree with another health system CEO who said, "My personal issue as a CEO is how to keep a strategic focus in the face of a tornado." Putting it another way, he said, "We are caught in a struggle between strategy and survival. We have to be concerned about both."

This chapter looks beyond what hospitals were doing in 1999 and 2000 to survive the impact of the BBA and focuses on strategies for the future. This does not mean that short-term strategies for survival are not important. However, our focus in this book is on the longer-term future. A key thesis of this chapter is that if hospitals do not look beyond their financial difficulties, they will lose the opportunity to position themselves as information brokers for consumers and physicians and will ultimately be relegated to a less influential role in the health care system.

A Framework of Hospital Strategies

Don Arnwine of McManis Consulting, who is a former CEO of VHA Inc. and a board member of two hospitals in Texas, suggests that the broad strategies of hospitals fall into eight categories. Arnwine's eight strategies, and the intensity of effort and investment he anticipates under each of four scenarios, are shown in Table 8.1. The importance of each strategy in each scenario is ranked on a scale of 1 to 10, where 1 signifies that the strategy is unimportant and 10 represents the greatest financial and management commitment.

"I don't see any of these strategies going away under any scenario for the future," Arnwine says. "However, the intensity of effort and investment could vary quite a bit. For example, centers of excellence, a revenue-generating strategy, would be ramped up if health care moved to a more consumer-driven stage." Arnwine suggests a strategy not included by most others—philanthropy. Philanthropy, he explains, "is a 3 now (on a 10-point scale) but because of the cost of acquiring technology, would reach 7 or 8 in a future dominated by information technology."

This chapter considers a number of strategies for hospitals and multihospital systems, taking the eight items listed in Table 8.1 into account. The specific strategies addressed in this chapter are summarized in Exhibit 8.1. In addition, we address some of the special challenges confronting rural hospitals.

Improving Overall Market Positioning

All types of acute care hospitals, including sole community providers, are rethinking their market position. With increased use of the Internet and greater consumer savvy about other alternatives, most hospitals will not be able to merely assume they can maintain market share in their service areas. Leland Kaiser, a health care futurist, believes hospitals will experience difficulties in defending their market areas: "With health care becoming more regional, national, and even international, locational advantage in a relatively small market area may not be sustainable" (interview, Mar. 31, 2000).

Table 8.1. Changing Strategic Emphasis for Hospitals in the Four Scenarios.

Strategy	Scenario 1: Incremental Change	Scenario 2: Constrained Resources	Scenario 3: Technology Dominant	Scenario 4: Consumerism and Technology (Retail)
1. Containing costs	6	8	6	6
2. Creating physician alliances	5	8	8	9
3. Divesting	5	8	4	7
4. Developing centers of excellence	5	6	7	8
5. Improving customer service	3	6	7	9
6. Consolidating	4	5	6	7
7. Expanding the market base	5	6	7	8
8. Pursuing philanthropy	3	7	7	7

Exhibit 8.1. Major Strategies for Hospitals and Multihospital Systems, 2000–2005.

1. Improving overall market positioning
2. Strengthening relationships with physicians
3. Improving the financial performance of hospital-owned primary care practices
4. Emphasizing mass customization
5. Developing or improving centers of excellence
6. Improving operating and financial performance
7. Networking, collaborating, and consolidating
8. Improving service and user friendliness
9. Building information systems
10. Gaining access to capital
11. Meeting community health care needs
12. Attracting and retaining clinical staff
13. Downsizing and divesting

Geographical Coverage

With growth in technology and consumerism, it will be important for hospitals to solidify their positions in their service areas and perhaps expand their geographical coverage. This would be especially true for tertiary care facilities, which would have greater opportunities to improve their reputation for providing excellent care for more seriously ill patients.

Reputation and Brand Name

Many community hospitals and smaller multihospital systems are fortunate in being well known in their market areas and having the equivalent of brand name advantage. Sioux Valley Health System (based in Sioux Falls, South Dakota, and serving parts of eastern South Dakota, northeastern Iowa, and southwestern Minnesota) is an example. It is also interesting that many hospitals have relinquished their local brand name advantage by changing their names as they have joined larger networks or systems.

Our focus group research with consumers, conducted in a wide variety of settings, has convinced us that many hospitals in the United States, perhaps well over half, have strong local reputations for quality, stability, friendliness, and service. Hospitals also benefit from their economic importance: they are typically one of the largest employers in the community, and local residents support them because of their many contributions to the community and region.

Strengthening Relationships with Physicians

A survey reported in *Modern Healthcare* (Bellandi, 1998, p. 30) showed that "physician distrust of our system" topped the list of major obstacles to increased organizational integration with physicians. Many hospital CEOs lack credibility among both primary care and specialty physicians. Among primary care physicians employed by hospitals, distrust typically stems from animosity generated during initial negotiations and from continuing perceptions that hospital leaders (both the board and management) have not kept their original agreements. Among specialists, who are rarely employed by hospitals, distrust usually arises from a perception that hospitals have turned their backs on them. One specialist told us, "A few short years ago all we heard about was primary care. Our hospital didn't care that much about us. It looks like the pendulum is swinging back toward specialists, who are major users of the hospital."

In the new health care marketplace, it will be particularly important for hospital CEOs and their management teams to find new and creative ways to work with physicians, both those in primary care and specialists. The "PHO of the future" discussed in Chapter Seven is one example. A continuing adversarial relationship between physicians and hospital leaders is almost surely a prescription for failure.

Differences Between Physicians and Administrators

The differences between physicians and administrators are difficult to reconcile. In their book *Trust Matters,* Michael H. Annison and Dan S. Wilford (1998, pp. 94–97) identify a number of differences between hospital managers and physicians that make it difficult to develop and sustain a trusting relationship:

- *Basis for respect.* A physician's reputation and respect among peers are based on professional capability, clinical skills, and ability to navigate the complex personal relationships among members of the medical staff. "Administration, by contrast, traditionally expect that respect will come with the job title" (p. 95).
- *View of systems.* Physicians tend to dislike systems, whereas most administrators enjoy working within an organization.
- *Allegiance.* Physicians feel an allegiance to their patients, their profession, and the practice of medicine. Conversely, managers usually have an allegiance to the organization.
- *Decision making.* Physicians make decisions quickly, whereas administrators take more time for analysis before making a decision.
- *Sense of time.* Physicians tend to have a greater sense of urgency than administrators do.

Our experience with integrated health care systems of the type led by physicians is that they have a greater understanding and appreciation for these differences and more patience in working through issues in order to build trust.

Competition from Physicians

In many communities physicians have become increasingly aggressive in establishing their own ambulatory care centers, including outpatient surgery as well as imaging, laboratory, pharmacy, and other ancillary services. This has led to major rifts with local hospitals and to the firing of more than one hospital CEO. In the future, consumers will decide which facilities—those owned by hospitals or those owned by physicians—provide the best value. The future of these sorts of outpatient and ancillary services will be decided by the marketplace.

New Relationships with Medical Specialists

Since the late 1990s there has been a developing trend toward elevating the status of many medical specialties. Some of this shift in emphasis was triggered by the growth and marketplace acceptance of single-specialty PPMs like MedCath and Pediatrix. Gain-sharing relationships between hospitals and physicians also opened up a number of possibilities for new types of relationships with medical specialists.

We believe that despite potential legal concerns about gain sharing, creative new relationships will evolve in a future dominated by consumerism and technology. In this type of health care environment, there will be much to be gained by combining financial resources to purchase technology and to jointly develop a strong market presence, including brand names. Centers of excellence will be an especially effective strategy.

Joint Physician-Hospital Learning Communities

We believe hospitals have a relatively small window of opportunity to become the primary sponsor of learning communities for their physicians. These learning communities need to experiment with new approaches to consumerism and technology. They need to compare results with other similar learning communities (that is, other markets). If hospitals do not do this, then someone else— e-health companies, health plans, or others—will.

Improving the Financial Performance of Hospital-Owned Primary Care Practices

Improving the financial performance of hospital-owned primary care practices continues to be one of the most widely discussed and misunderstood issues facing many hospitals. Our advice is not to rely on conventional wisdom and jump to a quick conclusion on this issue.

Reassessing the Objectives

Why did the hospital acquire physician practices in the first place? Because other hospitals were doing it? Because the hospital was trying to evolve into an integrated system? Because hospital leaders thought single-signature contracting was coming and primary care physicians would be the gatekeepers to the entire system? To fill hospital beds? To keep physicians from joining a PPM?

The situation has changed dramatically since the early to mid-1990s, when financial alignment with primary care physicians was the popular thing to do. In many cases, however, health plans and employers have spoken: they are not interested in contracting with a narrow panel of primary care physicians and a hospital. Consumers have let it be known that they prefer health plans that offer open access and broad panels of physicians and that they dislike having to go through primary care gatekeepers.

Reevaluating Primary Care Strategies

Where does this lead hospitals as they reevaluate their primary care strategies? Are the losses real? Can the financial performance of primary care physicians be improved? Does the strategy of hospital ownership of primary care practices make sense?

Are the Losses Real?

We are aware of many cases where primary care groups gave up most of their ancillary services (for example, X rays, treadmill tests) when they became part of a health system. We are also aware that increases in corporate overhead and in expenses for fringe benefits are sometimes ascribed to hospital-affiliated medical groups. But what about the additional business referred by primary care physicians to medical specialists affiliated with the hospital or the added income from inpatient and outpatient services that primary care physicians generate? We have seen very large numbers—over $1 million a year in some cases—representing the value of the additional revenues brought to a hospital by a single primary care physician.

However, there are few hospital-affiliated primary groups that have not suffered a decline in productivity following the sale of their practice. Their original contracts may have been flawed in the sense that they reduced physicians' financial incentives to work as hard as they had when they were on their own. Many primary care physicians viewed the new arrangements as an opportunity to spend more time with their patients and their own families.

Based on our experience, there are many situations where hospital boards and managers are comparing apples and oranges in evaluating the financial performance of their primary care practices.

The annual losses, frequently in excess of $50,000 per physician, receive the attention while other, positive financial contributions get lost in the shuffle. Before devising a plan of action, it is important to make a fair accounting of the added revenues and benefits, as well as the additional costs, associated with hospital-employed physicians.

Can the Financial Performance of Primary Care Physicians Be Improved?

There is hardly a situation anywhere in the country where it would not be possible to improve the financial performance of hospital-owned primary care practices. Based on our experience with medical groups, we believe the best opportunities for achieving a financial turnaround lie in increasing the number of patients served and improving physician productivity. It is unlikely that improvements in back-office operations can yield sufficient savings to put a serious dent in reported deficits.

Does Hospital Ownership of Primary Care Practices Make Sense?

Towers Perrin (1999a) observes that there are two very different motives for employing primary care physicians: economic and strategic. Large multispecialty group practices learned long ago that primary care practices, with their high overhead and low reimbursement, do not break even financially, yet many consider their primary care network to be one of their most valued strategic assets.

There are many hospitals that would like to undo their arrangements with primary care physicians and get back to the "good old days," when physicians were independent. Of course, this leads to an important question: Would these primary care physicians continue to be loyal to the hospital that dropped them? Another relevant question is whether the physicians might be acquired by a competitor.

It is perhaps even more important to determine the overall goal of the hospital or multihospital system in terms of its vertical integration strategy. Have circumstances changed sufficiently that this strategy no longer makes sense? Or is there a continuing need for physicians and hospitals to find ways to work together, particularly in a new era characterized by growing technology and consumerism?

Hospital-Owned Practices: Conclusions

We agree with Towers Perrin (1999b, p. 6) in its assessment of capitation and the future role of primary care physicians: "Because payer markets will not move to 'global capitation' as the preferred method of reimbursing providers, primary care physicians won't become the focal point of healthcare management. Their value in an overall health system strategy remains high, however, and they will retain an important role in health maintenance and preventive medicine."

The key to the economic viability of the strategy of employing primary care physicians goes back to the overall mission of the organization. On the one hand, if the mission is to fill beds and survive as a hospital or multihospital system, then employing primary care physicians may be of dubious economic value. On the other hand, if a hospital desires to take on the characteristics of an integrated system and approach the marketplace as a coordinated entity, aligning primary care physicians (and specialists) with the hospital will continue to make sense strategically.

Emphasizing Mass Customization

With the growth in consumerism, hospitals and multihospital systems will increasingly refine their skills in marketing and in customizing services. Several individuals we interviewed told us that developing a database to effectively segment the various markets that a hospital serves will be an especially important strategy for the future. (The same holds true for any other kind of health care system.)

What Is Market Segmentation in Health Care?

By *market segmentation* we are referring to identifying a number of groups of households or individuals with somewhat common characteristics who are likely to desire certain types of products and services. Market segmentation is just the opposite of the traditional approach of many hospitals that assumes "one size fits all."

Most hospitals have had experience in identifying women who are expecting children and in developing a variety of services directed to this market segment. But what about other market segments, such as individuals with certain chronic diseases—diabetes, congestive heart failure, or asthma, for example? Younger seniors who are focused on staying well are another example of a market segment that could be identified and targeted.

Can Hospitals Get the Job Done?

A survey by KPMG of 175 hospital and health system CEOs raised the question of whether hospitals have the infrastructure to market directly to consumers. Although 80 percent of the CEOs said consumers should and will be the ultimate market drivers, they admitted to sitting on the sidelines while health plans and insurance companies were in contact with consumers. KPMG partner Terry Newmyer said, "This may be the only industry where core business functions like marketing, sales and finance have been unintentionally turned over to a third party" (KPMG, 1998, p. 1).

Of course, lack of experience in marketing directly to employers and consumers is one reason cited by some health care systems for getting into the health plan and direct contracting business. One CEO told us, "It is valuable for us to have direct contact with health plan members; it gives us insights into the market that we wouldn't have otherwise."

Market Segmentation Will Be Essential to Customer Retention

Market segmentation is a necessary step in developing and marketing more specific and targeted health care programs. The consumers of the new millennium will want to be considered unique and will favor those hospitals (along with their associated physicians) that cater to their special needs. (Market segmentation as an overall strategy is discussed in more detail in Chapter Fifteen.)

Developing or Improving Centers of Excellence

Developing centers of excellence has been a popular strategy for hospitals of all sizes and in many different types of locations. As we look ahead, regardless of the scenario, developing or improving centers of excellence appears to be a useful revenue-generating, differentiating strategy for many hospitals.

What are typical centers of excellence for hospitals? We have observed over the years that it is possible for almost any hospital to identify and develop at least one center of excellence. For example, Routt Memorial Hospital in Steamboat Springs, Colorado, is known for its emergency room and orthopedic services. Many small hospitals in rural areas are adept at meeting the needs of the elderly, including joint management and colocation of long-term care and rehabilitation facilities. Many inner-city hospitals are well known for emergency services. Exhibit 8.2 lists several additional examples.

Realistic Assessment

Any hospital that hopes to develop one or more centers of excellence needs a realistic appraisal of its strengths and weaknesses and of how well the institution is positioned for the future. In some cases, focusing on one center of excellence may mean dropping an existing service. In others it may mean investment to build up

---

Exhibit 8.2. Examples of Hospital Centers of Excellence.

Hospital centers of excellence can be devoted to such specialties as these:

- Women's health
- Obstetrics, neonatal intensive care
- Oncology
- Cardiology
- Orthopedics
- Urology
- General surgery
- Emergency medicine
- Occupational health
- Mental health
- Alcohol and substance abuse prevention and care
- Rehabilitation
- Diagnostics
- Geriatrics

---

clinical services that have the potential to become centers of excellence.

Role of Physicians

Developing centers of excellence obviously calls for close relationships with physicians. Physicians must agree that the hospital needs to invest more in some clinical areas than in others and be willing to recruit new colleagues to build these centers. Our experience is that many specialists will embrace this strategy; there is usually an alignment of interests and financial incentives in centers of excellence.

The "Halo Effect"

One aspect of centers of excellence is the fact, supported by consumer research, that the reputations of a hospital for heart surgery or obstetrics and gynecology rub off on other product lines. "If they can do a good job in hearts, they have to be good in gallbladders and hernias." Of course, this is one reason for the proliferation of cardiac programs in many communities.

How Do Centers of Excellence Fit into the Future?

Centers of excellence would be especially important in the health care environment we anticipate. At present, consumers are swayed by their views on centers of excellence, and this would become even more powerful in the future that we envision. Even in markets where managed care is dominant, there is merit in investing in centers of excellence. One CEO pointed out to us that having two or three centers of excellence influences employees to sign up for health plans that include the hospital: "Our reputation in [obstetrics] and pediatrics is a major factor in health plans' wanting us—our physicians and the hospital—in their panel of hospitals and in employees' choosing a health plan that includes us." In other words, the halo effect works.

Improving Operating and Financial Performance

One physician leader we interviewed offered this observation: "Hospitals are like intensive care units; they can't look to the future until they stop the bleeding."

What Is Performance Improvement?

Performance improvement can mean many different things to hospitals. Is it full implementation of CQI? Reengineering? Is a hospital that employs a full-time industrial engineer investing adequate resources in performance improvement? Are across-the-board layoffs part of performance improvement? What about reorganizing and combining departments or better monitoring of how well the hospital is meeting its budget?

Performance improvement can be, and is, all of these things and more. It can include a department-by-department analysis of revenues, direct costs, and contribution to overhead, followed by initiatives aimed at improving departmental financial performance. It can include data collection and analysis of clinical product lines or services (such as cardiac or orthopedic services) in order to improve overall cost-effectiveness. It can include the development of clinical guidelines designed to optimize quality, lower costs, and reduce risks.

Potential Benefits of Performance Improvement Are Questioned

The Health Care Advisory Board said this about hospitals' efforts to reduce costs: "The chosen approach of most hospitals to cost reduction has been to launch a frontal assault on the problem, again and again and again. . . . The vast majority of CEOs have launched five or more cost-reduction campaigns over just the past 24 months" (Advisory Board Company, 1997, p. 10). The Advisory Board goes on to report that onetime efforts yield disappointing results: "More than 70% of these campaigns produced no significant FTE [full-time-equivalent] reductions and well over half produced less than 5% savings. Even the small savings realized often 'creep' back" (p. 11).

Performance Improvement Is a Strategy for the Future

Despite problems of follow-through, performance improvement efforts must continue. We know of many hospitals and health systems that have already reduced their expenses by several million dollars a year. We believe that performance improvement relates closely to quality of care and service levels in the hospital, both matters of special emphasis under a scenario where consumers take charge.

Networking, Collaborating, and Consolidating

Most hospitals are part of a local or regional network of hospitals or part of a large national alliance, such as VHA Inc. In addition to imparting economic advantages through group purchasing and the sharing of development costs of new technology, networking also helps hospitals gain market clout with managed care companies.

Hospital Networking

Most of the hospital networking we have evaluated over the years has been for the purpose of managed care contracting, usually with PPOs. Most of these networks are not organized to accept financial risk. The Health Care Advisory Board (1994, p. 46) found that loose affiliations, or networks, of hospitals were all but useless in reducing system costs: "The hallmark of most effective systems is a single governance structure including one corporate board, one CEO, one income statement; highly integrated hospital systems able to dissolve individual hospital boards operate as a single unit with multiple locations." Our experience is that many hospitals are not willing to go this far; however, constrained resources brought about by an economic downturn and less money in Medicare would push them in this direction.

Collaboration with Other Hospitals

Our research into collaborative relationships among hospitals suggests that collaboration in the following areas can yield major benefits:

- Helicopter service
- Ambulance service
- Hospice care
- Laboratory services
- Imaging centers
- Joint ownership of rural hospitals

- Community health education
- Child care
- Blood banks
- Information systems

Weaknesses in Collaborative Efforts

At the same time, weaknesses have appeared in some collaborative efforts. One chief financial officer of a hospital involved with another hospital in a fairly elaborate collaborative effort told us, "Religious issues are tough to deal with. We can't seem to overcome them. Also, the turnover of board members and management of both hospitals makes it difficult to hold our collaborative efforts together."

Another factor making it difficult to collaborate is fear of violating antitrust laws. More than one collaborative arrangement has come under intense scrutiny by both the Federal Trade Commission and state regulators. The fear of violating antitrust laws (a criminal offense) is not underestimated by most hospital CEOs. In many respects it seems counterproductive to subject hospitals to such intense scrutiny when they are trying to take costs out of their systems and at the same time offer area residents a service that might not otherwise be available. There are mixed signals from various payers and regulatory agencies on this issue.

On balance, however, we expect hospital collaboration to continue. Competing hospitals will increasingly be forced into finding ways to work together to eliminate duplication and reduce expenses. With the increasingly high costs of technology, there may be motivations for hospitals to collaborate in developing and acquiring information systems. We have examples of this in many other industries, including large retailers, financial institutions, newspapers, and airlines.

Establishment of Networks with Medical Groups and Integrated Systems

Hospitals, particularly those in rural areas, have established tight relationships with multispecialty clinics and integrated systems. This enables these hospitals to maintain their share of the market, offer more physician services to residents of their service area, and compete for managed care contracts.

We see hospitals networking with large medical groups and integrated systems as an especially relevant strategy for the future. As technology becomes increasingly important, networking with integrated systems might lead to a reduction in investment requirements. Growth in consumerism will motivate hospitals to network in order to offer a broader array of services and achieve greater geographical coverage.

Merger or Sale of the Hospital

With poor economic conditions and constrained resources, which would include continuing problems with reimbursement from Medicare, many hospitals would be forced to sell or merge. With consumerism and technology growing in importance, the capital investment required to stay competitive may exceed the resources of many independent hospitals.

Improving Service and User Friendliness

For most hospitals there is much room for improvement in service levels. Nearly every person we interviewed cited the need to improve service and user friendliness of hospitals (and other segments of health care as well) as a top priority for the future.

We know, based on research conducted over the past two decades, that consumers believe that service is important, and its visibility often overshadows quality of care. Even with dramatic improvements in the ability to measure and report clinical quality of care, we expect service enhancements to be critical for hospitals during the first five years of the new century. Service encompasses such aspects of health care delivery as the admission and discharge processes, emergency department procedures, nursing care, friendliness of staff, communication between physicians, patients, and patients' families, and insurance claim and other paperwork processing.

Becoming User Friendly

User friendliness depends on more than just friendly staff; it involves the systems in place and whether or not they make it relatively easy to navigate through a hospital.

Gaining Competitive Advantage Through Better Service

Northwestern Memorial Hospital in Chicago built a $580 million facility that opened in 1999. If consumers are increasingly involved in making health care decisions, the design of this new facility should give Northwestern a competitive advantage. Here is one description of the new facility:

> Every patient admitted to Northwestern has a private room with windows; less visibly, the hospital has gathered labs and diagnostic services that were scattered throughout 22 old buildings and placed them near the staff and patients who need them.
>
> Besides visions of bedside cappuccino, the first novelty to hit new patients entering the shared base of the hospital's twin skyscrapers comes when they head for the admitting department. It isn't there. Instead, an aide with a laptop computer registers a patient at bedside in his or her own room [Fischman, 1999, pp. 68–69].

Many U.S. hospitals would like to emulate Northwestern Memorial but do not have the financial resources to do so. However, we anticipate more of these sorts of state-of-the-art facilities in the future.

Implementing Service Strategies for the Future

One health system CEO told us that improving service is a never ending challenge: "You have to continually educate existing employees and make a special effort with new employees. I personally handle this part of new employee orientation; they need to know that I think it is important to our success."

Building Information Systems

We see the development of more IT as one of the most important issues facing hospitals over the first five years of the new millennium. Don Arnwine, who proposed the eight broad strategies for hospitals referred to earlier in this chapter, does not view investment in IT as a strategy. "I see information systems as an enabler," he says. "You are going to have to invest in information technology, and probably many more dollars than in the past. This is going to be part of the price to stay in the game." We have included the development of new IT as a strategy primarily because of the required financial and human resources. Most hospitals are behind businesses in other industries in their use of IT, and catching up will be tremendously expensive.

We have noted in our studies of large integrated systems that these systems have invested more in IT than the typical hospital or multihospital system. Integrated systems typically have the challenge of providing a centralized database for patients that use both a multispecialty clinic and hospital services and of providing "seamless" care for patients. This is a substantially more complicated, and more expensive, IT challenge than the one facing most hospitals.

We have also noted that integrated systems tend to be larger users of e-mail and that their physician-to-physician communication is far ahead of that of the typical fragmented, independent medical community. Although there are many advocates of "virtual" integration (that is, staying away from ownership of medical groups), one of the fixed costs of achieving virtual integration will be substantial investment in IT.

Gaining Access to Capital

Gaining access to capital includes planning to ensure the long-term economic viability of the hospital or multihospital system.

What Are the Major Capital Needs of Hospitals?

In addition to IT, a capital strategy includes plans for rehabilitating or replacing aging facilities. Many hospitals have fallen behind in modernizing patient rooms and other patient care areas, and the needs are mounting. Of course, this adds to the financial burdens facing many hospitals.

Poor Earnings and Cash Flow Are Limiting Hospitals' Access to Capital

Not a week goes by without a story in one of the health care magazines or newsletters about the downgrading of the debt, or credit worthiness, of a hospital. Without relief from the BBA, it is unlikely that the situation will improve; in fact, it will probably get worse.

Many Hospitals Have Become Dependent on Nonoperating Income

There are many hospitals and several very large multihospital systems that are dependent on earnings and gains from their investments. Operating income is marginal or negative and not expected to improve. In lamenting the difficulty of achieving a positive margin on operations, the chief financial officer of one large health system said, "And this is in a strong economy. If the bottom falls out, where will we be?" This viewpoint was echoed by many chief financial officers and other hospital executives we interviewed.

How Can Hospitals Increase Their Access to Capital?

Increasing access to capital begins by improving the financial performance—the cash flow—of the hospital or hospital system. This involves the performance improvement initiatives discussed earlier and finding new revenue sources. In our view both finding new revenues and lowering costs are important, but the greatest potential is on the revenue side, especially in a market dominated by consumerism and technology.

Philanthropy Can Attract Venture Capital

We are continually impressed with the community support for not-for-profit hospitals, especially in rural areas or two-hospital communities. In a health care environment characterized by rapid growth in technology and consumerism, pursuing opportunities to seek local funding for new initiatives should yield big payoffs.

One of the advantages of funds raised by hospital foundations is that these dollars can often be viewed as the equivalent of venture capital. These monies can be used to purchase technology and initiate new services where there are risks involved. Venture capital for hospitals will be an extremely valuable resource in any conceivable health care future.

Meeting Community Health Care Needs

Almost every acute care hospital has something in its vision or mission statement about improving the health status of the community. Are these statements serious? Will any of the changes in the health care marketplace of the future encourage hospital boards and managers to invest more resources in meeting this objective?

Hospitals' Unique Roles in Communities

Despite the serious issues facing hospitals as they position themselves for the future, the local hospital is often the safety net of health care. This has become clear as the BBA has negatively affected long-term care and home health; hospitals have been left to make up the difference.

Larry White, president of St. Patrick Hospital in Missoula, Montana, explains it this way: "We were blindsided by the impact of the BBA on nursing homes. They wouldn't accept patients that we wanted to discharge. This drove up our average length of stay by one day." The BBA also affected home health care in Missoula and put more of the load on the two hospitals in the community. White concluded, "Hospitals seem to be the safety net. When [the Health Care Financing Administration] cracks down on other types of providers, we end up carrying a disproportionate share of the burden" (interview, July 1999).

An Outstanding Example of a Hospital Meeting Community Needs

Although most hospitals give lip service to meeting the needs of the community, there are hospitals around the country that are taking this seriously. The seventy-bed Franklin Memorial Hospital in Farmington, Maine, is a prime example. (Farmington is in south central Maine, about an hour's drive north of Portland.)

The hospital took the lead in creating the Franklin Community Health Network in 1991. The network has four affiliates: the hospital, Pine Tree Medical Associates (nine primary care physicians), Evergreen Behavioral Services (a joint venture with St. Mary's Regional Medical Center in Lewiston), and the Healthy Community Coalition. The coalition, which became a part of the Franklin Network in 1993, is committed to improving the health and well-being of the people of the region.

There are at least two unique features of the Franklin Network. The first is that 250 people from the region are involved in governance and committees. One board member said, "We have strong community buy-in. Also, we listen and act upon what we hear." He added, "The people in Farmington have a lot of pride in this community and its hospital." Based on our work with hospitals in small communities, this is not an unusual perspective; it points to one of the strengths of hospitals.

The second unusual feature of the Franklin Network is the all-day visioning conference, held every other year, involving individuals from the community and region. Richard Batt, the CEO, said, "This is an effective way to get a first-hand community assessment. When two hundred fifty people, including nearly all of our physicians, are willing to spend a day thinking about the future and what we need to do to improve the health status of the community, this is truly impressive" (BBC Research & Consulting, 1997, p. 11-6).

These are some of the programs coming out of the efforts in Farmington:

- Farmington has an organized wellness program that has achieved impressive success in smoking cessation and cardiovascular risk reduction.
- A healthy families program includes home visits for first-time parents and identification of high-risk parents.
- Occupational health programs for major employers in the region are highly developed and have produced demonstrable results. One paper company reported that its annual bill for occupational health was reduced from $900,000 to $40,000.

Is the Vision of Meeting Community Health Needs Still a Viable Strategy?

In a sense, meeting community needs is what we are talking about in the new health care marketplace. In this type of market the emphasis will be on meeting the needs of increasingly demanding consumers who will have more choices than ever before, even more than in the days before managed care.

Although more hospitals talk about meeting the health care needs of the community than have effective programs for doing so, we believe that this is still an ideal worth seeking. Many in health care would advise hospitals to stick to their inpatient and outpatient programs and not get carried away with diversification and vertical integration. However, we think this approach can be shortsighted. Particularly in more sparsely populated areas, hospitals need to see themselves as integral to meeting the total health care needs of the communities and regions they serve. This is where many hospitals should make their stand, and it will pay off in the future.

Attracting and Retaining Clinical Staff

Given a healthy economy, there are continuing concerns about being able to attract and retain sufficiently trained and motivated staff for the hospital. This includes nurses, nurse's assistants, technicians, and lower-level staff. We hear this concern expressed by almost every hospital CEO and physician leader we interview or work with.

Mary K. Wakefield, director of the Center for Health Policy and Ethics at George Mason University, told us that a serious shortage of nurses could develop over the next five to ten years: "Many nurses are approaching retirement age, and there are many more career opportunities for young people, especially women, than there were twenty or thirty years ago. Consequently, applications for nursing programs are down. There is also the question of quality; we may not be getting the very best like we have in the past" (interview, Aug. 1999).

We anticipate problems with attracting and retaining staff to be especially important in a market where consumerism and technology are the drivers. The human resources departments of most hospitals have their work cut out for them.

Downsizing and Divesting

If the current economic climate for hospitals continues or worsens, discontinuing financially marginal services and downsizing the hospital will be necessary strategies for many organizations. The BBA has already forced many hospitals to divest themselves of their home health services. As discussed in more detail in Chapter Ten, many integrated systems are divesting themselves of their health plans. Given the fact that hospitals do not normally experience significant economies of scale, downsizing may be a viable alternative for many organizations. In fact, almost every hospital in the United States has had experience in downsizing its inpatient capacity.

Special Challenges for Rural Hospitals

It is difficult to be encouraged about the prospects for rural hospitals under any of the scenarios. Poor economic conditions and the lack of relief from the provisions of the BBA would be especially damaging. If technology dominates, many rural hospitals will experience difficulties in financing the needed advances in medical technology and information systems. This would force them to either network or join larger hospital systems.

Clark Fork Valley Hospital

Larry White discussed his experience with the sixteen-bed Clark Fork Valley Hospital in Plains, Montana (population one thousand, located seventy-five miles from the next nearest hospital), where he is a board member: "In Plains, we had a smooth-functioning integrated system revolving around the hospital. We have three outreach clinics, employ a few primary care physicians, offer a twenty-eight-bed nursing home, and provide home health care. In other words, the hospital offers a continuum of care that really meets the needs of the community" (interview, July 1999).

Because of changes brought about by the BBA, White said, Clark Fork Valley Hospital was recently advised that it owed the Health Care Financing Administration $160,000 for overcharging. "This is money that the hospital doesn't have," White said. "They will either have to miss a payroll or turn over the hospital to a larger system that has deeper pockets" (interview, July 1999).

Critical Access Hospitals

Critical access hospitals are hospitals in small communities that agree to certain restrictions (such as limitations on the number of beds and the length of time they will keep patients) in order to be reimbursed by Medicare on a cost basis. Larry White said, "This may be the best hope for a number of small hospitals in Montana" (interview, July 1999). Don Wilson, president of the Kansas Hospital Association, agrees: "We expect to have thirty critical access hospitals in Kansas by the end of the year, with the potential for this number to go to forty" (interview, July 1999).

Conclusions: A Balancing Act for Hospitals

One of the objectives of this chapter has been to identify the best strategies for hospitals. If a specific strategy works well under varying scenarios, it should receive a high priority in terms of investment of capital and management resources.

Revenue-Generating Strategies

We favor strategies that generate revenues over those designed to cut costs. These revenue-generating strategies include:

- *Expanding or improving centers of excellence.* This is an especially attractive strategy under any scenario for the future.
- *Expanding the extent of geographical coverage and gaining increased market share within the service area.* This relates to the growing desire on the part of many consumers for increased convenience.
- *Improving service.* With the growth in consumerism, there is no choice but to improve convenience and service. There are plenty of opportunities, and costs are low.
- *Strengthening relationships with primary care physicians and specialists.* This is obviously a high priority for almost all hospitals.
- *Investing in IT.* If a hospital is unable to make significant investments in IT, it will need to collaborate with or be part of a network or multihospital system that is making these investments. Avoiding the need for IT upgrades is not an option for any hospital, regardless of its size.
- *Segmenting the market.* The ability to identify specific market segments and design services for these segments will become increasingly important.

Investment-Leveraging Strategies

In the early 1990s hospitals sought to dominate health care. They invested in proprietary information systems, employed primary care physicians, and even started provider-sponsored health plans. If this approach did not work in the early 1990s, when hospitals were doing relatively well financially and were receiving a greater share of the health care dollar, then it certainly will not work now. Hospitals have to anticipate and leverage the investments of others—including pharmaceutical and e-health companies.

For many hospitals, we recommend partnering with physicians and working as fast as possible to brand local providers as the best, most accessible, most trustworthy sources of information for consumers. This means monitoring, contracting with, and leveraging investors in new consumer-oriented CAM and e-health services.

Defensive Strategies

Several strategies need to be pursued under any of the scenarios:

- *Collaboration and networking.* We expect the pressures to cut costs to lead to significant increases in the willingness of competing hospitals to collaborate on certain services.
- *Performance improvement.* This is an area where hospitals are investing heavily, which will continue. When performance improvement is combined with investing in IT and developing new relationships with physicians, the payoff should be high.
- *Reduction of losses associated with primary care networks.* This will be accomplished in two ways: by terminating contracts with employed physicians and by changing the incentives for those physicians who continue to be affiliated with a hospital.

We are not pessimistic about the future of hospitals or multihospital systems. In many communities across the country, hospitals remain the most trusted and valued health care organizations. Although their role has changed substantially over the past two decades and will continue to change, most hospitals will have a bright future if they adjust to the new health care marketplace. However, they have to move fast and must leverage investments made by others.

Chapter Nine

Strategies for Academic Medical Centers and Specialty Hospitals

Our strategies are designed to differentiate our organization in this competitive marketplace. We either differentiate our services or we will be viewed as a commodity and compete on price.
CEO OF LARGE HEALTH SYSTEM IN THE MIDWEST, Summer 2000

This CEO's comments are especially apropos for academic medical centers and specialty hospitals. Almost by definition, these are unique institutions, either in their service areas or nationally. The new health care marketplace, with its emphasis on consumerism and technology, presents many opportunities—and challenges—for specialty medical centers.

Related to the need for service differentiation, Dennis C. Brimhall, president and chief executive officer of University of Colorado Hospital, told us, "By virtue of our close relationship with university physicians, they bring us new products and services. We are different from other Denver-area hospitals in the services we provide and the types of patients we care for. One of our challenges, however, is communicating these differences to the public and the payers" (interview, Jan. 1999).

This chapter focuses on three types of specialty hospitals and medical centers: academic, children's, and rehabilitation. Other types of specialty hospitals touched on more briefly include cardiac and psychiatric facilities. Of all the different types of specialty hospitals, however, academic medical centers are the largest and most influential. We discuss them first.

Academic Medical Centers: Strategies for the Future

In reviewing a 1999 book about academic medical centers, Steven Schroeder (2000), M.D., president and CEO of the Robert Wood Johnson Foundation, writes, "For most of the twentieth century academic medicine was the jewel in the crown of the U.S. health-care system. Our 125 medical schools and their affiliated teaching hospitals were the major focus for innovation in bio-medical science, as well as for the introduction of the dazzling array of diagnostic and therapeutic technologies that (insured) American patients enjoy in such abundance." He goes on to say that academic medicine seems to be in full rout: "Prestigious teaching hospitals hemorrhage red ink, faculty are demoralized, and academic clinical research is in serious jeopardy."

Robert Dickler, senior vice president for health care affairs at the Association of American Medical Colleges, has a somewhat different view on the status of teaching hospitals. "Many academic medical centers," he told us, "were doing quite well. A number have experienced increases in market share, and until the recent hits by the BBA, Medicaid, and private-market forces, many had been doing reasonably well financially" (interview, Feb. 2000).

Mission

Writing in the *New England Journal of Medicine,* Wendy Levinson and Arthur Rubenstein (1999, p. 840), state, "The mission of academic medical centers typically includes three distinct goals: providing patient care, educating future doctors, and acquiring new medical knowledge." They go on to say that most academic medical centers seek to distinguish themselves in all three of these areas.

Our research indicates that many academic medical centers are struggling with balancing these three missions. Economic pressures are pushing the emphasis toward patient care and research (where the money is) and away from teaching. Related to this change in emphasis, Robert Kuttner (1999, p. 1092), a frequent contributor to the *New England Journal of Medicine,* writes, "Teaching hospitals are no longer able to bill at rates that reflect the extra costs of their academic role—traditionally representing a premium of about 30 percent." Kuttner points out that the federal government's share of the costs of medical education at teaching hospitals is close to 50 percent—about $8.5 billion of the $18 billion total. Tuition has dwindled to less than 5 percent of medical school income. Of course, the BBA funding levels are not keeping up with cost increases for most teaching institutions.

Strategic Initiatives

The major strategies of academic medical centers include the following:

- *Expanding faculty practice plans.* The goal of this strategy is to generate more income from patients and to obtain better-paying referrals to the medical center for both inpatient and outpatient services.
- *Capitalizing on prestige and the reputation of physicians.* For example, the University of Colorado Hospital advertises that its physicians "practice what they teach." Branding is becoming an increasingly important strategy.
- *Consolidating.* This has been a strategy of the 1990s, and the results have been mixed.
- *Improving operational efficiency.* With current and pending reimbursement cuts from Medicare, all university medical centers are pursuing this strategy, many of them more aggressively than in the past.
- *Modernizing and expanding facilities.* Many teaching hospitals are in run-down inner-city areas with inadequate parking for outpatient services. One of the issues, of course, is whether "bricks and mortar" are the place to invest financial resources.
- *Developing IT.* This is especially important for teaching hospitals and at the same time a particularly challenging and costly strategy.
- *Seeking more funding for research and clinical trials.* Although most of the funds for research and clinical trials typically go to

physicians and pay for support of research, academic medical centers also benefit indirectly from rent paid, overhead absorbed, and services purchased by medical researchers.

- *Capitalizing on the results of research.* Some medical centers are considering patents, royalties, and opportunities to establish new technology-based for-profit businesses. (The profits would be used to further the educational mission.)
- *Heightening the emphasis on philanthropy.* There is no alternative but to pursue development programs more aggressively and, in many cases, to coordinate these efforts with the medical school and university.
- *Increasing the political pressure on state and federal governments for equitable funding.* The CEO of a university medical center told us, "We have a major educational program ahead of us on this one. Neither Congress nor our state legislators want to hear about our problems."

Expanding Faculty Practice Plans

According to Robert Dickler, faculty practice plans accounted for about 35 percent of the income of medical schools. How much more can faculty practice plans be expanded to generate additional income to support the patient care mission of academic medical centers without jeopardizing the teaching and research components of their mission? Robert Dickler told us, "Some physicians are wondering why they are in academic centers if they don't have time to spend with students" (interview, Feb. 2000).

It appears to us that without a major change in funding for academic medical centers, these organizations have to work more closely with faculty practice plans to generate additional patients and business. This would include joint advertising and marketing and generating referrals from community primary care physicians. At the same time, medical schools and faculty practice plans will have to find creative new ways to work with medical students and residents, perhaps through increased use of distance learning or other technology-oriented teaching methods.

Capitalizing on Prestige and Reputation

Capitalizing on prestige and reputation appears to be an excellent strategy for many academic medical centers. This strategy pressures health plans into including a region's teaching hospital and faculty physicians in order to market managed care to employers and consumers.

Robert Dickler noted that many of the members of the Association of American Medical Colleges are considering this strategy. "But this is more difficult than first meets the eye," he said. "There is a lot of competition for the minds of health care consumers" (interview, Feb. 2000). Dennis Brimhall agreed, noting that the University of Colorado Hospital's market research indicates that a relatively high proportion of consumers do not know what university the hospital is associated with and cannot differentiate between the physicians and the hospital (interview, Jan. 1999).

Consolidating

In the 1990s two premier hospitals long affiliated with Harvard, Brigham and Women's Hospital and Massachusetts General Hospital, combined to form Partners HealthCare System. As Kuttner (1999, p. 1095) writes, "Partners was organized not primarily to reduce capacity or to combine clinical programs, but as a business strategy to maximize referrals and bargaining power with insurers." Partners pursued a strategy of affiliating with physicians' practices.

Kuttner also describes another consolidation in the Boston area:

> Literally across the street from Brigham and Women's Hospital, a merger of two other Boston teaching hospitals is faring far worse. Beth Israel Hospital and Deaconess Hospital combined in 1996 under the name CareGroup. CareGroup acquired outlying hospitals, increasing its debt. By 1998, the two teaching hospitals were suffering from serious over-capacity, and they began to consolidate clinical departments and close some inpatient units, causing widespread bitterness and demoralization among the staff. In the first six months of 1999, CareGroup's flagship Beth Israel Deaconess Medical Center had an operating loss of about 12 percent [1999, p. 1095].

Kuttner says that blue-chip teaching hospitals serving affluent, well-insured populations are better able to face the future. For example, Northwestern Memorial Hospital (which has a strong reputation in its service area) and its new facilities have a superior bargaining position with insurers. Operating profit margins were

12.3 percent in fiscal year 1997 and 8 percent in 1998 (Kuttner, 1999).

Improving Operational Efficiency

Dennis Brimhall told us that the University of Colorado Health Sciences Center has been reducing costs for years but that with the even greater spending cuts from Medicare, the efforts have to become even more determined and effective. "We have to look to the Internet as a way of reducing the costs of scheduling and registering patients," he said. "We can save $20,000 to $30,000 a year by doing patient-satisfaction surveys using e-mail, and have the results immediately. We have to reduce the number of transactions that require people to talk on the telephone. Automation is part of the answer." Robert Dickler said, "Most medical centers are approaching cost reduction incrementally, but a few have gone to the extreme of calling in the Hunter Group or a similar type of organization!" (interview, Sept. 1999).

Modernizing and Expanding Facilities

Most academic medical centers are in crowded locations with little parking, and their facilities are antiquated. Many of these centers are in downtown areas, where adequate space is often not available for new facilities. Therefore, despite concerns about spending on "bricks and mortar," many academic medical centers have a desperate need to build new facilities.

The University of Colorado Health Sciences Center is solving its facilities problem by moving to the former Fitzsimons Army Hospital campus and will be transferring nearly all of its activities to this site over the next twenty years. The Fitzsimons location is ten miles east of the present campus in Denver. Dennis Brimhall, who is in charge of the new campus, said, "We are fortunate to have this as an alternative. Many teaching hospitals have no place to go" (interview, Sept. 1999).

In the late 1970s Dartmouth-Hitchcock Medical Center, which includes Dartmouth Medical School, Mary Hitchcock Memorial Hospital, and a large multispecialty clinic, faced a similar problem in downtown Hanover, New Hampshire. The Dartmouth-Hitchcock Medical Center purchased a 225-acre wooded campus in neighboring Lebanon and constructed a $228 million building that provides top-rate facilities. Furthermore, the design of the building has encouraged the further clinical and administrative integration of the medical school, hospital, and clinic.

Over the next five years facility modernization and expansion will become an increasingly important issue and strategic opportunity for academic medical centers. Of course, if the BBA and other payment shortfalls severely damage academic medical centers' bottom line, they may not have the financial strength to modernize, expand, or relocate.

Developing Information Technology

Many academic medical centers are behind other large health care systems in installing information systems, including an EMR. For academic medical centers the high cost of IT—spending $10 to $20 million a year is not unusual for large medical centers—is a significant barrier to catching up to developments in single-specialty and multispecialty medical groups, community hospitals, and large integrated systems. Robert Dickler told us that progress on the EMR among academic medical centers is slower than anticipated. "The problem isn't so much the technology," he explained, "as it is the cost and the human side of it. There is a lot of resistance to change among physicians in academic medical centers" (interview, Feb. 2000).

In our view, being strong in IT is consistent with being an academic medical center. The databases that can be created lend themselves to research, and medical students need to be trained with the latest information systems. This appears to us to be a high-priority strategy, especially in the new health care marketplace, where consumerism and technology will increasingly dominate. Perhaps some academic medical centers will find ways to collaborate with other teaching hospitals to accelerate progress and reduce costs.

Seeking More Funding for Research and Clinical Trials

Almost every academic medical center is seeking more external funding for clinical research programs and clinical trials. One physician CEO told us, "We need to have more funded research for a variety of reasons. First, research is part of our mission, and we need to do more. Secondly, it is one of the factors that differentiates us from community hospitals. Third, we simply can't generate the funds to pay for more research ourselves; we have to develop more outside sources." Even though the dollars available for medical research are growing, the competition is becoming severe. Robert Dickler told us, "I have talked to forty different academic medical centers who all say they want to be in the 'top ten' in research funding" (interview, Feb. 2000).

Capitalizing on the Results of Research

Robert Dickler observed that a number of academic medical centers are relying on their ability to stay at the leading edge of medical technology as a strategy for the future. "I wouldn't be surprised to see new businesses, or spin-off companies, coming out of this," Dickler said (interview, Feb. 2000). We believe that this is an excellent strategy for academic medical centers, and one that holds promise. Route 128 in the Boston area provides an example. This high-tech corridor developed as a direct result of university-based aerospace and electronics research, which led to the formation of a large number of high-tech companies.

Heightening the Emphasis on Philanthropy

Charitable contributions are a potentially much more important source of funding for some strong regional academic medical centers and those that have established a national reputation. For example, the Mayo Foundation (a 146-student medical school with one thousand residents and clinical fellows) has plans for raising $600 million over the next few years.

Dartmouth-Hitchcock Medical Center and Scott & White provide two other examples. Dartmouth-Hitchcock has a $350 million endowment, and Dartmouth Medical School is attempting to build its financial reserves. Scott & White, which runs the third and fourth year of medical school for Texas A&M University, is attempting to raise $30 million for education and research and $25 million for capital needs.

The affiliation of many academic medical centers with well-known national or regional universities is also a benefit. Given a continuing strong economy and the aging of the population, additional funds should be available from multiple funding sources.

Increasing the Political Pressure for Equitable Funding

With their high dependence on federal funding, particularly from Medicare, one of the strategies of most academic medical centers is participation in lobbying efforts to either restore funding cuts or devise alternative financing programs. Robert Dickler said, "We have no choice but to keep fighting this battle, especially funding for graduate medical education. There are a number of special interest groups that want to cut this out entirely" (interview, Feb. 2000).

At the state level there needs to be continuing pressure to maintain adequate funding for Medicaid recipients and for the uninsured. At University Hospital in Denver, for example, the deficit from the uninsured was $26 million in 1999. Dickler told us, "Many teaching hospitals have no choice but to try to find ways to minimize the amount of free care they provide. They can no longer bear the financial burden of this type of care" (interview, Feb. 2000).

Despite all of the strategies available to academic medical centers, there appears to be no solution to their problems without equitable federal and state funding. The burdens of financing medical education plus caring for the uninsured and those on Medicaid place an almost impossible burden on many of these institutions.

Strategies for Academic Medical Centers: Conclusions

Kuttner (1999, p. 1096) concludes his review of the future of academic medical centers by saying, "[B]usiness strategy is not what academic institutions are all about. But academic medical centers now find their very survival dependent on their commercial position and clinical income—and this cannot be good for teaching."

Because academic medical centers cannot count on increased state and federal funding, it appears that these types of organizations will have to pursue many of the same strategies as large community hospitals and integrated systems. These include reduction of operating costs, differentiation and branding of products, an emphasis on philanthropy, networking with physicians, increased application of IT, and in some cases consolidation.

It is not appropriate to end this discussion of academic medical centers on a negative or alarming note. Robert Dickler, who has worked with these types of organizations for more than two decades, offered this positive observation: "Academic medical centers and physician practice plans are highly innovative and adaptive. There are lots of smart people in these organizations. They are accustomed to working under difficult situations and being under all kinds of pressure. If any group of hospitals can survive, it will be the academic medical centers" (interview, Feb. 2000).

Children's Hospitals: Strategies for the Future

Children's hospitals are different from other hospitals because they serve only a defined subset of the total population—generally children from birth to seventeen years old. Children's hospitals provide an environment, services, and expertise tailored to meet the unique needs of children and their families. In addition, as Larry McAndrews, president and CEO of the National Association of Children's Hospitals and Related Institutions (NACHRI), notes, "Children's hospitals and related institutions are committed to caring for every child, regardless of their ability to pay" (interview, Apr. 2000). Serving all children—and only children—in an environment that is designed to best meet their needs is what makes a children's hospital special.

Mission

NACHRI defines the mission of children's hospitals and related institutions to include "service/care for children and their families, training for the future pediatric work force, research in pediatric health care and community service/advocacy" (National Association of Children's Hospitals and Related Institutions, 1999, p. xiii). Each children's hospital assesses the specific needs of its community and the availability of organizational expertise and resources to determine the appropriate proportion of attention to give to each of these mission components. Whereas patient care is an important part of the mission of all children's hospitals, advocacy, teaching, and research receive varying degrees of attention.

NACHRI has 162 members, including 66 freestanding children's hospitals and 96 children's hospitals within acute care hospitals. Although these children's hospitals serve a defined population and have a unique mission, this has not insulated them from many of the typical challenges to health care providers, including increasing competition and insufficient reimbursement.

Donna Shelton, director of child health financing for NACHRI, observed, "Adult hospitals are aggressively marketing their pediatric services" (interview, Apr. 2000). Family practitioners and adult specialists and subspecialists are also showing more interest in serving pediatric patients. As all providers struggle to attract more patients and increase revenue, the once inconspicuous pediatric population now receives plenty of attention. In addition, while children's hospitals struggle to receive adequate reimbursement (which is especially challenging given the severity of illnesses of their patients), other hospitals and physicians are finding Medicaid reimbursement to be more attractive as their traditional commercial reimbursement continues to be ratcheted down.

Strategic Initiatives

To address market pressures and accomplish their mission, the major strategies of children's hospitals include the following:

- *Creating specialty and subspecialty satellite clinics.* Such clinics improve access and convenience for patients.
- *Developing referral relationships with primary care physicians.* These providers continue to be vital links to the larger patient community.
- *Developing relationships with other providers.* This enables specialty hospitals to gain access to additional patients or resources.
- *Determining appropriate managed care contracting strategies.* Maintaining or gaining access to patients through managed care plans is critical to success.
- *Increasing the political pressure on state and federal governments for equitable funding.* Advocacy efforts are directed at achieving sufficient reimbursement.
- *Improving operational efficiency.* Reducing expenses and improving profitability through additional economies is a key strategic thrust.
- *Modernizing facilities.* Facilities must be convenient and attractive to patients and their families.

- *Seeking more funding for research and clinical trials.* It is important to diversify sources of revenue and complement patient care.
- *Maintaining an emphasis on philanthropy.* Spreading out revenue sources and maintaining connection and visibility in the community leads to continued support.
- *Communicating the unique role and identity of a children's hospital.* Reinforcing why the hospital is different and valuable will help to gain additional patients.

Creating Specialty and Subspecialty Satellite Clinics

Many children's hospitals are located in urban neighborhoods. These locations are not always convenient or attractive for families with children. As a result, a number of children's hospitals have developed satellite clinics to make access to their services more convenient for patients. For example, Children's National Medical Center in Washington, D.C., has six regional outpatient centers in the District of Columbia, Maryland, and Virginia where patients can see children's specialists. This is an especially relevant strategy in the new health care marketplace.

Developing Referral Relationships with Primary Care Physicians

The unique expertise of children's hospitals is usually thought of as the range and depth of specialty and subspecialty services they provide for children. However, a number of children's hospitals are also developing relationships with primary care pediatricians. For example, Cook Children's Health Care System in Fort Worth, Texas, has developed Cook Children's Physician Network, which employs 250 pediatricians and specialists.

Others, like Children's National Medical Center, have developed a network of affiliated physicians. These and other approaches are designed to strengthen relationships and develop referrals between primary care pediatricians and the specialists and subspecialists practicing at the children's hospital. In addition, these relationships can facilitate contracting with managed care firms.

Developing Relationships with Other Providers

In response to market pressures, children's hospitals are developing relationships with other providers, such as adult-focused health care systems, other children's hospitals, and other providers serving children and physicians. For example, some children's hospitals manage the pediatric units, pediatric intensive care units, and neonatal intensive care units in community hospitals. Other children's hospitals have joined large regional adult-focused systems to gain access to capital and corporate expertise.

Two-thirds of respondents to a NACHRI member survey reported that they were part of a system, network, or alliance. Of those reporting development of a formal relationship with another health care delivery organization, 69 percent formed a relationship with an adult-focused organization and 30 percent formed a relationship with another children's hospital or system (National Association of Children's Hospitals and Related Institutions, 1999). Developing relationships that support the accomplishment of their mission, while maintaining their unique identity, will continue to be a challenge and a priority for children's hospitals.

Determining Appropriate Managed Care Contracting Strategies

Managed care makes up 32 percent of all Medicaid and 59 percent of all commercial insurance payments to freestanding children's hospitals. In addition, because of contractual adjustments or discounts, bad debt, and charity care, freestanding children's hospitals only collect 68 percent of their gross patient revenue (National Association of Children's Hospitals and Related Institutions, 1999).

Although the types of contracts and reimbursement rates vary from community to community, children's hospitals generally contract with all payers and attempt to negotiate higher reimbursement based on the severity of the illnesses of their patients. In some cases, if a children's hospital is part of a larger system with its own managed care product, the system may not allow the children's hospital to contract with competing health plans. However, regardless of the scenario for the future, attracting a critical mass of patients through fair contractual relationships with all payers will continue to be in the best interests of most children's hospitals.

Increasing the Political Pressure for Equitable Funding

Selling a product or service at a price that is less than the cost of producing it is a formula for failure for any business. However, this is the challenge children's hospitals face as reimbursement for their services continues to fall. Given their strong commitment to serving all children regardless of their families' ability to pay, children's hospitals will continue to look to fundraising to make up the shortfall. However, in the long run, children's hospitals will need to persuade government payers that if their reimbursement continues to decline to even less manageable levels, the children's hospital industry will no longer be able to provide the quality and depth of care that parents and consumers have come to expect.

Improving Operational Efficiency

Insufficient reimbursement and growing competition have increased pressure on children's hospitals to reduce expenses. However, this is a challenging undertaking, given the high staffing ratios, expensive technology, and specialized services that characterize children's hospitals. It is likely that, rather than pare back services, children's hospitals will become increasingly dependent on philanthropy to support the development and maintenance of specialized services that are not independently financially viable. In addition, the need to be more cost effective will require children's hospitals to work more closely with other organizations to reduce unnecessary duplication of specialized services.

Modernizing Facilities

Many children's hospitals are older facilities in urban neighborhoods that are not convenient or inviting for children and their families. Other children's hospitals are located within larger hospitals that were not designed specifically to accommodate the unique needs of children. Children's hospitals in either of these circumstances are increasingly focusing on enhancing their facilities to be more appealing and convenient for children and their families. For example, Babies and Children's Hospital in New York City, on the campus of New York Presbyterian Hospital, is planning for a major construction and renovation project that would both modernize and enhance the feeling of separateness of the children's hospital facility.

Seeking More Funding for Research and Clinical Trials

Conducting research is an important part of the mission of many children's hospitals. In addition, children's hospitals with employed faculty are increasingly finding that additional research funding lessens the impact of poor patient care reimbursement. Competition for research funding will increase both because of its positive financial impact on children's hospitals and because of its ability to help differentiate children's hospitals from their competitors.

Maintaining an Emphasis on Philanthropy

Children's hospitals have long been aware of the importance of philanthropy to both the financial well-being and community support of their organization. Children's hospitals have been successful in raising money and continue to rely on philanthropy to support new program development and, in some cases, to offset operational losses.

Ninety-four percent of freestanding children's hospitals report having dedicated staff for fundraising and development. Ninety-one percent of freestanding children's hospitals report having one or more foundations for fundraising (National Association of Children's Hospitals and Related Institutions, 1999). The challenge is the growing competition for limited fundraising dollars, from other organizations serving children, other health care providers, university patient care, and teaching and research initiatives.

Communicating the Unique Role and Identity of a Children's Hospital

Although other providers also care for children, only children's hospitals provide an extensive range of services for children in an environment tailored specifically to meet their needs. If children's hospitals are to continue to effectively serve this market segment, they must attract a significant proportion of pediatric patients to ensure the delivery of high-quality, cost-effective care. If children's hospitals are not visible and valued in the community, other providers will siphon off pediatric patients, which will dilute the effectiveness and viability of children's hospitals, especially in smaller markets.

Strategies for Children's Hospitals: Conclusions

Larry McAndrews concludes, "The market forces that create regionalization are reinforcing the role of children's hospitals" (interview, Apr. 2000). For example, the shift from inpatient to outpatient care, greater emphasis on utilization and disease management, and centralization of tertiary services are all approaches that are consistent with how children's hospitals seek to deliver care. If children's hospitals can demonstrate that they provide higher-quality, more cost-effective care and if this is valued by the community and by adult-focused providers, children's hospitals will continue to play a vital role in meeting an important community need.

Rehabilitation Hospitals: Strategies for the Future

Dennis O'Malley, CEO of Craig Rehabilitation Hospital, a nationally known spinal cord injury facility in Englewood, Colorado, believes that Medicare funding is the key for most rehabilitation hospitals: "Medicare payment is fundamental to the way rehab people view the future. Medicare pays 75 percent of all rehabilitation services." It follows, then, that the BBA would dominate the thinking of CEOs of rehabilitation facilities. "Under the BBA," O'Malley said, "there are severe limits on spending per year per beneficiary. There is no way that we can perform adequate rehabilitation on patients for the amounts allowed by Medicare unless some relief is given" (interview, July 1999).

O'Malley believes that under a business-as-usual scenario most rehabilitation facilities would struggle: "I see more demand for services, which for most hospitals is very much related to age. This isn't going to change. The question is: How are we going to respond? If funding from Medicare is not increased, rehabilitation facilities will have no choice but to move more aggressively into private pay. Consumers are going to have to dig deeper into their pockets for all types of health care services, including rehabilitation," O'Malley said (interview, July 1999).

Strategies for a Future Characterized by Constrained Resources

In terms of preparing for a future characterized by constrained resources, Denny O'Malley observed, "There isn't much we can do to prepare. If resources are limited, and we want to survive, we will have to reduce staff and cut service levels." If this were to happen, many acute care hospitals might get out of the rehabilitation business, and this would be favorable for specialized rehabilitation hospitals like Craig and others. "That would be a benefit," O'Malley agreed, "but going through the trauma of constrained resources would be a tough way to achieve this result" (interview, July 1999). In poor economic times many of the for-profit organizations, like

HealthSouth, might get out of the rehabilitation business. Profit margins would not be attractive to Wall Street. All rehabilitation facilities would be under tremendous financial pressure.

Strategies for a Future Dominated by Technology

Technology could have a major impact on rehabilitation. Denny O'Malley said, "If product developers create better joints and make older people feel better, there will be more demand for rehabilitation." O'Malley believes a technology-driven future is the most promising future for rehabilitation. However, as O'Malley pointed out, "Rehabilitation is about laying hands on people. This isn't going to change. The Internet and other technology will facilitate communication, and this is important, but it is unlikely to change the basics of rehabilitation" (interview, July 1999).

Raymond Uhlhorn, president and CEO of MossRehab, part of the Albert Einstein Healthcare Network in Philadelphia, believes that a future dominated by technology is the most likely and that it will present both challenges and opportunities for rehabilitation organizations. "For example," he said, "we can expand our market area through telemedicine and better manage satellite facilities in communities some distance from our main campus." Uhlhorn described how MossRehab has opened up communications with people with disabilities through launching a special Web site that provides a variety of information for individuals with physical disabilities. "In late 1999," he noted, "we were averaging over fifty thousand hits a month on this Web site" (interview, Jan. 2000).

Additional Strategies

Ray Uhlhorn cited a number of additional strategies that rehabilitation hospitals might consider, especially in a future dominated by technology and consumerism (interview, Jan. 2000):

- *Satellite beds in acute care hospitals in the region.* "I am talking about twelve- to sixteen-bed units," Uhlhorn explained. For example, MossRehab has a fourteen-bed rehabilitation unit at Sacred Heart Hospital in Allentown.
- *Geographical coverage.* The MossCare Network has twenty-three

locations for outpatient rehabilitation in five counties in eastern Pennsylvania.

- *Diversification*. Uhlhorn noted, "Specialty hospitals of all types, including rehab facilities, are going to have to develop niche products and seek new markets and dollars. This points to the suburbs, where people are more likely to have discretionary dollars."

- *Centers of excellence*. "With its expertise in traumatic brain injuries and neuro-orthopedic injuries," Uhlhorn said, "MossRehab is a center of excellence. Other rehab facilities will have to find centers of excellence."

- *Marketing*. As Uhlhorn pointed out, "Rehabilitation hospitals are going to have to dramatically improve their expertise in consumer marketing and market segmentation. This is not something we've had a lot of experience with in the past."

- *Wellness and fitness*. Uhlhorn reported that MossRehab has already partnered with fitness centers: "We have become an equity partner in a group of aquatic and fitness centers. Not only does this provide a place for some of our patients, but it positions us to get patients from some of the regular users of these facilities. For example, we can help people recover from sports injuries."

- *Willingness to accept risk*. The MossCare Network has 150,000 covered lives for outpatient rehabilitation services. Uhlhorn told us, "Even though capitation may not be growing in many markets and for more traditional medical services, we find that employers and health plans like us to go at risk for outpatient rehab services. With our geographic coverage and network of providers, we find that it is feasible."

- *Close relationships with health plans*. For some types of rehabilitation facilities, developing a close relationship with insurance companies is a useful strategy, particularly when the rehabilitation organization has a track record of getting people back to work or back into the community quickly.

Labor Shortages: An Increasingly Important Issue for Rehabilitation Hospitals

Dennis O'Malley believes that within the first five years of the twenty-first century, the dominant issue for rehabilitation providers will be skilled labor, or lack of it: "This will be particularly critical if the economy continues to be strong." Uhlhorn agrees. "We are going to have to find ways to replace some of the more labor-intensive activities, like speech therapy, with technology. We are working on this now through the use of computer-assisted interactive hardware," he said.

Many hospital CEOs we interviewed also expressed concern about the pending shortage of personnel, particularly nurses and nurse's aides as well as other clinical workers, that they expect to develop over the first few years of the new millennium. One CEO of a Catholic system in New England that operates both a rehabilitation unit and nursing home put it this way: "The changing demographics—more older people and fewer in the working ages—spell trouble for health care in more ways than one. We hear a lot about increasing demand, but what about shortages of labor? Furthermore, we are going to have to pay more, and this will further drive up health care costs."

Strategies for Rehabilitation Hospitals: Conclusions

The outlook for rehabilitation hospitals is unfavorable without overall health care market growth and expansion. Growth in consumerism and technology, however, would provide an environment in which rehabilitation hospitals could prosper. Given the close relationships rehabilitation facilities and their staff develop with patients and patients' families, a consumer-oriented health care environment would be especially favorable.

Other Types of Specialty Hospitals

This section presents a brief overview of the challenges and strategic opportunities for two other types of specialty hospitals: heart hospitals and psychiatric hospitals.

Heart Hospitals

MedCath, established as a PPM in 1989, typically partners with cardiologists and cardiovascular surgeons to build specialized heart hospitals. These hospitals are often referred to as "focused factories," the term used by Regina Herzlinger in her 1997 book *Mar-*

ket Driven Health Care. MedCath has established heart hospitals in a number of cities (the year each was opened is shown in parentheses): McAllen, Texas (1996), Austin, Texas (1998), Little Rock, Arkansas (1997), Tucson, Arizona (1997), Phoenix, Arizona (1998), Dayton, Ohio (1999), Albuquerque, New Mexico (1999), and Bakersfield, California (1999). Others are under development.

The heart hospitals, which are full-service facilities (including emergency rooms, operating rooms, labs, a pharmacy, food service, imaging services, and so on), range in size from 52 to 112 inpatient beds. In Dayton and Albuquerque the heart hospitals are three-part joint ventures: an acute care hospital, cardiologists and cardiovascular surgeons, and MedCath.

MedCath heart hospitals represent a resurrection of an old idea, the physician-owned hospital, which went into decline after World War II. As one observer points out, "Under the MedCath model, physicians become shareholder-owners with MedCath, helping to raise funds to build and equip a new heart hospital (averaging $50 million), and sharing equally in the profits, when and if they occur. It's a model the investors love, but one that has come under heavy attack from competitors, who say MedCath is ruthless" (Heimoff, 1999, p. 4).

Strategies Heart Hospitals Use

Cardiologists and cardiovascular surgeons who are shareholders of these hospitals are not required to refer patients to the heart hospitals in which they own an interest; however, they usually do. As a result, in every market MedCath has entered, its heart hospitals have been able to attract the majority of patients within a short period of time (Heimoff, 1999).

In addition to partnering with physicians, the strategies of heart hospitals are to achieve economies of scale, be cost effective, provide the highest-quality care in the region, offer new facilities and state-of-the-art equipment, and achieve high levels of patient satisfaction through private rooms, above-average staffing ratios, good food, and a pleasant environment. Some rooms can accommodate an overnight guest. Meals are typically at the patient's convenience, and visitors are served along with patients. The same nursing team cares for a patient from admission to discharge (Robinson, 2000).

The Future of Heart Hospitals

As consumers increasingly dominate health care decision making, heart hospitals should prosper. They are designed and operated to be focused on a specific type of patient; this is market segmentation in action. Given their partnerships with leading cardiologists and heart surgeons, they should be able to develop strong brand name awareness in their markets and deliver high quality (in heart surgery, like many medical procedures, quantity and quality go hand in hand). These kinds of hospitals should also rank high in service, convenience, and patients' ability to establish a close relationship with a clinical team.

We anticipate that heart hospitals will also perform reasonably well regardless of what health care future unfolds. The pattern of MedCath's heart hospitals is to dominate their markets. Partnering with leading physicians in the region facilitates their success.

Psychiatric Hospitals

Both private and public psychiatric hospitals have experienced dramatic drops in utilization over the past two decades. Part of this has been due to the new drugs and treatment protocols, and part has been due to substantial overbuilding during the late 1980s and early 1990s and a subsequent downsizing, including closure of many old-line psychiatric facilities.

Psychiatric Hospitals Experience an Unfounded Growth Spurt

Part of the problem for private psychiatric facilities is that beginning in the mid-1980s, several of the for-profit chains expanded rapidly into many metropolitan areas. We estimate that at the peak of the mental health boom in the late 1980s, there were several hundred psychiatric hospitals in the United States. This growth was facilitated by the removal of certificate-of-need laws in many states. In our view this opened the floodgates of new competition and overbuilding of inpatient capacity.

During this same time period, the mid-1980s, mental health costs were rising more rapidly than other types of medical expenses. As a result, it was commonly believed that psychiatric hospitals and mental health care had a bright future as the most rapidly growing sector in health care. Many acute care hospitals considered branching out into mental health, and a number converted part of their capacity to caring for psychiatric patients.

Health Plans Curb the Increase in Utilization

In 1985 most health plans limited hospital stays for psychiatric episodes to thirty days. (As it turned out, thirty days was the average length of stay!) Within a few years, owing to the growth of managed care, more careful patient management, pharmacological advances, and changed financial incentives, the average length of stay dropped substantially.

Spending on mental health also dropped dramatically. For example, the Hay Group estimated that behavioral health benefits fell from 6.1 percent of all employer health benefits in 1988 to 3.1 percent in 1997. Another study reported that alcohol and drug rehabilitation and mental health costs fell from 9 percent of all health care costs in 1989 to about 4 percent in 1995 (Mechanic and McAlpine, 1999).

This drop in spending and a shift in utilization away from inpatient care essentially broke the backs of many psychiatric hospitals, both for-profit and private. Charter and other for-profit chains exited the business as fast as they had entered during the mid-1980s. The surviving hospitals, of course, have had to downsize their inpatient facilities and focus on outpatient services. This has made it almost impossible for most freestanding psychiatric hospitals to survive financially. Some have been taken over by acute care multihospital systems.

What Does the Future Hold for Psychiatric Hospitals?

It is difficult to be optimistic about the future of psychiatric hospitals, given the flow of new drugs expected in the new millennium and the growing ability of psychiatrists and other mental health professionals to manage patients in an outpatient setting. Psychiatric hospitals would certainly suffer if economic conditions deteriorated and fewer dollars were available for health benefits. It is possible that a limited number of psychiatric hospitals could position themselves as centers of excellence (such as Menninger Clinic in Topeka) and survive. If they are able to establish strong brand names and reputations for quality, service, and consumer friendliness, a limited number of psychiatric hospitals will have their best opportunities for survival in a future where consumerism is key.

Specialty Hospitals: Conclusions

The BBA is having a dramatic impact on university and rehabilitation hospitals and is forcing increased emphasis on cost reduction. Cost pressures on Medicaid and the growing number of the uninsured are having the same effect on children's hospitals. Growth in consumerism would offer some relief to children's hospitals, as the proportion of the uninsured would be the lowest in that scenario.

Despite the BBA and other problems experienced by academic medical centers, we expect many of them to perform well in the years ahead, especially with the convergence of consumerism and technology. They have the opportunity to establish strong brand names, and centers of excellence, that should appeal to increasingly discriminating consumers.

With managed care continuing to be the dominant payment source, teaching hospitals will have continuing problems in justifying their inclusion in the networks of health plans. Constrained resources and poor economic conditions would hit academic medical centers—with their obligation to care for the uninsured and their heavy reliance on Medicare, Medicaid, and government-funded medical research—especially hard.

Heart hospitals appear to have a bright future. The market is far from saturated, and the initial heart hospitals appear to be successful in dominating their local markets for cardiac services. They claim to be cost effective, and they offer high levels of service designed to optimize patient and family satisfaction. We expect these kinds of hospitals to perform well regardless of the shape of the health care market of the future.

It is difficult to be optimistic about psychiatric hospitals. This category of health care facility was almost obliterated by gross overexpansion in the mid-1980s and then dramatic drops in inpatient utilization beginning in the late 1980s and early 1990s. At the same time, it is obvious that there continues to be a need for some inpatient capacity; most of it will probably fall on the shoulders of state government and state behavioral health hospitals.

Chapter Ten

Strategies for Integrated Health Care Systems

Several years ago we were certain that vertical integration was the way to go—the strategy of the future. We acquired some primary care practices and for a while even owned a share of a health plan. We sold out of the health plan, but not before losing several million dollars. Now we are wondering what to do with our primary care offices.
HOSPITAL CEO IN THE MIDWEST

Vertical integration was one of the most controversial health care strategies of the late 1990s. The envy of the early to mid-1990s, a number of these systems have been unable to increase market share and demonstrate positive financial performance. The "experts" are calling for virtual integration and an end to the type of integration where all elements of the system—physician practices, hospital, and health plan—are owned by a single entity.

This chapter deals with future strategies for integrated health care systems under alternative future scenarios. We believe certain types of integrated systems have a bright future, especially if consumerism and technology are dominant. After defining integrated health care and describing the characteristics of two different types of integrated systems, we identify and discuss several strategies for the future. We begin the discussion of strategies by presenting an analysis prepared by the management team of Methodist Community Hospitals Indianapolis of the impact of each of the four scenarios for the future that we propose.

What Is Integrated Health Care?

Our definition of vertical integration is shown in Figure 10.1. This definition is based on an examination of the vision and mission statements of a number of advanced integrated systems. In these statements there is an emphasis on teamwork, quality of care, cost-effectiveness, and meeting the needs of people in the communities and regions served.

For many of the integrated systems we studied, the definition would also include this sentence: The medical care we provide will be enhanced by a commitment to education and research.

Another approach we have used in defining integrated health care is to describe the characteristics of these systems. We developed ten broad criteria, and a number of subcategories, which we have found useful in measuring the extent of integration among various types of health care organizations. The ten characteristics are shown in Exhibit 10.1.

We have taken our definition a step further and developed weighting factors for each of the criteria and a checklist for evaluating the extent of integration in various organizations. For example, the Mayo Foundation and Kaiser Permanente would receive more than ninety out of one hundred possible points, and we would consider these organizations to be highly integrated. On the other hand, the typical community hospital that has acquired primary care practices would receive a rating in the twenty-five to thirty point range. As a general rule, organizations led by a multispecialty clinic tend to rank much higher in terms of their degree of vertical integration. Two broad types of integrated systems are discussed next.

Figure 10.1. Definition of Integrated Health Care Systems.

An integrated health care system provides a comprehensive spectrum of high-quality, well-coordinated health care services on a cost-effective basis to residents of its service area. To accomplish this, physicians, hospitals, and other health care providers work together for the benefit of customers.

Coddington, Ackerman, Fischer, and Moore, 2001, Chapter 1.

Two Broad Types of Vertically Integrated Systems

There are at least a dozen different types of integrated systems, but for the purposes of this book, we consider two broad types: those led by multispecialty clinics and those initiated by hospitals or multihospital systems.

The biggest difference between the two types of integrated systems is how they began: physicians played a key leadership role in one type, and hospital executives were usually leaders in the other. Where an integrated system has been formed under the leadership of a hospital, there are usually efforts made to place physicians in leadership roles, ranging from physicians in key positions on the management team to joint CEO-physician leadership.

We do not contend that one type of integrated system is superior to another. However, in our view, it is more difficult for a hospital to form a successful integrated system that has most of the characteristics listed in Exhibit 10.1. At the same time, we are beginning to see hospital-led systems displaying many of the integration characteristics and successfully serving their markets.

Exhibit 10.1. Ten Characteristics of Integrated Health Care Systems.

1. Comprehensive scope of clinical and health-related services.
2. Total focus on meeting the needs of patients.
3. Physicians organized.
4. Strong physician leadership.
5. Increased emphasis on quality improvement.
6. Strong governance structure that includes physicians and community representatives.
7. Geographic coverage of the service area or region.
8. Development of IT to support coordination and integration.
9. Financial plan for meeting investment needs and maintaining economic viability.
10. Strong reputation in the marketplace.

Source: Coddington, Ackerman, Fischer, and Moore, 2001, Chapter 1.

Integrated Systems Led by Multispecialty Clinics

The most prominent examples of integrated systems led by multi-specialty clinics are Mayo in Rochester, Jacksonville, and Scottsdale; Marshfield in Wisconsin; Park Nicollet Health Services in Minneapolis; the Cleveland Clinic in Ohio and Florida; Dartmouth-Hitchcock in New Hampshire and Vermont; Carle in Urbana, Illinois; Scott & White in Temple, Texas; and Fallon in Worcester, Massachusetts.

All of these integrated systems began as multispecialty clinics. They took on the characteristics of integrated systems when they developed regional networks of primary care physicians, owned or had a special relationship with a hospital, and, in some cases, established their own health plans. All of these organizations continue to place a high priority on clinical integration.

Integrated Systems Led by Hospitals

Examples of hospital-led integrated systems include Aurora in eastern Wisconsin; Advocate in Chicago; Sutter in northern California; Intermountain Health Care in Utah and southern Idaho; Scripps in San Diego; Stormont-Vail in Topeka, Kansas; and Inova in the Virginia–Washington, D.C., area. Most hospital-led integrated systems make a serious effort to promote medical groups and physician leadership. Many develop primary care networks, own health plans (or have in the past), and maintain a close relationship with a variety of physicians and medical groups.

In many respects, it is less complex to make integration work from the starting point of a multispecialty clinic. Physicians are already in leadership positions, they have had years of experience in governing themselves, and they are accustomed to making strategic and management decisions. However, many of the hospital-led integrated systems often have better access to capital, enjoy greater community support, and may be more stable over the long term.

Virtual Integration

The question frequently comes up as to whether an integrated system should own all of the key elements—medical groups, hospitals, and health plans—or whether the various components should be tied together contractually. The latter is often referred to as "virtual" integration.

In reality, most of the large and successful integrated systems include elements of virtual integration. For example, Marshfield Clinic does not own hospitals, but it has a close relationship with Ministry Corporation, Sisters of the Sorrowful Mother, based in Milwaukee. Over 99 percent of the admissions to Ministry's St. Joseph Hospital, in Marshfield Clinic's service area, are patients of Marshfield Clinic physicians. Naturally, Marshfield Clinic and Ministry Corporation have developed a close working relationship.

Park Nicollet Health Services was formed as the result of a merger between the Park Nicollet Clinic and Methodist Hospital. Park Nicollet Health Services does not own its own health plan but contracts with a number of health plans and is a "care system" for the Buyer's Health Care Action Group, a coalition of thirty-five employers in Minneapolis–Saint Paul.

Even Kaiser Permanente of Colorado, an advanced integrated system that combines the five-hundred-physician Permanente Medical Group and the Kaiser Foundation Health Plan (with over four hundred thousand subscribers in the Denver and Colorado Springs metropolitan areas), does not own a hospital. Kaiser Permanente contracts with the five-hundred-bed Saint Joseph Hospital, part of the Sisters of Charity of Leavenworth, Kansas, for inpatient and other hospital-related services. (Saint Joseph Hospital, along with Lutheran Medical Center and physicians associated with both hospitals, is also part of Exempla Health System.)

Strategies of Integrated Systems: Overview

Our research indicates that the strategies of integrated systems led by multispecialty clinics differ somewhat from the strategies of hospital-led integrated systems. For example, hospital-led systems often have problems in dealing with independent physicians who continue to use the hospital but are not part of the core medical group (or groups). In our research and experience, we have found that hospital-led integrated systems may also be more concerned about the "poor" financial performance of their primary care practices.

For their part, integrated systems led by multispecialty clinics may be more likely to experience financial problems. Some of these organizations do not have direct access to the tax-deferred debt markets that are readily available to most hospital systems. Carle Clinic, for example, considered merging with Carle Foundation, owner of Carle Hospital (which is colocated with the clinic), primarily to improve its access to capital. (Another reason for merger is to reduce potential problems associated with self-referral and private inurement.)

William Corley, CEO of Methodist Community Hospitals in Indianapolis, a hospital-led integrated system, defined nine core strategies for his organization. These are shown in Table 10.1 along with his opinion on the degree of emphasis each strategy should receive under each of our four different scenarios for the future of health care.

Some of these strategies—patient satisfaction, cost containment, the uninsured, investment in information systems—would be the same for an integrated system led by a multispecialty clinic. However, most clinic-led integrated systems would not have a strategy with regard to physician integration. They might very well have other strategies, such as enhancing their corporate culture, developing more seamless delivery of care (or "microsystems of care"), and ensuring sufficient financial resources. The discussion that follows combines the strategies of the two major types of integrated systems.

Growth and Improved Market Positioning

Although not specifically mentioned by Corley, integrated systems of all types are concerned about maintaining or improving their market position. Almost every integrated system is focused on growth or at least on gaining sufficient size to achieve economies of scale and balance within the system—for example, the right number of primary care physicians to generate the referrals needed for specialists and for the hospital or an adequate base to support teaching and research.

Geographical Coverage

In our experience, clinic-led systems tend to have larger service areas, and their markets often include small communities in rural settings. The service area of one clinic-led system, Scott & White, and the locations of its care centers, are shown in Figure 10.2.

Table 10.1. Overview of Strategies.

Major Strategy or Health Care Player	Scenario 1: Incremental Change	Scenario 2: Constrained Resources	Scenario 3: Technology Dominant	Scenario 4: Consumerism and Technology (Retail)
Managed care	Continue present strategies	Sell PPO and other insurance products	Continue present strategies	Continue present strategies
Patient satisfaction	Increase emphasis	Meet basic needs, cut back on personnel	Increase emphasis	Make a major emphasis
Physicians	Continue integration (care management across continuum)	Do not pursue integration	Continue integration	Increase emphasis on integrated care management
Merger	No	Yes	Probably (because of capital needs)	No
Cost containment	Emphasize	Lay off staff	Make a major emphasis	Make a major emphasis
Medicare and Medicaid	Emphasize	Limit number of patients	Emphasize	Take on healthy Medicare patients
Uninsured	Take fair share	Limit significantly	Take fair share	Limit significantly
Employers	Pursue partnership	Pursue partnership	Pursue partnership	Avoid
Information systems	Invest 2% to 4% of net revenues	Cut back significantly	Invest 5% to 8% of net revenues	Focus on EMR and customer database

Source: Bill Corley, interview, Feb. 1999.

Figure 10.2. Scott & White Regional Clinic Locations.

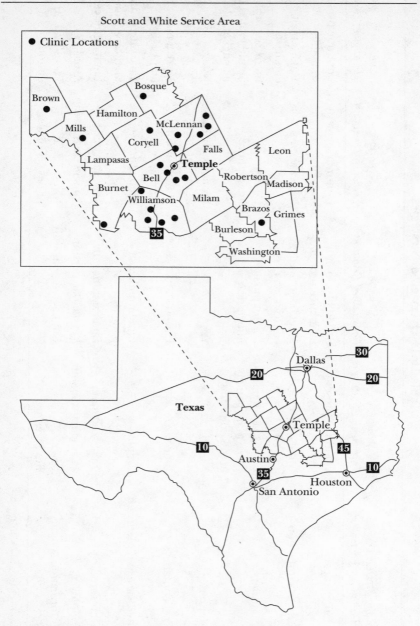

Source: Provided by Scott & White.

MeritCare, which involved the former Fargo Clinic, has a large service area including parts of northwestern Minnesota, eastern North Dakota, and northeastern South Dakota. MeritCare has thirty-five locations, plus its main campus in Fargo.

As part of its efforts to solidify and expand the boundaries of its service area, Carle Clinic in Urbana, Illinois, played a lead role in forming Stratum Med, an organization of fifteen multispecialty clinics in central Illinois and parts of Iowa. Robert Parker, M.D., former CEO of Carle Clinic and a founder of Stratum Med, stressed the importance of this alliance to Carle. He said, "Under a future where consumerism and technology dominate, we might sell off some of our assets in order to have money to invest in strengthening our regional network. This is where we would maximize our market position, especially with consumers" (interview, Feb. 2000).

Market Clout with Managed Care Plans

Even if an integrated system owns a health plan or has a partnership relationship with a managed care organization, these types of plans seldom account for a majority of the patients and revenues of the system. Therefore it is important for most integrated systems to develop a strong position vis-à-vis other health plans.

Developing market clout is not necessarily about higher payment rates. Avoiding exclusion from a health plans' panel of providers could be more important. Most integrated systems, especially those that serve rural areas where they may be the only providers, give priority to making their services available to all residents living in these areas.

Despite criticism of primary care as a strategy, a primary care network is one of the most fundamental ways for an integrated system to develop and maintain market clout with health plans. Without these networks, some health plans would be tempted to exclude some specialists and hospitals..

Brand Name and Reputation for Quality

Establishing a brand name and a reputation for quality is a priority for every integrated system, and many systems have been successful in developing both of these in their service areas. Not every integrated system can be a Mayo Clinic, with a national and international reputation. But most integrated systems can develop strong reputations within their regions.

Among the clinic-led integrated systems we have studied, most have strong regional reputations. These include Lovelace, Merit-Care, Park Nicollet, Deaconess-Billings Clinic in eastern Montana and northern Wyoming, Dartmouth-Hitchcock, and Scott & White.

Hospital-led integrated systems have more than held their own in developing brand names and strong reputations in their service areas. Examples include Aurora, Intermountain Health Care, Sutter, Scripps, Sisters of Providence on the West Coast, Allina in Minnesota, and Baptist Health System in Alabama.

Growth Imperatives

Robert Waller, M.D., former CEO of the Mayo Foundation, told us that stopping growth was not an option for Mayo. Several years ago Mayo considered its alternatives, including a no-growth strategy, and concluded that one strategy that should be pursued was to expand nationally. The main reason for this decision was patient mobility—Mayo needed to position itself to be convenient to its patients (interview, Sept. 1999).

We have observed many large integrated health care systems pursuing growth strategies. One goal of these strategies is to build the capacity to serve more patients. Another goal is to maintain a balance between primary care physicians and medical specialists; without growth the systems might end up with too many specialists. As noted earlier, economies of scale are a factor, particularly for integrated systems that run medical schools.

Regional Networks

Establishing or operating primary care offices in their service areas or regions continues to be among the most fundamentally important yet controversial strategies for integrated systems. We are continually struck by the dichotomy between the many hospitals that shed their primary care practices (or drastically restructure their agreements with physicians) and the hospitals that expand their primary care networks. Many integrated systems continue to report that their regional primary care networks are among their most valuable assets.

Related to this last point, the CEO of a hospital-based integrated system in New England told us, "Our thirty-five primary care physicians are valuable. They directly and indirectly account for over half of all admissions to the hospital and [contribute] to our outpatient volume. Sure, we have to subsidize this group, but on a systemwide basis the benefits far exceed the costs."

Regional Care Centers Offer More Services

It is becoming increasingly clear that regional offices must offer more than primary care services—patients want access to medical specialists. Often, obstetrician gynecologists, otolaryngologists, general surgeons, pediatricians, and other specialists from the main campus of an integrated system make half-day or one-day visits to a satellite office on a weekly or monthly basis. This is an important consumer-friendly strategy, and one that is likely to pay off, especially in the new health care marketplace.

Regional Networks: Conclusions

We believe that under almost any scenario of the future, integrated systems will benefit from their regional networks of primary care centers augmented by visiting specialists. With consumers valuing convenience, specialized services at the local level, and the personal touch, this type of networking strategy will be successful regardless of how the future of health care unfolds.

Quality Improvement

Every mature, successful integrated system has invested heavily in quality improvement—a key aspect of added value, as described in Chapter Two. These investments in time and effort have often been in the form of clinical guidelines, or information systems and analysis, that identify and promote best practices. Integrated systems that have been national leaders in the development of clinical process improvement include Intermountain Health Care, Dartmouth-Hitchcock, Lovelace, and the Mayo Clinic. These organizations, and most other integrated systems, have long recognized that the extreme clinical variation existing across the country is becoming unacceptable to employers, health plans, Medicare, and consumers.

Kevin Fickenscher, M.D., former chief medical officer of Catholic Healthcare West and senior vice president of CareInsite, told us that developing clinical guidelines is only part of the story. "These systems," he said, "have to finish the job by putting in place the clinical and administrative processes to make sure these guidelines are implemented. This may be the toughest part, but until it happens, the payoffs will be minimal" (interview, Sept. 1999).

Frank Villamaria, associate medical director for quality and board member at Scott & White Clinic, told us that guidelines have to be designed so that they can be easily implemented. As he noted, however, "This is not always possible." He added, "When the guidelines are too complicated, or take too much time to understand, the chances of their being used are greatly diminished." Scott & White had reduced the number of guidelines to fifteen in late 1999 and was focusing on developing retrospective measures of physician performance and overall quality. Villamaria said, "We have found that providing physicians data showing how they compare with their peers works well in improving practice patterns and reducing clinical variation" (interview, Nov. 1999).

At Dartmouth-Hitchcock the focus is on continuing to encourage physicians and other clinical practitioners to develop "microsystems of care" that are based on careful analysis of patients' needs, best clinical outcomes, and cost-effectiveness. A physician leader told us, "This is slow work, and it is difficult. We have to have champions who really believe in these kinds of models. However, we can see progress over the past decade, and we are encouraged that clinical process improvement is critical for improving health care."

Investment in Information Technology

In our analysis of various types of health care organizations over the past decade, we have found that integrated systems have been leaders in investing in and developing comprehensive information systems. Furthermore, the efforts of most of these systems have been ambitious, spanning the medical group, hospital, and often the health plan and incorporating the Internet.

Examples of Paperless Systems

Robert Waller, M.D., of the Mayo Foundation told us that the Mayo site in Jacksonville is paperless: "Physicians can pull up a medical record from anywhere in the clinic. Physicians in Jacksonville would never go back to the paper medical record" (interview, Sept. 1999). However, given the much larger size of the medical enterprise in Rochester, Minnesota, the Jacksonville information system is not scalable up to the much larger Rochester clinic.

Kaiser Permanente in Colorado has a paperless medical record. This $160 million system was created in a joint venture with IBM. As of early 2000 this paperless medical record was being introduced in other Kaiser Permanente regions, beginning with Hawaii. Toby Cole, M.D., former head of the Permanente Medical Group in Colorado, told us, "There are no paper records except in storage. Physicians keyboard their notes into the electronic system" (interview, Jan. 2000). Kaiser Permanente expects significant productivity improvements and better service to members.

Partial Development of Information Technology

In many integrated systems, IT is a work in progress. For example, at Dartmouth-Hitchcock in New England, an EMR is partially developed. Peter Johnson, chief information officer of the IT group, said, "In addition to the electronic medical record, our definition of information systems includes telephone systems, the Internet, our intranet, e-mail, physician notes, pharmacy, and laboratory. We are proceeding on all fronts and at a pace that meets the needs of our physicians. Ours is definitely an incremental approach." Development of an EMR at Dartmouth-Hitchcock is facilitated by the fact that hospital and clinic medical records have been combined for decades. Johnson said, "We don't have to fight that battle, and that makes it easier." Johnson also noted that Dartmouth-Hitchcock had benefited from the investment in IT by other large systems, including Intermountain Health Care (interview, Jan. 2000).

Some of the large integrated systems say that the high capital investment required for full implementation of IT is beyond their means, and they are seeking partners, such as IBM (which partnered with Kaiser Permanente) and 3M (which partnered with Intermountain Health Care). The CEO of one system told us, "It is critical that we move in the direction of a paperless system, but we can't afford it on our own. We are going to have to have a partner."

Our conclusion is that gaining economic benefits (such as reduced costs of dictation), achieving time savings for physicians and nurses, replacing telephone calls with automated systems, increasing consumer satisfaction, and gaining physician acceptance are the drivers of the development and adoption of IT in integrated systems.

Clinical Integration, or Seamlessness

Most integrated systems have the goal of improving clinical integration, "which can be defined as the seamless delivery of care to patients, or the right care at the right place at the right time" (Young and McCarthy, 1999, p. xi). We have heard about seamlessness time and again in our ongoing research into integrated systems. What seamlessness really means is total coordination of patient care—eliminating duplication of effort and ensuring the smooth transition of patients among physicians. At Dartmouth-Hitchcock this is accomplished through dozens of microsystems of care within the overall organizational structure.

Gigi Hirsch, M.D., CEO of IntelliNet, based in Boston, said that the biggest challenge for the future is creating true care teams and involving patients in these teams. "Our collective adversary is illness and its related suffering," Hirsch said. "We need to work on involving physicians in these types of change processes" (interview, July 1999).

Unfortunately, the health care market does not reward seamlessness as much today as it likely will in the future. Therefore we do not anticipate that clinical integration is a strategy that would pay large dividends for integrated systems under a business-as-usual scenario or under poor economic conditions. However, we fully expect integrated systems to pursue clinical integration even if the financial rewards are not immediately evident.

However, when consumers take charge, supported by greater access to information and technology, we expect interest in clinical integration to increase dramatically. The same would be true of the "first cousin" of clinical integration: chronic disease management. Stories of consumers being inconvenienced, being asked the same questions over and over, undergoing duplicate tests, and suffering poor coordination of care (for example, when medical staff does not administer beta-blockers to heart attack victims) are common. We do not believe that consumers will tolerate a lack of coordination when they find there are better ways.

Corporate Culture

Among integrated systems, the development and enhancement of corporate culture are a top priority. Of all the health care organizations we have worked with and studied over the years, the major integrated systems, usually led by multispecialty clinics, have the most impressive corporate cultures. Indeed, they could not function without strong corporate cultures.

Corporate culture primarily refers to core values, which can include a commitment to patient care, quality, service, research, medical education, teamwork, mutual respect, and loyalty to the organization. Related to this aspect of core values, one physician leader of a large integrated system (a surgeon) told us that although he personally would prefer spending his time performing surgery, taking on management and leadership responsibilities was more important. "I love this organization, and I will do anything I can to make it successful," he said. Expressions of strong loyalty to the organization are not uncommon in many of the more advanced integrated systems.

However, over a period of time, the stresses and strains on many integrated systems, especially those led by hospitals, tend to create divisiveness and mistrust. Many coalitions formed between hospitals and physicians fall apart. The personal relationships that are a necessary part of a strong corporate culture never have a chance to develop and mature.

We believe that when consumers increasingly take charge, health care organizations with strong core values will enjoy a significant competitive advantage. These values almost always put the interests of the patient above all other interests. Organizations with these kinds of core values can move quickly in response to changing consumer needs. And they can do so in a unified manner, with physicians working together and with the medical group and hospital coordinating their efforts.

Development of Physician Leadership

F. Kenneth Ackerman Jr., a longtime leader of the Geisinger System in Pennsylvania and a vice president of McManis Consulting, believes that developing physician leadership continues to be a major strategic issue for integrated health care systems. He said, "There is some progress being made, but it is going to take a number of years before we have a large supply of proven physician leaders" (interview, Oct. 1999).

Based on our research, we believe that physician leadership tends to develop more naturally in integrated systems led by medical groups. In these types of organizations, there is a culture of physicians willingly spending time on management and leadership. For example, the seven physicians on the board of the Scott & White Clinic spend at least five hours a week (7 A.M. to noon every Wednesday) governing and managing the clinic. Physician members of the boards of governors of Mayo and Dartmouth-Hitchcock make substantial time commitments.

One physician leader of an integrated system, a cardiologist, told us that he makes an effort to read books on management and leadership and participates in professional organizations that focus on leadership issues. "In effect," he said, "I have burned some bridges in my medical practice; I no longer do invasive cardiology. But I believe that I can impact the health of more people by taking a leadership position in this organization."

We believe that physician-led integrated systems, more than any other type of health care organization, have the best chances of developing physician leaders. This kind of leadership will be especially important as consumerism and technology become more important. The new health care marketplace will involve massive shifts in the way health care is organized and delivered, and we expect physicians to lead these efforts.

Improvement of Financial Performance and Access to Capital

Improving financial performance has emerged as one of the most important issues for health care systems of all types, and integrated systems are no exception. Despite doing many things right from a market and clinical perspective, the financial results have often been disappointing. Just as a number of hospitals and health plans posted significant operating losses in the late 1990s, including some of the most prestigious in the country (Kaiser Permanente and Harvard Pilgrim among them), integrated systems have had difficulty demonstrating profitable operations. This kind of inconsistency leads to problems in ensuring long-term access to adequate capital.

Responding to Pricing and Reimbursement Pressures

Pricing and reimbursement were key issues for integrated systems in the late 1990s, and the pressure is unlikely to abate—particularly if resources are limited because of weak economic conditions. In late 1999 at a meeting we participated in with twelve CEOs of integrated systems, coping with the BBA was the most important issue. One CEO said, "We anticipate some additional relief, but not enough to really solve the problems we are facing and expect to face in the future. We are going to have to cut programs." The chairman of the board of one large integrated system told us that the system had lost $30 million in 1999—"We were blindsided on this one," the chairman said—and that it was all attributable to poor Medicaid reimbursement. Furthermore, the losses were expected to be higher in subsequent years.

The reasons for the poor financial performance of some integrated systems run the gamut: being squeezed by health plans and Medicare, poor medical management, information system errors (underreporting of costs), acquisition of medical practices that do not perform up to expectations, poor rate setting for health plans, high administrative overhead, high costs of outlying primary care clinics, merger with another organization, and (sometimes) undoing a merger.

Reducing Operating Expenses

Like hospitals and medical groups, integrated systems have experienced difficulty in controlling their operating costs. One CEO told us that his system would be cutting its costs by 10 percent in the coming two years. "But," he added, "we aren't sure that will be enough, given the constraints of the BBA and the pressures of managed care." The CEO of a metropolitan-area integrated system that experienced significant operating losses in 1998 and 1999 told us, "I would like to believe that revenue enhancement would be the answer for us, but we can't count on it. We have to do everything we can to cut costs."

The chief financial officer of an integrated system led by a multispecialty clinic in the Upper Midwest said that one of the advantages of an integrated system, as compared with a stand-alone hospital, is that an integrated system is somewhat protected from the impact of the BBA: "In some ways, physician reimbursement comes out ahead. We don't have home health, a skilled nursing facility—and very few interns. While the BBA has had a negative impact on the hospital, these other considerations minimize the overall effects."

Another CEO disagreed with placing too much focus on the cost-cutting strategy, saying, "If our only strategy is to cut costs, we will disappear." In our interviews with the leaders of integrated systems, we often heard statements such as, "You can't downsize your way to survival. This is a one-way street."

Propping up Primary Care

Long before the current concern over subsidizing primary care practices, the leaders of integrated systems recognized that primary care offices rarely cover their full costs. One physician leader of an integrated system told us, "We don't think of it as a subsidy. If we didn't have our regional network, overall system profitability would suffer. You can't look at the financial performance of just one piece of an integrated system."

While showing patience with the financial performance of their primary care networks and reaffirming the importance of those networks, most integrated systems are searching for organizational and technological approaches that will reduce costs and, they hope, lead to something close to break-even operations for these regional networks. Their approaches include using an MSO model, working more closely with small community hospitals, adding ancillaries (for example, a laboratory or pharmacy), improving information systems, achieving economies of scale by eliminating very small practices, and enhancing specialty services in the field.

Merging with Hospitals

Mergers with hospitals have been a partial solution to the problem of weak financial performance and lack of access to capital. A number of multispecialty clinics and hospitals that have been partnering in virtually integrated systems have merged, or are considering merger, in order to streamline the care process and improve access to capital. The desire to eliminate duplication, lower costs, and reduce complexity is also a motive for these types of mergers. Here are four examples of such mergers:

- Billings Clinic, a 120-physician multispecialty clinic, merged with the 306-bed Deaconess Medical Center, in Billings, Montana.
- In 1993 Fargo Clinic, with 250 physicians at the time, merged with the 311-bed St. Luke's Hospital in Fargo, North Dakota, to form MeritCare. According to MeritCare executives, the immediate-term impact on the bottom line was highly beneficial.
- In 1995 Q&R Clinic, comprising 90 physicians, in Bismarck, North Dakota, merged with Medcenter One, a 230-bed hospital.
- Since the mid-1980s the Mayo Foundation has acquired two hospitals in Rochester and one in Jacksonville and has built its own hospital in the Phoenix area.

At the time of this writing, a number of other for-profit multi-specialty clinics were seriously considering merging with not-for-profit hospitals, primarily to improve access to capital and reduce concerns over inurement. One clinic administrator told us, "We are getting tired of spending so much time on internal negotiations between the hospital, clinic, and health plan. By becoming a single entity, we can focus on meeting the needs of people in our area and on being more competitive."

Gaining Access to Capital

Although a limited number of large integrated systems have deep pockets and few financial worries, most are concerned about their ability to finance the new technology (with IT at the head of the list) and infrastructure (or teaching and research programs) needed to be successful during the first five years of the twenty-first century. The BBA has created enormous problems and challenges for these types of systems.

A future characterized by constrained resources would be a financial disaster for many integrated systems. An incremental-change scenario would not be particularly favorable either, in that the marketplace would be unlikely to reward the more coordinated, comprehensive systems of care. However, a scenario in which technology and consumerism dominate would provide the kind of environment where integrated systems could perform well financially and therefore be able to attract the capital they need to develop technology and provide a wider variety of services.

Conclusions

Despite reports to the contrary, integrated health care is far from dead. In fact, true vertical integration is not on the defensive or declining. It may appear to be in decline because of the wide publicity given to the many hospitals with a 1990s-type vision of integration that have dropped their health plans, severed their mergers with other hospitals, and either reduced or eliminated the number of employed physicians. Many of these hospitals have rejected the integration strategy, deciding instead to "get back to the basics."

By the end of the 1990s most integrated systems had long since made the decision to focus on consumers, employers, and health plans as their primary customers. By contrast, many hospitals had decided to focus on physicians as their customers. *In the more advanced integrated systems, physicians and hospitals are both leaders and partners in meeting consumer needs.* This is an important point that must be taken into account in order to understand the true focus of vertical integration and to understand why we believe those systems that are faithful to their vision and core values will succeed in the future.

Nearly everyone on the boards or management teams of integrated systems realizes that those systems have to improve their financial performance in order to generate investment dollars and secure their future. The focus has to be on doing a better job of meeting the needs of consumers, and at a lower cost. This is especially important for integrated systems. If they cannot demonstrate substantially greater added value for their customers, they will not survive in their present form.

We believe that most integrated systems will thrive in the new health care marketplace, where consumerism and technology will be the key drivers. The more that technology dominates and consumers make their own decisions and control their own care, the better the chances of success for organizations that focus on coordinated care.

Chapter Eleven

Strategies for Other Types of Health Care Services

Don't focus all of your attention on medical groups and physician networks, acute care and specialty hospitals and integrated systems. There are lots of other important players out there, and they are growing in importance.
LEADER OF A DISEASE MANAGEMENT ORGANIZATION,
July 2000

This chapter summarizes strategies and opportunities for a number of important players in health care that have not been discussed so far, including long-term care, home health, vision care, dental care, CAM, and disease management. Figure 11.1 shows estimates of spending, for 2000 and 2005, on five of the six categories of health care discussed in this chapter. (Data are not available for disease management or for certain elements of long-term care.)

Long-Term Care: Expanding the Continuum of Care

Among the various sectors making up the gigantic U.S. health care industry, long-term care is one of the largest and fastest growing. This section briefly reviews spending on long-term care services, discusses the continuum of long-term care, and defines strategies that make sense under various future scenarios.

The long-term care industry encompasses a wide array of services, largely for the elderly but also for younger individuals with

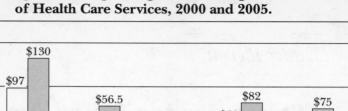

**Figure 11.1. Spending on Five Categories
of Health Care Services, 2000 and 2005.**

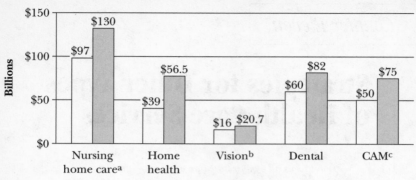

[a]Independent living, congregate care, and assisted living are not included in total health care spending statistics. These three categories of long-term care cost more than nursing home care and are growing more rapidly.

[b]Vision excludes physician services in eye care.

[c]CAM is not included in total health care spending statistics.

Sources: Health Care Financing Administration; authors' estimates based on Coddington, Fischer, Moore, and Clarke, 2000, chaps. 3–4.

disabilities. This continuum of care is illustrated in Figure 11.2 and includes the four major categories defined in Exhibit 11.1.

Over the years, *long-term care* has often been used synonymously with *nursing homes*. Major payer sources for nursing homes have traditionally been Medicaid and private pay, and to a lesser extent Medicare. The nursing home sector has evolved into a highly regulated business. It is a sizable industry with over 1.8 million beds throughout the country (American Health Care Association, 1998). Most nursing homes are for-profit, nearly the reverse of the ownership structure of hospitals.

At the beginning of the twenty-first century, the nursing home sector was in transition. Nursing homes were considered by the public to be a last resort for custodial care. Many nursing home operators sought to build up their rehabilitation capacity to make up for a diminishing traditional clientele. The higher rates paid

Figure 11.2. Service-Housing Continuum of Care.

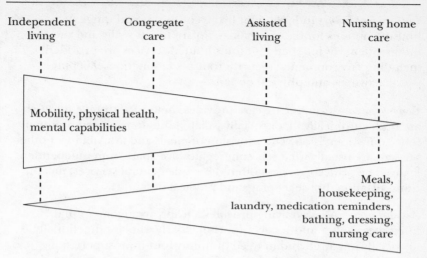

for restorative care often offset declining revenues from patients elsewhere in the facility.

Nursing homes have tried to reinvent themselves as affordable alternatives to costly hospital stays. Hospitals, operating under DRGs, were quick to discharge patients to these less costly alternatives for post-acute care. Medicare pays for most post-acute care on a cost basis. Medicare+Choice plans also seek out favorable contracting arrangements to direct members to select certain facilities for restorative care. When the market was strong in the early 1990s, some of the larger national chains, including Vencor, Mariner Post-Acute Network, and Sun Healthcare Group, invested heavily in this strategy.

However, the introduction of prospective payment in nursing homes, brought about by the BBA, sharply curtailed expenditures for post-acute care. Prospective payment systems wreaked havoc on a sector that flourished under cost-based reimbursement. By the end of 1999 several major chains (including Vencor, Mariner Post-Acute Network, and Sun Healthcare Group) declared bankruptcy. Their reliance on a single strategy—cost reimbursement from government sources—left them particularly vulnerable to changes in

Exhibit 11.1. Long-Term Care: Definitions.

Independent living: Independent living covers a broad range of housing options for older persons who are functionally and socially independent. In independent units limited services are provided, including environmental security, transportation, housekeeping, social activities, and physical design.

Congregate care: Congregate care provides shelter for those elderly who are frail, chronically ill, or socially isolated but do not need twenty-four-hour supervision. The provision of meals and availability of other services are usually what sets congregate care apart from independent living. The primary services offered include general services, meals, transportation, housekeeping, and physical design.

Assisted living: Assisted living provides a living arrangement that integrates shelter and services for frail elderly who are functionally or socially impaired and in need of twenty-four-hour supervision. The primary services include daily living assistance, meals, medicines, safety, and physical design.

Nursing home care: Nursing home care provides living arrangements that integrate shelter with medical, nursing, psychological, and rehabilitation services for persons who require twenty-four-hour nursing supervision. Seniors in nursing home care cannot function on their own.

government policy. Nursing homes were also under increasing pressure from lawsuits brought by patients and their families. In one example of the growing force of consumers in health care, these patients and families were asserting their demands in the courts—and winning.

New Approaches to Nursing Home Care

Future strategies for nursing homes will include recasting their image and becoming more involved in case management within the framework of prospective payment. We also anticipate that nursing homes will distinguish themselves by offering niche services, including dementia and Alzheimer's care. We expect occupancy levels to continue to plummet in some markets—not because the elderly population is not increasing but because other alternatives are emerging to replace or delay placement in nursing homes.

More recently these alternatives have included in-home health services (discussed later in this chapter) and assisted living. Len Fishman, former CEO of the American Association of Homes and Services for the Aging, noted, "I think one of the most significant trends in our industry is the growing role of consumers. That's one of the reasons that there has been such growth in assisted living and that the number of [continuing care retirement communities] last year reportedly increased by 40 percent" (Nakhnikian, 1999).

Growth in Assisted Living

The long-term care industry has been at the forefront of recognizing consumer demands and responding with products and services to meet these expectations. For example, assisted living has emerged as a new industry segment that offers the frail elderly an alternative to institutional nursing home care.

The concept of assisted living is grounded in providing a home-like environment for individuals who need assistance with activities of daily living, such as bathing or dressing. Assisted living appeals to frail elderly who do not want to go to a nursing home. This form of care is also attractive to the adult children of aging parents who are often uncomfortable with, and feel guilty about, sending a parent to a nursing home.

Assisted living now exists throughout the country and has spread from large metropolitan areas to communities of all sizes. The industry is composed of over thirty thousand units. It is estimated to be a $15 billion industry and is projected to grow to $56 billion by 2010 (Jensen, 1999).

Future Strategies

We expect that in the future, assisted living will continue to evolve and respond to marketplace needs. This may mean that some facilities will accept increasingly frail seniors and provide more services. Other long-term care facilities are developing niche markets, including care for individuals with Alzheimer's or dementia. This segment will also seek out opportunities to expand the breadth of the market. Because most of the assisted living in this country has been targeted at the wealthy, private-pay market, there is a significant opportunity to reach moderate-income seniors through developing affordable housing and service packages.

State and federal government agencies are also encouraging the development of assisted living as a means of replacing costly nursing home care for Medicaid recipients. The Department of Housing and Urban Development is supportive of programs that enable housing developments for the elderly to convert to assisted-living models of care as residents of these developments age.

Lessons Learned

The development of assisted living (and other retirement housing options), which grew directly out of consumer demand for alternatives to nursing homes, provides several lessons:

- *Innovators may come from outside the industry.* The innovators in long-term care came from outside the industry. Although many nursing home chains have since added assisted living to their portfolios, they did not lead the effort—and many initially resisted it. New entrants who listened to the market seized the opportunity.
- *Freedom from regulatory and reimbursement pressures may soon be diminished.* Because it has functioned in the private-pay marketplace, the assisted-living segment has enjoyed relative freedom from external regulatory and reimbursement pressures. However, this may change if the government emerges as a payer. Furthermore, as the assisted-living concept has taken hold, a significant variability in the quality of care has developed; this has often led to consumer outcries and the desire for more regulation to weed out low-quality providers. Several efforts are under way to create greater regulatory oversight and an accrediting body for assisted living.
- *Branding is an effective strategy.* The rapid growth and fragmentation in the long-term care industry has favored branding as a strategy. Marriott is an example of an organization using

branding as a key strategy in its senior living communities. Adult children who are seeking options for their aging parents identify with a national brand name like Marriott.

Home Health: Operating at the Mercy of Government Payers

As the twentieth century ended, home health moved from a period of unprecedented growth to a near implosion. Between 1980 and 1998, national expenditures for home health grew by 12.8 percent a year, reaching $33.2 billion by 1998 (Schlesinger and others, 1998). Medicare accounts for roughly 60 percent of payments to home health agencies (Hoechst, 1999). Home health became a viable and important source of income for many health systems, especially for small rural hospitals seeking to diversify their revenue base and spread out fixed overhead costs. However, the BBA changed all that.

The BBA sharply curtailed payments to home health agencies, forcing many out of the business. Total reductions to home health constituted $16 billion of the five-year $115 billion in BBA reductions (HCIA, 1999). One in ten home health agencies has closed since the BBA was enacted.

Relatively high levels of fraud and abuse have also plagued the home health industry. Further regulations related to reporting requirements and limits on utilization have turned the sector upside down. Although home health agencies received some financial relief from the BBA in late 1999, it remains a financially vulnerable business. It is also a very popular service among consumers, especially the elderly and their families.

What will the future hold? The future of home health services is predicated on Medicare policy and reimbursement. In a sector dominated by a single payer, one stroke of the pen can create massive change. Home health is likely to undergo more changes as the Health Care Financing Administration introduces a prospective payment system for home health services. Hospitals and health systems are likely to continue to struggle to provide financially viable home health services.

In working with clients who provide home health services, it has been remarkable to observe the steep decline in volume that most agencies have been experiencing since 1999. If they are financially

able, many large and comprehensive health care systems will continue to subsidize home health because it provides a valuable service to the community. Others will cut their losses and get out of
the home health business. This is an especially likely outcome where
multiple home health agencies are serving the same market.

Advances in technology might also affect home health services.
Electronic communication and the sharing of information via the
Internet (telehealth) are likely to reduce actual home visits while
still allowing for monitoring and assistance of homebound patients.
Patients could check in with home health via the Internet and report vital signs, caloric intake, and other factors. It will be some
time, however, before computers can draw blood, give a bath, or
change dressings, so the need for direct patient care will persist.

Home health might also evolve to increasingly serve those in
the private-pay market who can afford private nursing. Given the
high cost of this service, however, it will largely target wealthy seniors or their children.

Dental Care: Operating Under the Influence of Private Pay Consumers

About 4.5 percent of all U.S. health care dollars are spent on dental
services, including general dentistry, dental surgery, and orthodontics. A high percentage of consumers make at least two visits a year
to their dental professional. This volume of contact is high—at least
twice as many visits as to primary care physicians and CAM providers.

Insights into the Future Gleaned from Dentistry

If you want to anticipate the future of health care, it is instructive to
evaluate past and present trends in dentistry. For example, most
patients have freedom of choice in selecting a dentist. In addition,
personal relationships with dentists are extremely important, as are
convenience of location and the friendliness of dental assistants
and office staff. Consistent with this emphasis on consumerism,
consumers pay a large portion of total dental costs out of pocket.
Even if families have dental insurance, they pay a substantial share
of the cost themselves. And most orthodontics is private pay.

Dentistry emphasizes prevention. Although this may have
reduced revenues in the short term, the routine checkup once or

twice a year has become commonplace. Dentists also make heavy use of dental assistants and hygienists—the equivalent of nurse practitioners and physician's assistants in medicine.

Most dentists are providers in the same dental plan. In other words, in most markets health plans have not fragmented dentists. Some independent dentists form associations for joint advertising and purchasing of supplies. There are also franchised dental groups in which independent dentists have access to a brand name and receive support in running their offices.

New payment methods are emerging. An increasing number of employers are offering "direct reimbursement" for dental bills. Employees pay their bills and then submit them to the employer for reimbursement, up to a specified amount per year. This sounds similar to defined contributions.

Many dentists and small groups target specific market segments, such as those with high incomes who can afford to pay a premium. These patients are pampered and often purchase additional services, such as teeth whitening or braces. Financing services are usually available for big-ticket items.

As with medical groups, dental groups based on a for-profit practice management model (a type of PPM) were common in the 1990s; however, many failed. Most dental PPMs paid too much for the practices they acquired and could not retain the owner or staff. The value of services provided by these management firms did not live up to the firms' promises. (Does this sound familiar?)

But what about strategies for the future in dentistry? Tom Oberle, former executive director of the Colorado Dental Association, suggests these strategies (interview, Mar. 2000):

- *Creation of dental associations.* These are similar to IPAs except that they are not formed for the purpose of managed care contracting. Dentists come together for joint marketing, branding, and purchasing and to offer convenience for patients through geographical coverage.
- *Franchising.* The franchisee is an independent dentist who wants the benefits of a brand name, local advertising, back-office assistance in billing and record keeping, and help in purchasing equipment.
- *Financing for expensive procedures.* Financing is already available

for higher-cost procedures and for orthodontic work, and
we expect financing options to continue to develop.
* *Continued emphasis on prevention.* Dental offices continue to
become even more sophisticated in advising patients on how
to avoid dental problems and in providing new products to
assist in prevention.

Strategies in Dentistry: Summary

The dental industry has succeeded in giving consumers high value
for dollars spent. A high proportion of the population, even the
uninsured, are willing to pay for routine dental services. As we move
into a future dominated by consumerism, dentistry provides a useful model of how providers might respond.

One area of IT that appears to be ideally suited for dentistry is
the Internet—for appointments, reminders, and communication
between the patient and dental office via e-mail. We anticipate that
dentistry will be a pioneer in these kinds of e-mail applications.

Another important finding relevant to the future of health care
is that consumers are accustomed to paying a relatively high proportion of the cost of dental services out of their pockets. They do
it without much complaining because dental services have traditionally functioned this way. In fact, the broad availability of dental insurance benefits is a recent phenomenon.

Vision Care: Operating Within a Burgeoning Consumer Market

Vision care is a $16 billion industry. Excluding physician services,
vision care represents just over 1 percent of all health care spending. Over the past five years, as new technologies have become available, vision care has become a more consumer-oriented business;
as a result, the industry is growing rapidly.

Strategies for Ophthalmic Practices

The strategies of ophthalmic physicians have included internal
growth through physician recruiting, opening new offices, merging with and acquiring other practices, marketing directly to consumers, introducing new revenue-producing services, and selling
the practice to a PPM. The fundamental motivation underlying

these strategies has been the desire to secure and expand market share, increase revenues, improve economies of scale, and obtain managed care contracts (Wolper, 1999).

For many ophthalmic practices, as with other medical specialties, selling to a PPM has not worked well. If the ophthalmologists accepted stock in the PPM for all or part of their payment, the stock almost always declined in value. Also, in many cases the PPM did not provide the kind of practice management expertise that ophthalmologists had anticipated.

Shift in the Mix of Services Provided

As a result of declining Medicare reimbursement, the revenues and profits from cataract surgery that once placed ophthalmologists' income second among all medical specialties have virtually disappeared. As one observer points out, "Cataract surgeons are paid less than 40 percent of what they received just a few years ago" (Dewey, 1999, p. 47).

One of the attractions of refractive eye surgery is that because they consider it elective surgery, managed care organizations do not pay for it. And "[t]his means cash on the barrelhead from patients: No claims to file, no waiting for checks to arrive, and no arguing with a voice on the telephone whose job it is to question physicians' decisions" (Dewey, 1999, p. 47). About one-quarter of the eight thousand ophthalmic surgeons in the United States perform refractive eye surgery, and this number is expected to increase to three thousand by 2002. An estimated 1.5 million refractive eye surgery procedures will have been performed in 2000, and the demand for this type of surgery is growing rapidly.

Shifting an ophthalmic practice to refractive eye surgery requires a change in marketing—from older patients, many on Medicare, to consumers between the ages of twenty-five and forty-five. It also requires changing the aesthetics of the practice site, offering more convenient locations, and training a more service-oriented staff.

The Future of Vision Care

In the new health care marketplace, the number of vision correction surgeries will increase dramatically. A growing number of ophthalmologists will shift the focus of their practices to this type of private-pay surgical procedure. Although declining, payment for cataract surgery by Medicare will continue to be attractive. The aging of the population will drive up demand for this type of service under any of the four scenarios for the future.

In a scenario where resources are constrained, eye care practices that focus on the private-pay sector are likely to experience a serious slowdown. Doing cataract surgery for Medicare patients will be more attractive. Those ophthalmologists expecting a recession and significant stock market decline should not give up their Medicare business.

We expect ophthalmologists to employ a number of market-friendly approaches, such as adding offices in retail or mall locations, spending more on marketing and advertising (their ads blanket the airways today), developing networks of eye care specialists, integrating with optometrists, and improving the operating efficiencies of their practices. These strategies will be especially appropriate in the new health care marketplace.

Disease Management: Establishing Its Role in Health Care Delivery

With as many as one hundred million Americans—one-third of the population—suffering from one or more chronic illnesses, disease management programs have been growing rapidly. For a number of reasons, including the fragmented nature of health care, the future of disease management appears to be bright.

In this section we focus on five questions:

- What is disease management?
- How do specialized disease management programs compare with the disease management services of physicians and medical groups?
- What are the implications of IT for those with chronic diseases?
- Is disease management worthwhile for patients, providers, and health plans?
- How will disease management play out in the future?

What Is Disease Management?

Major pharmaceutical companies were the first to coin the term *disease management,* applying it to programs they developed for the continuing treatment of patients with certain chronic diseases, such as diabetes, congestive heart failure, and asthma. More recently a number of specialized companies, such as CorSolutions, have formed around the development of disease management programs.

David Goodman, founder of Lifemasters, defines disease management this way: "The systematic, coordinated, and integrated approach to managing chronic disease, resulting in better outcomes and lower costs." Goodman said that 19 percent of the population suffers from one or more chronic diseases and that this population accounts for 59 percent of all health care spending (Goodman, Feb. 8, 2000).

Pharmaceutical Companies: Pioneers in Disease Management

According to Thomas Bodenheimer, M.D., of the University of California at San Francisco School of Medicine, the boom in disease management was initiated by the pharmaceutical industry. "By 1995," Bodenheimer (1999c, p. 1202) writes, "most pharmaceutical manufacturers had unveiled a variety of disease-management programs."

Bodenheimer (1999c, p. 1203) summarizes how one pharmaceutical company's program works:

> Merck-Medco Managed Care sells its diabetes disease-management program to the employers and managed-care organizations for which it provides pharmaceutical-benefit services, identifying patients with diabetes through its 51-million-person pharmacy data base. The patients are sent a self-assessment questionnaire, and those who respond are divided into high-risk and low-risk groups. . . . High-risk patients may receive counseling calls from Merck-Medco pharmacists, in most cases from call centers in Ohio. Merck-Medco charges its clients a monthly capitation payment per enrolled patient with diabetes. Employers and HMOs purchase the program to reduce health care costs.

Bodenheimer (1999c) warns that the "carve-out models" used by drug companies may emphasize medications rather than exercise, diet, or a lower-cost generic drug. He says they may also promote their own drugs rather than those of a competitor. He argues that the carve-out model may have negative consequences for American health care.

Access Health: An Outsourced Disease Management Program

Access Health provides disease management services for employers and health plans. The diseases covered include asthma, diabetes, congestive heart failure, and coronary artery disease. Of the more than thirty-five million employees and family members included in the organizations served by Access Health, between five thousand and six thousand individuals are under active management during a given month. Access Health is paid by a combination of per member per month payments and fees based on utilization. The firm maintains a record of every telephone call, and telephone interventions and outcomes are reported to health plan clients.

Rufus Howe, former vice president for product integration at Access Health, said that there are five or six stages of "readiness to change" on the part of those with chronic disease. "Nurses are trained to pick this up," he told us, "and they know how hard they can push" (interview, Mar. 1999).

In terms of potential payoffs, Howe used diabetes as an example: "For every one hundred individuals with diabetes, the probabilities are that 3.2 percent will have a heart attack in the next twelve months. The average cost of a heart attack is $30,000. If we can help prevent one heart attack, we have saved the health plan or employer a significant amount of money. You multiply these dollars times the number of people with diabetes, and you can see the potential. Plus, life is a lot more pleasant for those consumers who have avoided a heart attack" (interview, Mar. 1999).

Howe also emphasized that Access Health makes a concerted effort to work with primary care physicians. "Bedraggled doctors need help; they like prompts," Howe said. "We work mainly with primary care physicians and try to get them involved with patients with chronic illnesses" (interview, Mar. 1999).

Physician-Based Disease Management

Bodenheimer (1999c) favors disease management programs that bolster primary care. He believes that these types of programs have the potential to improve outcomes for patients with chronic diseases. He cites Group Health Cooperative of Puget Sound (a group-model HMO) as an example of a physician-driven disease management program:

> Group Health's electronic information system allows primary care physicians to view a spreadsheet of information on patients with diabetes, including when they were last seen, glycohemoglobin levels, dates of eye examinations, microalbumin determinations, and medications. The system periodically notifies practitioners about patients who have not received all appropriate services, and patients are called to arrange needed services. Three days each week, an endocrinologist and a nurse specialist travel to Group Health's medical centers, coaching the primary care teams on how to make the best use of a 10-to-15-minute visit for the management of diabetes [p. 1204].

As a result of Group Health's program, initial data show that the rate of regular foot examinations for patients with diabetes increased from 18 to 56 percent and that the rate of annual retinal examinations increased from 46 to 64 percent. "In contrast to the carve-out approach," Bodenheimer (1999c, p. 1204) explains, "Group Health focuses on improved care rather than reduced costs, and it targets all patients with diabetes, not only those at highest risk."

Impact of Technology on Disease Management

The Internet has the potential to expand the scope of disease management programs at both the carve-out and physician-based level. Consider, for example, the following story from the *Wall Street Journal* about the "virtual house call":

> From her accounting office here in the heart of Silicon Valley, Lena Diethelm gets her diabetes checked without ever leaving her desk. Five miles away, at a medical complex in Atherton, J. Joseph Prendergast monitors her blood-sugar readings over the Internet.

"It's easy," says Ms. Diethelm, a 46-year-old tax practitioner. After pricking her finger and squeezing a drop of blood onto a glucose meter the size of a wallet, she hooks the meter up to her PC with a cable. Then, with a few mouse clicks, she beams every reading from the past two weeks to Dr. Prendergast and his staff for review.

Such virtual exams take place daily at DiabetesWell.com, which treats more than 700 patients across the U.S. by making it possible for doctors and nurses to collect data from patients online, then send back evaluations and treatment instructions, DiabetesWell is inventing a new kind of Web business: the e-clinic [Weber, 2000].

Cost Savings Associated with Disease Management: A CorSolutions Study

In a study of the effectiveness of disease management, CorSolutions compared data on 143 individuals in a control group that received traditional care for coronary artery disease with 148 people enrolled in a disease management program. Seventy-two percent of both groups were male, and the average age in the groups was fifty-four. Over a one-year period the group enrolled in the disease management program had 73 percent fewer emergency room admissions and 40 percent fewer hospital admissions. Total medical costs for those in the disease management program were 30 percent lower than the costs for those in the control group (Humana, 1999b).

The Future of Disease Management

Disease management appears to have an excellent future as a way of more efficiently caring for the needs of individuals with chronic illnesses and as a means of improving their quality of life. As discussed in Chapter Twelve, we anticipate that disease management programs and the early identification of those with chronic disease will become part of the way health plans are structured.

We also believe that disease management is a natural step for larger medical groups and integrated health care systems. In fact, many of the large systems that were pioneers in clinical guidelines are now incorporating the guidelines into their disease management programs (see Chapter Two).

Whatever the merits or flaws of pharmaceutical company disease management programs, niche programs like Access Health, and programs based in physicians' offices, we believe that physicians and medical groups should consider maintaining relationships with their patients rather than defaulting to outside disease management programs. This is in the best interests of both the patient and the medical group.

In summary, because of several interrelated factors—the aging of the population and the corresponding increase in chronic illnesses, the ease of communication with consumers via the Internet, and the financially favorable cost-benefit ratio of disease management—disease management programs appear to have an excellent future in the new health care marketplace.

Complementary and Alternative Medicine: Becoming Mainstream

Our discussion of CAM focuses on the potential for integration of CAM into traditional medicine by physician practices, medical groups, and hospitals.

What Is Complementary and Alternative Medicine?

What do we mean by CAM? Exhibit 11.2 lists a number of examples of products and services that would fall within the definition of CAM.

Inclusion of Complementary and Alternative Medicine in Health Plan Benefits

Here are three examples of health plans that offer CAM:

- *Group Health Cooperative in Washington.* Group Health, a staff-model HMO, pays for acupuncture, naturopathy, massage therapy, and chiropractic care for specific conditions (Grandinetti, 1999).
- *Blue Cross and Blue Shield of California.* These two health plans offer CAM programs. Blue Cross has offered acupuncture and chiropractic care to large groups, has announced that it would

**Exhibit 11.2. Examples of Complementary
and Alternative Medicine.**

---

1. Acupuncture
2. Acupressure
3. Nutrition
4. Herbal medicine
5. Guided imagery
6. Hypnotherapy
7. Aromatherapy
8. Meditation
9. Homeopathy
10. Biofeedback
11. Chiropractic
12. Therapeutic massage
13. Yoga
14. Spirituality
15. Music therapy
16. Vitamin therapy
17. Stress management
18. Naturopathy
19. Reflexology

---

be instituting its own discount program, and has begun providing all enrollees with access to massage therapists, yoga teachers, and the like (Grandinetti, 1999).

- *Blue Cross and Blue Shield of Massachusetts.* This health plan offers members discounts on massage therapy, acupuncture, and nutritional counseling (Daily, 1999, p. S6).

Incorporation of Complementary and Alternative Medicine into Traditional Medical Practices

Judging from the number of articles on the subject and from interviews with physician leaders of medical groups, interest in incorporating CAM into traditional medical practices is not new.

Tri-Rivers Surgical Associates

In 1998 Tri-Rivers Surgical Associates, a seven-physician orthopedic practice in Pittsburgh, opened the Institute for Alternative Medicine. While recognizing an ethical responsibility to provide patients with accurate information, practice leaders believed that alternative care could complement its approach to musculoskeletal care.

Martha Hamilton, executive director of Tri-Rivers Surgical, said, "We felt patients would be best served if we could bring orthopedic surgeons and alternative practitioners together in a mutually inclusive way." Tri-Rivers hired a chiropractor to serve as medical director for the institute, as well as a massage therapist and a nurse practitioner, who provides nutrition and lifestyle counseling. On the financial side, Hamilton said, "We're growing every day, but the growth has been slower than we projected. We had initially thought it would take six months for the institute to break even. It now appears it will take nine months" ("Does Alternative Medicine Fit?" 1999, pp. 16–17).

Advocate Medical Group

Advocate Medical Group opened the Center for Complementary Medicine in August 1998 in Chicago. The center had a staff of independent contractors that included two chiropractors, two massage therapists, two homeopathic physicians, and an acupuncturist (Baldwin, 1998).

Mercy Regional Health System

About fifteen thousand square feet of Mercy Hospital Fairfield's health complex in Cincinnati are devoted to CAM—acupuncture, reflexology, nutritional counseling, massage, and biofeedback. A nearby retail store sells aromatherapy and homeopathic products, and a resource center offers books and tapes on wellness topics (Tokarski, 1998).

Writing in the *MGM Journal,* two authors come to this conclusion about CAM and medical groups: "There are business opportunities for medical groups although careful planning is required. CAM represents the opportunity to grow practice revenues, expand a group's tool kit for assisting patients with health care issues, and retain or increase market share by proactively responding to consumers" (Hofgard and Zipin, 1999, p. 20).

Arizona Centers for Health and Medicine: An Unsuccessful Attempt

The Arizona Centers for Health and Medicine began in the early 1990s as the private practice of Sam Benjamin, one of the first physicians in the country to combine conventional and alternative medicine. In 1994 Benjamin's clinic was acquired by St. Joseph's Hospital and Healthcare System, a Phoenix-based affiliate of Catholic Healthcare West (CHW).

However, in January 1999 CHW announced it was shutting down or selling the Arizona Centers. In April ten physicians and twenty staff members were looking for jobs elsewhere. Why? The main reason was inadequate reimbursement that led to financial problems. Also, Benjamin left the practice. Phyllis Biedess, former CEO of the Arizona Centers, says, "We should applaud CHW, because they did try. They believed integrative medicine was a better way to deliver care, and they funded it. Finally they reached a point where overwhelming financial and programmatic priorities pointed them in other directions" (Zablocki, 1999, p. 71).

Complementary and Alternative Medicine Strategies for Hospitals

Hospitals once turned their backs on all forms of CAM. One of the authors was on the board of a hospital fifteen years ago when the local society of chiropractors threatened to sue for staff privileges. This was shocking to the hospital board and the medical staff. That same hospital now allows chiropractors to see patients.

Here is an example of a hospital in California that has assimilated CAM:

> Outside the entrance to California Pacific Medical Center, a highly regarded acute-care hospital in San Francisco, patients in bathrobes are often seen making their way, in meditative silence, around a spiral painted walkway called a labyrinth. Sometimes they are joined by family members and even hospital staff, all of whom are seeking the healing power and inner peace of this ancient form of walking meditation, used in early Christian rituals and currently enjoying a revival in this country.
>
> No, this is not some scenario concocted by a New Age dreamer. California Pacific is one of dozens of U.S. hospitals seeking to integrate alternative and complementary healing therapies with mainstream medicine [Stevens, 1999].

Here are examples of two other acute care hospitals offering CAM:

- *Via Christi Regional Medical Center, Wichita.* Beginning in 1996, this hospital built its complementary healing services around therapeutic touch, finally finding open acceptance of the procedure from physicians by offering it with other relaxation response therapies, such as guided imagery, relaxation tapes, massage, and music therapy (Larson, 1998).
- *Presbyterian Hospital, New York City.* The Complementary Care Center, which opened in 1996, serves cardiac, oncology, orthopedic, and neurology patients using therapeutic touch, hypnotherapy, music therapy, massage, and other therapies (Larson, 1998).

Herbal Medicines and Traditional Pharmacies

Aurora HealthCare, a large integrated system in eastern Wisconsin, owns close to one hundred retail pharmacies. According to Dennis Rakowski, president of Aurora Pharmacy, the system incorporated herbal medicine in early 1998. Aurora Pharmacy has a standardization committee for herbal formulations to evaluate all new products for safety and efficacy (Egger, 1999b).

Valley Medical Center in the Seattle area began an herbal medicine program at one of its pharmacies in May 1999. According to a consultant who helped Valley establish this program, the major reason for the project was to satisfy the demands of baby boomer customers who avidly seek CAM therapies (Egger, 1999b).

Integration of Complementary and Alternative Medicine into Mainstream Medicine

CAM continues to grow rapidly and is becoming mainstream. Despite some financial problems, such as those of CHW in Arizona, it appears that the integration of CAM into conventional medicine will continue. In a health care future dominated by consumerism, CAM could become a common element in the array of services available from traditional primary care physicians and medical specialists. Although some types of CAM will increasingly be covered by health plans, most of the cost of products and services will continue to be paid directly by consumers. This is one of the attractive features of CAM for medical groups and hospitals; because CAM is a cash business, they do not have to deal with managed care.

Conclusions

The six types of health care services highlighted in this chapter account for more than one-fifth of all health care spending, an amount equal to the total dollars spent on physician services. Furthermore, these types of services are expected to grow rapidly. Many of the medical specialties discussed here—especially dental, vision, assisted living, home health, and disease management—are already perceived by consumers as distinct health care segments that mix private pay and third-party payer reimbursement. At the same time, skilled nursing and home health in particular face difficult financial challenges. It appears that proponents of these two types of health care services will continue to encounter difficulty in justifying the costs of these services relative to perceived benefits.

Chapter Twelve

Strategies for Health Plans

There is a confluence of forces, including consumers, technology, and employers, wanting out of the health benefits business. This is going to fuel individual purchasing of health care coverage.
ROBERT VERNON, SENIOR VICE PRESIDENT,
AON MANAGED CARE, FORT WORTH, TEXAS

Among the different types of health care organizations discussed in Part Two, health plans face perhaps the greatest challenges in developing strategies for the future. For example, in a health care market experiencing growth in individual insurance and defined contributions, employers would be largely out of the business of providing health care coverage for employees, and consumers (or consumer coalitions) would be responsible for purchasing their own health plan coverage.

Other challenges that will face health plans during the first few years of the new millennium include the following:

- Developing new health plan products that cover increasingly expensive drugs and medical technology
- Offering consumers a greater variety of health plan choices
- Determining how to offer added value to employers and purchasing coalitions that desire to contract directly with providers
- Finding ways to lower both medical loss ratios and overhead
- Regaining credibility with the public and physicians

One health plan executive believes that the only hope for managed care, and for health care in general, is to move toward individual choice. Eric Sipf, president and CEO of PacifiCare in Colorado, says, "There's no way we are going to make health care more affordable and more consumer friendly under the current system." He feels that "as long as the healthcare system is employer-based, consumers will have no incentive to control their own use of healthcare and utilization will continue to climb" (Egger, 1999a).

Richard Huber, former chairman and CEO of Aetna U.S. Healthcare, believes that the health care system would be better if we moved to a defined-contribution model. "But as I look five or ten years out," he says, "we must be prepared for the market to move to a defined-contribution system. What if employers shifted to something like the Federal Employees Health Benefits Program, where in essence you get a voucher and you can choose from a menu of health plans? If the plan you want costs more than your voucher or the sponsor's defined contribution, you dip into your pocket" (Robinson, 1999, p. 90).

Health plans have had a unique and often untenable role—that of an arbiter between employers, consumers, and providers. This is illustrated in Figure 12.1. This chapter identifies and evaluates possible strategies that health plans might pursue as they attempt to strike the right balance for each of the four scenarios for the future. We start with the left-hand side of the scale shown in Figure 12.1: meeting the demands of consumers and employers. Then, moving to the right-hand side of the scale, we focus on strategies aimed at moderating increases in health care costs.

Capitalizing on the Growth of Consumerism

By 2000 health plans were focused on increasing premiums while at the same time repositioning their products and benefit designs to be more responsive to the market. An example was United-Health's decision in late 1999 to cease using prospective reviews and leave referral decisions up to physicians.

Many of the changes in health plan design have meant relaxing provisions regarding out-of-network care. Health plans offering open access (without primary care gatekeepers) and POS options experienced the most rapid growth in enrollment in the late 1990s.

**Figure 12.1. The Challenge for Health Plans:
Managing the Balance.**

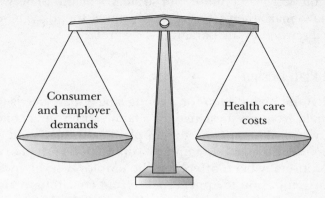

In addition, many health plans sweetened their benefits design by including a provision for CAM—a direct response to consumers' demands.

These incremental changes by health plans acknowledge the growing role of consumers. We expect more of these types of changes under a business-as-usual scenario. Under this scenario health plans would tinker with their products within the framework of an expected continuation of the employer-based system while simultaneously raising premiums in an attempt to restore profitability. (Some would contend this is in tune with the six-year underwriting cycle, maintaining that it is time to raise premiums.) But what strategies should health plans pursue under the more radical scenarios? Do health plans have a future in a scenario where consumers dominate?

The health plan experts we interviewed were quick to admit that consumers are playing a greater role than ever before. Even though the principal point of contact and "first customer" is usually the employer, it is consumers' demands for wider access and greater choice that have led to the multitude of open-access products that barely existed a few years ago. Further, as more and more employers institute cafeteria-type benefits plans and shift toward a defined-contribution model, consumers will play an even larger role in health plan decision making.

Exhibit 12.1 lists a number of strategies health plans will need to pursue to make themselves more consumer friendly. These strategies are discussed in the paragraphs that follow.

Flexible Plan Design

Given that the plan design for a young single male needs to differ substantially from one designed for a family with young children or for a fifty-year-old empty-nester couple, health plans will need to appeal to discrete market segments. Although health plan designs have traditionally been offered at the employer level, more individual customization to appeal to different consumer market segments will be required in the future. For example, those consumers who want access to a full range of CAM might pressure employers to include more of these services as part of their covered benefits.

Richard Huber anticipates a mind-boggling array of new health plan products. Huber says, "We see our goal very clearly as working with plan sponsors to help them satisfy their employee benefit needs, using whatever products suit them the best" (Robinson, 1999, p. 90). Successful health plans of the future might well use an approach resembling that of Dell Computer, which allows consumers to purchase over the Internet, choose which features they want, and check the status of their order on-line. Both consumers and employers will also receive much of their service and administrative support on-line.

The Complexity of Mass Customization

Some health plan executives contend that the idea of mass customization is overrated. They are concerned that customizing their benefits for individuals will be too complex. "I expect a number of standardized plans to emerge," Robert Vernon told us. He went on to note, however, that these plans will appeal to various market segments: "Only a certain number of consumers can afford the Cadillac, most will buy the Chevy, and there are some out there who will want to buy a Yugo" (interview, Oct. 1999).

Dennis Horrigan, vice president of managed care development at Independent Health, a regional not-for-profit plan serving great-

Exhibit 12.1. Consumer-Friendly Strategies for Health Plans.

- Flexible plan design
- Accessible care
- Improved customer service and easier administration
- Accessible health information
- New marketing approaches
- Better management of health care costs

er Buffalo, New York, likened the concept of customization to education. "There are some people out there who choose private schools," he observed, "but for the most part, the vast majority use the public education system. Many people want to keep things simple and inexpensive" (interview, Oct. 1999).

As market segments become more discrete and refined, defining and combining risk pools will become more challenging. This suggests that health plans will need to be large enough to profile the overall community in order to effectively price products and spread the risk. In other words, there will be changes in underwriting strategies.

The Direct-Pay Market

On a related note, health plans may be forced into the retail market simply because of the growing number of individuals who do not have access to employer-based health plan coverage but instead have voucher-type plans, MSAs, or individually purchased insurance. We know from the experience of the Buyer's Health Care Action Group (BHCAG) in Minneapolis–Saint Paul that a relatively small number of individuals can dramatically influence the shape of the provider community and the competitive environment.

At a time when there is growing evidence of consumers playing a larger role in selecting and purchasing their health plan coverage, many health plans are leaving the retail market (such as Medicare+Choice) or significantly raising the premiums on individual policies. But will health plans be able to afford to drop out in the future, when a large portion of the population is likely to control its own health plan purchasing decisions?

Accessible Care

The ability of health plans to continue to market limited panels of providers is questionable. Consumers' desire to choose their own physician or hospital is much greater than anticipated even five years ago. (This has been a particularly important issue for provider-sponsored health plans, which have a vested interest in directing subscribers to their own physicians and hospitals.)

In the future a growing number of consumers will not tolerate limitations on their access to care. Even today, employers routinely assess the amount of overlap between the provider network of their existing health plan and the provider panel of any new health plan being considered. If the overlap is limited, employers are often reluctant to switch plans and require employees to go through the upheaval of selecting new physicians.

Another dimension of access, beyond choice of providers, is ready access to desired physicians and hospitals. In a world with more demanding consumers, waiting is no longer acceptable. For example, Kaiser Permanente in Colorado has restructured its scheduling system to ensure that a member who calls and needs to see a physician that day will be able to do so.

Independent Health in New York launched a pilot program in conjunction with the Institute for Healthcare Improvement, in two primary care physician sites, in which members are able to schedule an appointment the same day they make the call. Dennis Horrigan said, "We use industrial management theory to enable physicians to provide more immediate access to membership. Open access scheduling allows physicians to do today's work today." (interview, Oct. 1999). MeritCare in Fargo is implementing a similar policy throughout its network of primary care sites.

Improved Customer Service and Easier Administration

Consumers and employers are demanding less administrative complexity in their health plans. From a consumer perspective, this has generally been one of the advantages of HMOs—patients have not had to bother filing claims, and they simply pay their copayment at the time of the physician or hospital visit. Until recently, however, consumers have found themselves caught in the administrative tangles of preauthorizations, referral requests, and exemptions from the formulary. As consumers increasingly have the ability to choose among health plans, or purchase their own insurance, administrative simplification will gain significance.

Further, if business and government employers move to defined contributions or vouchers or otherwise offer more choice, employers will not be willing to take on more of the costs of administering their benefits plans. Therefore health plans will need to ensure their infrastructure readily supports a greater variety of options.

Achieving administrative simplicity may be easier in theory than reality. For example, information systems are usually designed to fit one HMO model, and they can be difficult to retrofit to accommodate different models. Group- and staff-model health plans, such as Kaiser Permanente (KP), find this to be a particular dilemma. One KP executive noted, "Our systems were built around a closed-panel HMO. It is amazingly time consuming and costly to deal with a wide variety of options. With something as simple as a change in copay from $15 to $25, all our contracts need to change, our membership cards have to be modified, and our front-office personnel trained to understand all the variations we offer."

In fact, some health plans are limiting the range of options in order to gain administrative efficiencies. Plan executives have determined that it costs less to offer an employer a $20 copayment than to alter information systems to offer a $25 copayment. However, this could prove a risky strategy in a consumer-dominated future. Plans that are not able to offer customization at the employer level—to say nothing of the consumer level—are likely to lose market share.

Accessible Health Information

Many consumers crave information about their health and the health of family members. Some health plans are moving to the forefront of providing consumers with health-related information. Self-help handbooks and other resources are often sponsored by health plans; this benefits consumers and the health plan alike. More recently Web sites have begun to replace handbooks, but the principle is the same. There are still a few plans that prefer not to give out too much information for fear of fueling greater demand for services.

Kaiser Permanente Online: A New Form of Patient Access

KP Online is an example of expanding information and services to consumers through Web-based technologies. By clicking on this Web site, consumers can access Healthwise Handbook, a registry of pharmaceuticals (including information about every drug available), a schedule of wellness classes, a provider directory, and other health information. Members receive additional services, including the ability to renew a prescription on-line, learn the results of lab tests, schedule appointments, and, ultimately, communicate with their personal physician electronically.

KP Online's approach of making some of its services available to nonmembers illustrates the opportunities for health plan branding of consumer-directed health information. What health plan would not want both its enrollees and nonmembers to log on to its Web site to learn about physicians, hospitals, drugs, and other sources of health information?

Given the unfavorable public image of most health plans, however, they are unlikely to be a trusted resource for information when competing with established health systems or medical groups. Nonetheless, health plans clearly have the information to build effective Web sites. As one health plan executive commented, "We should be able to outpace the ability of hospitals and medical groups to provide valuable health information because we will have larger and more detailed databases on disease patterns throughout the community and region."

Concern over Those Left Behind

Kate Paul, retired president of KP's western division, commented, "I am concerned about the segment of the population that is not computer literate, the elderly, the poor, minorities. They might be left out, and more than ever we may create a two-tiered system of care in this country" (interview, Sept. 1999). In our past research and publications, we have often addressed the challenges for providers of operating in a health care market split between fee-for-service compensation and capitated payment. This analogy may be shifting to those consumers who are deeply involved in an Internet-based world versus those who are part of a computer-illiterate world.

Access to Information on Provider Quality

Another dimension of the distribution of health information is ensuring consumer access to information on plan and physician quality measures to help them make informed decisions. Quality report cards, the Health Plan Employer Data and Information Set, and the results of consumer satisfaction surveys are the early manifestations of this effort. Steve Wetzell, executive director of BHCAG, said that after three years of receiving these kinds of information on the care systems available in the market, consumers are increasingly relying on quality and satisfaction indicators when selecting their coverage options (interview, Jan. 2000). The experiences of BHCAG are indicative of the future direction of consumerism in the health care marketplace.

New Marketing Approaches

IT will make it possible to meet and exceed employers' and consumers' expectations from health plans and their networks of physicians and hospitals. Web-based technologies will make it easier to sell health insurance over the Internet. As the Internet takes hold in the health care world, health plans will need to retool their marketing departments and change their distribution channels, putting greater emphasis on e-commerce and less on direct marketing representatives or brokers. Although some employers might still prefer a personal relationship with their broker, others will opt for the increased efficiency of dealing directly with health plans via the Internet.

This change in the methods of marketing health plans to both employers and consumers raises questions about the future of benefits consultants. One managed care executive noted, "I see very little role in the future for benefits consultants or brokers who focus on health care, because they can be replaced by Internet resources."

Better Management of Health Care Costs

Health plans are often accused of controlling medical expenses rather than managing care. The principal strategies health plans have used to control costs are contracting with limited panels of physicians, hospitals, and other providers, using capitated payment to physicians, and creating economic incentives or requirements for enrollees to use the lowest-cost alternative first (for example, the requirement to go through a primary care gatekeeper first). To execute their strategy health plans have attempted to shift financial risk to physicians and medical groups in order to give them financial incentives to manage the costs of care. However, the strategy of shifting risk to physicians, especially through capitated payment, is fraught with challenges and is falling out of favor in most parts of the country.

Meeting the Demands of Consumers and Employers While Lowering Costs

What can health plans do in the future to manage the right-hand side of the scale and ensure that annual increases in health care costs are acceptable to both consumers and employers? Exhibit 12.2 illustrates strategies health plans might pursue to gain a semblance of control over health care costs. We discuss those strategies in this section.

Aligning Financial Incentives with the Marketplace

Contracting strategies among health plans and providers are in chaos. In some parts of the country, capitation has predominated. Many physician groups organized into IPAs, PHOs, group practices, and other contracting entities to be able to take on risk through capitation. However, in the late 1990s a number of physician networks collapsed, leaving physicians unpaid and the courts to decide if the health plan that already reimbursed the IPA was liable to pay physicians for the unpaid claims of the IPA. The magnitude of financial failures of medical groups and networks has far exceeded expectations.

As the twentieth century closed, we witnessed a significant retrenchment in capitation in many parts of the country. A headline story in *Modern Healthcare* in mid-1999 was titled "Decapitation." Health systems have struggled to generate sufficient capitated revenue and are holding out for per diem or other limited-risk payment arrangements. Providers have consolidated to the point that they have sufficient market clout to not accept risk if this is what

Exhibit 12.2. Strategies for Enhancing
Health Plan–Health System Relationships to Lower Costs.

- Align financial incentives with the marketplace
- Collaborate on clinical guidelines and disease management
- Address the drug and medical technology crisis
- Harness the power of information systems
- Consolidate

they prefer. An executive of a major national insurance firm noted, "For the first time in years, there has been a big drop-off in applications for stop-loss policies"—further evidence of the decline in capitated contracts.

Health plans, for their part, are reluctant to pass on risk to medical groups that do not have adequate information and payment systems in place or the experience to manage financial risk. Health plans are more willing to contract with IPAs that have substantial capital reserves, but not with networks lacking financial resources. Unfortunately, there are not many IPAs that meet this criterion.

If capitation is disappearing, what will replace it as the preferred payment mechanism for physicians and hospitals? The care system concept used by BHCAG in Minneapolis–Saint Paul, for example, pays physicians and hospitals based on services rendered, but within the framework of budget estimates developed at the beginning of each year.

Max Brown, senior vice president of WellPoint in California, says, "The public doesn't grasp capitation, and we ought to give up on it. There is no reason that we can't make fee-for-service work." His approach would be to maximize care management and focus on the small portion of the population who consume most of the health care resources (interview, Sept. 1999).

James Hertel, president of Healthcare Computer Corporation of America and publisher of widely read managed care newsletters in Arizona and Colorado, believes the answer lies in retrospective review, closer examination of claims, slow payment to providers who are viewed as stretching the limits, and deselecting some physicians and medical groups (interview, Jan. 2000).

Dennis Horrigan of Independent Health noted, "Global capitation has not worked, but we are having success with three-way risk-sharing arrangements involving physicians, hospitals, and a health plan." In Independent Health's market area, capitating hospitals and physicians for their portion of the medical budget has been effective in controlling utilization and costs (interview, Oct. 1999).

It is difficult to generalize about future payment arrangements because there will continue to be significant regional variations. Capitated payment, especially for physicians, will continue in some markets. Other markets, like Minneapolis–Saint Paul, will move more to a fee schedule with limited risk sharing based on overall budget targets. Still other markets will eliminate risk for physicians and hospitals as they revert to fee schedules and focus on managing overall utilization through other means, including better retrospective data on utilization patterns, disease management, and the management of critical cases.

We expect the contracting function to become less of a focal point in health plan–provider relationships. Instead of contracting, the focus will become analysis of data generated by more sophisticated information systems, dissemination of more health information to consumers, disease management for those with chronic illnesses, and better monitoring of the performance of individual physicians, medical groups, and hospitals.

Collaborating on Clinical Guidelines and Disease Management

The emphasis on clinical guidelines and care process improvement that became commonplace in many large health care systems in the mid-1990s appears to be evolving into disease management programs for chronically ill patients (such as those with diabetes or congestive heart failure). In other words, the clinical guidelines are being extended to serving the needs of patients beyond the time they are in the hospital.

Max Brown of WellPoint noted that according to his organization's data, 8 percent of members account for 71 percent of all health care costs, an average of $12,000 per member per year. The next 24 percent account for 22 percent of the costs, averaging $1,300 per year. The remaining 68 percent consume 7 percent of the resources, for an average of $150 per year. Brown cited the 1996 claims experience of a Fortune 100 company: "Of salaried employees, the 1 percent with catastrophic illnesses consumed 25 percent of the claims expense. Another 17 percent with unstable chronic disease accounted for 63 percent. Those who were healthy or had stable chronic illnesses (82 percent) consumed only 12 percent of health-related expenses" (interview, Sept. 1999).

Brown's conclusion was that managed care has been designed as a program to apply to 100 percent of the population when in fact it would be more appropriately directed at the limited number of individuals who are heavy utilizers. "What is the point," he asked, "in restricting choice of providers for two-thirds of the population who are spending less than $150 annually?" He also observed, "Why do we subject most employees to managed care? We don't need to do it, and they don't need it" (interview, Sept. 1999).

The main issues become (1) identifying employees and family members with serious medical needs and (2) effectively and aggressively managing the care of these individuals. Plans can be designed to provide wide access and choice for all enrollees but, when significant medical needs arise, to create economic incentives for those enrollees to enter into more comprehensive managed care options. These alternatives would offer more comprehensive benefits and include utilizing a smaller panel of physicians who have proved themselves to be the best clinicians in handling a particular disease. As Brown stated, "You put your best providers on the most serious cases and don't worry too much about which physicians are used by the rest of the members" (interview, Sept. 1999).

James Hertel, however, questioned the feasibility of this approach: "We have known for years that just over 10 percent of the patients use 90 percent of health care resources. However, these are often the patients who scream the loudest in the press and to their elected officials. They often resist being moved into smaller panels of providers" (interview, Jan. 2000).

Our conclusion is that health plans have little choice but to focus on controlling the costs of the high utilizers (often individuals with serious chronic illnesses). This will be especially important if financial resources for health care are constrained and there is more willingness on the part of employers and the public to accept tough measures to control health care costs.

Addressing the Drug and Medical Technology Crisis

One health plan executive told us, "Most health plans have no clue about what to do about drug costs. They are using their old bag of tricks." This may be true today, but we expect changes in the future.

Alternatives for Controlling Drug Costs

Indemnity plans rarely paid for drugs. Drug coverage has been associated with HMOs as they sought to maintain or restore the overall health of their members. However, few (if any) health plans foresaw the huge growth in the cost of providing drug coverage. One health plan executive noted, "Our drug costs had been very predictable for years and not a major cost factor, but all that changed in the past year."

As drug costs mount, we can expect health plans to become more sophisticated in how they price and market the drug benefit. Riders for drug coverage will become commonplace, with co-payment levels and premiums tied to specific formularies. A typical health plan will offer three-tiered pricing with the lowest copayments for generics, the next level for drugs on the formulary, and the highest copayment for drugs not on the formulary.

Rising drug costs will mean excluding certain expensive drug-intensive treatments from covered benefits. One health plan executive reported, "We presently cover a growth hormone treatment that costs $30,000 a year. I doubt that we will be able to offer that in the future." Rising drug costs will also be a principal factor behind further consolidation among health plans. Only large health plans can extract the heavy volume discounts and rebates from drug manufacturers that are part of the ability to control drug costs.

Strategies for Dealing with New Medical Technology

Medical technology also poses challenges for health plans in an environment where consumers are exerting more influence. Related to this, one health plan executive told us, "Until recently, we did not have a gamma knife in our market. Physicians tended to use an alternative (and inferior) treatment rather than giving up care of the patient to an out-of-town provider. Now that consumers are doing their research, there has been a marked increase in the demand for the gamma knife, prompting our physicians to pressure the local hospital into acquiring this technology."

When it comes to advances in medical technology, there will be even more debate about the medical necessity versus the elective nature of various procedures and equipment. For example, will health plans cover a wheelchair that climbs stairs, operates on the beach, and can be elevated to reach grocery store shelves or kitchen cabinets? Should employers and health plans (or the government) pay for this $25,000 piece of equipment?

Harnessing the Power of Information Systems

Richard Huber predicts, "The ability to invest in information technology is going to be the determining factor in success" (Robinson, 1999, p. 94). We have already discussed how Web-based technologies could significantly reduce direct marketing costs and at the same time appeal to consumers. IT also holds enormous potential for reducing health plan administrative expenses.

"In the not too distant future, all our interfaces with physicians will be electronic," noted a health plan CEO. Health plans are developing systems that will make it easy for the physician's office to interact with the health plan electronically and that will enable the physician's office to conduct eligibility verification, retrieve information on covered benefits and formularies, receive referral authorizations, and obtain access to a host of other relevant data—all on-line. Access to disease management programs, electronic record keeping, and billing and collections would offer significant advantages to physicians who have been struggling with the higher administrative expenses of dealing with multiple health plans.

Humana's Approach

Humana has embarked on an initiative with the TriZetto Group, a provider of application services and Web portals for the health care industry. According to a press release (Humana, 1999a), Health-Web will offer these benefits:

- *Members* will be able to enroll in Humana health plans, select a primary care physician, request identification cards, and view the status of their claims.

- *Physicians* will be able to verify patient eligibility and benefits, view claims status, and submit specialist referrals for approval.
- *Employers* will be able to monitor the enrollment process to mitigate errors and gauge employee enthusiasm for plan offerings.

Support for Medical Groups' Web Sites

Another strategy for health plans seeking to align themselves more closely with physicians and medical groups will be to offer health information resources to practices that are creating their own Web sites. Health plans have the advantage of being the major repository of demographic and clinical information on consumers in general and on patients in particular. Increasingly, physicians will need ready access to this information to effectively manage the care of their patients.

Consolidating

Although consolidation has been in full force over most of the 1990s, it is a strategy that is likely to continue in the future. The arguments favoring further health plan consolidation are compelling. Consolidation allows health plans to spread the cost of IT development and administrative expenses over a larger member base.

But plan administration is only one of the forces driving consolidation. Another is the market clout available to health plans that gain control of a significant share of the market. As consolidation continues and two or three dominant plans emerge in many major metropolitan markets, leverage with providers increases. There is also significant leverage to be gained, with suppliers and other vendors, for those plans that establish themselves on a national basis. Finally, a large national presence is particularly advantageous in serving major employers that operate in multiple states.

Health plan consolidation appears to run counter to the growing trends of consumerism and demand for more choice and more customized service. If large health plans find they are unable to move from being a wholesaler to a retailer, there will be opportunities for niche players. More likely we will see the major health plans acquiring the capabilities they need for adapting their organizations to new market realities. We need look no further than the financial services industry to find numerous examples of stalwart traditional firms like Merrill Lynch or A.G. Edwards making the move to on-line trading.

Reconsidering the Provider-Owned Health Plan Model

"S.C. Systems Shutting Down Joint HMO." "End of the Line for Fla. System's HMO." These were the headlines of two stories that appeared on the same page of *Modern Healthcare* in 1999. One story told of three South Carolina hospital organizations that said they could not afford to continue subsidizing the money-losing three-year-old health plan. Executives of the three systems did not expect the financial condition of the health plan to improve for another two years (Burda, 1999). The essence of the other story is captured in this quote from the article: "One of Florida's largest healthcare systems has pulled the plug on its money-losing HMO. The 15,600-enrollee Community Health Care Systems racked up losses of $8.2 million over the past 18 months" (Taylor, 1999).

These stories are representative of articles that appear weekly in many health care publications. This leads to a question: What is the future of provider-owned health plans? Many health care providers entered the health plan business for one or more of these reasons:

- To gain a share of the premium dollar
- To get closer to their customers
- To take advantage of their brand name and reputation in their service area
- To learn how to manage care under a budget and align financial incentives
- To control their own destiny rather than being a vendor for multiple health plans
- To operate more efficiently from an administrative standpoint (time and again, we have heard hospital CEOs and physician leaders say, "We can do this for a lot less than the 15 percent in administrative expenses of an HMO")

However, many of the reasons for initially getting into the health plan business are no longer valid. Payment systems have not moved toward capitation. Health systems found that they could not manage health plans at lower administrative expenses, and their enrollee base was too small to generate significant economies of scale. Many plans could not withstand pricing pressure from larger, better-capitalized, and better-known competitors.

As we move into the future, the role of provider-sponsored health plans seems tenuous. Established health plans that have captured a sizable share of their market and have a well-known provider network are likely to survive and thrive. For example, Security Health Plan owned by the Marshfield Clinic in northern Wisconsin, Scott & White Health Plan in central Texas, and the Geisinger Health Plan in Pennsylvania have all achieved prominence in their regions and have a strong association with well-regarded multispecialty clinics.

However, plans that have failed to gain market advantage often find themselves struggling. If resources are constrained in the future, they are likely to be unable to compete with larger players on the basis of price. In a new health care marketplace, they may find it difficult to offer the broad network and wide array of choices that consumers demand. Provider-owned plans may find it prohibitively expensive to keep up with the information systems and applications of technology that the market will expect.

In summary, it appears to us that the prospects for provider-owned health plans are bleak. James Hertel told us, "These types of plans are swimming against the current, and I don't expect many to survive" (interview, Jan. 2000). We agree; none of the scenarios for the future that we envision is particularly promising for provider-owned health plans.

Setting the Stage for the Future

Without regaining credibility with physicians, hospital boards and CEOs, policymakers, and the public at large, health plans' ability to pursue any of the strategies just described will be compromised. An increasingly tough legislative and regulatory environment, a result of losing the public trust, is one of the biggest challenges facing health plans. Repeated calls for a patient's bill of rights, more regulatory oversight of managed care plans, mandated benefits, and increased reserve requirements are among the pressures on the industry. Dennis Horrigan noted, "Regulatory demands will make it increasingly difficult for small IPAs and regional health plans to survive" (interview, Mar. 2000).

These challenges are unlikely to disappear. In fact, the intensity of regulatory pressures may grow unless managed care can turn the tide of public opinion. Accomplishing this will require more choices for consumers, better service by health plans, changes in the way providers are paid (capitation, for example, is a serious deterrent to public understanding of what health plans are trying to accomplish), and an all-out effort to regain the support of physicians.

Conclusion: A New Look for Health Plans

Perhaps no single component of the health care delivery system will be called on to change as much in response to consumerism and technology as the health plan. Health plans will have to change their image (away from refusing care), their product offerings (to be more flexible and tailored), their operations (to be more automated), and their supply chain management (to be less adversarial, particularly with physicians). Meanwhile, they will need to respond to new Internet-based competitors and to the forces of consolidation and commoditization. Health plans have a key role to play in the transition to the new health care marketplace. It will not be easy, and they will not come out looking the same.

Part Three

Positioning Health Care for the Twenty-First Century

Our system of medical care, for the most part, is fragmented and uncoordinated. Patients and families are left to make decisions from a confusing array of treatment options. Furthermore, there is a great need to do something about the billing nightmare patients and their families experience.

RICHARD L. CLARKE, PRESIDENT AND CHIEF EXECUTIVE OFFICER, HEALTHCARE FINANCIAL MANAGEMENT ASSOCIATION

In this third part of our book, we focus on what health care leaders can do to ensure the future of their organizations and meet the needs of the dramatically changing health care marketplace. We are not talking about passive reaction but about opportunities to initiate and take advantage of change.

Management for the Future

Assuming we can envision the future health care system, how will leaders successfully guide their organizations toward that vision? We can anticipate that the next several years will see some of the most dramatic change ever in the health care industry. Meanwhile, we can say with near certainty that this will be one of the most difficult periods in which to manage health care organizations. What managers need to do to adjust themselves and their organizations in order to have the best chances of success is the topic of Chapter Thirteen.

Governance for the Future

The old ways of governing and managing will not work much longer. The kinds of issues facing governing boards have changed dramatically over the past decade and will shift again even more substantially during the next five years. Chapter Fourteen describes how governance must change in order to be successful in the new health care marketplace.

Marketing, Mass Customization, and Branding

There is substantial agreement among health care leaders that to be successful in the future, hospitals, medical groups, health plans, and other organizations will need to become more adept at market segmentation. The consumer-dominated health care market of the future will be more fragmented and more demanding. To be successful, organizations will need strategies to meet the needs of these varying segments through mass customization of services. In addition, with consumers playing a more important role in decision making about health care, new marketing approaches will be required. One effective approach is branding of health care organizations, products, and services. Marketing, mass customization, branding, and other marketing-related matters are analyzed in Chapter Fifteen.

Chapter Thirteen

Leadership and Management in the New Health Care Marketplace

Creating the right vision is obviously helpful. However, the hardest act by far—and for several years to come— is managing our organizations toward that vision.
JOHN KOSTER, M.D., VICE PRESIDENT, CLINICAL AND PHYSICIAN SERVICES, SISTERS OF PROVIDENCE HEALTH SYSTEMS

For some leading health care organizations, the next five years may well be both the best of times and the worst of times. We may look back and say that this was the time when some of our most advanced organizations began to chart the course for delivering next-generation health care. Meanwhile, we can already look ahead and say that this will likely be one of the most difficult periods ever for health care managers. Whereas most of this book is about developing the right strategies and vision, this chapter is about managing health care organizations toward the right vision.

Managing Toward a Vision

We have had the privilege of working with and observing two health system CEOs who have a joint vision. These two CEOs believe that, together, they can create a new organization that will surpass their current capabilities. Their joint vision is not an "easy to see, easy

257

to implement" vision. For example, the distance between their facilities is too great for cross-referrals to be practical. However, their joint vision includes many of the issues discussed in this book—for example, innovative approaches to IT and consumers and close joint decision making with physician groups. Ultimately, their two organizations may merge, but in the meantime, the CEOs must tease out the details of this new vision. They must move their boards, physicians, management teams, staffs, other community leaders, parent system managers, and other key constituencies in this new common direction.

It has been a pleasure to watch these two CEOs work. There is an art to what they do. They repeatedly bounce back and forth between their several constituencies—articulating the latest version of their vision, trying out new ideas with those who would need to be involved in implementation, asking questions, probing for problems, being willing to be told they are wrong. They are constantly learning and revising their vision, even as they are consistently inching their organizations toward it.

As with most other systems today, these two CEOs must wring more costs out of their current organizations while imposing more requirements for change. In other words, the tensions naturally associated with change must be superimposed on the tensions associated with cost cutting. There is no other way. Therefore the two CEOs continue to gently but steadily push and prod. They pause frequently to defuse the tension and uncertainty with humor. And they pause to take care of themselves—taking time off when they need it—but often refuse to show tension when they feel it themselves. These CEOs understand intuitively what they have to do; and they manage themselves, their associates, and their organizations based on this intuition.

Getting Results While Building a Change-Oriented Culture

Management observers know more than they used to about the art of managing change. Originally, there was the theory that, to achieve change, one just "went for it"—analyzing problems and shaping solutions, managing change from the top down, motivating through financial incentives. Then came the theory that in order to achieve continuing improvement, one must cultivate the organization's capability to change—building supportive structures in which organizations continually experiment and evolve while managers themselves identify the key changes. Michael Beer and Nitin Nohria (2000) call these two approaches "Theory E" and "Theory O." Table 13.1 shows the approaches taken to various aspects of change in each of these theories.

Management gurus today say what some managers have known intuitively for a long time: the most successful change and the most sustained improvement come about when both approaches are pursued, in balance, simultaneously. The greatest successes are achieved when CEOs consciously mix top-down, results-oriented efforts with bottom-up, culture-building approaches.

Cutting Costs While Making New Investments

We sat in on a meeting between a health plan CEO and one of his business unit heads two weeks before the annual planning meeting.

The CEO began, "These are great ideas! We should have done this three years ago. But now our medical loss ratio is sky high. This meeting is going to have to be about cutting costs—period. I can't be seeking cuts everywhere then turn right around and talk investments."

The unit head answered, "I know it sounds weird, but that's exactly what I think you need to do. First, look at it from a morale perspective. I'm not going to keep my good people if they don't see we have a vision beyond cost cutting. They have to be for something, to anticipate improvement, to see investment in the future. Second, the truth is, if we wait, we will be too late; we will miss the window of opportunity."

The CEO initially rejected the idea but continued to think about it and talk it over with others. Ultimately, the company, which simply had to cut $6 million out of operating costs, found a way to cut $8 million and reinvest the other $2 million.

Similar scenarios have been played out in several executive suites this year. They will likely be played out many more times in the years to come.

Recently, we have seen a convergence in investment strategies among health care organizations that started out miles apart. For example, we have seen CEOs who started with a clear vision and a plan to invest heavily in gaining market share but who then decided to pull back, recognizing the absolute necessity of cost cutting. They

Table 13.1. Theory E and Theory O.

Dimension of Change	Theory E	Theory O	Theories E and O Combined
Goal	Maximize shareholder value	Develop organizational capabilities	Explicitly embrace the paradox of economic value and organizational capability
Leadership	Manage change from the top down	Encourage participation from the bottom up	Set direction from the top and inspire participation from below
Focus	Emphasize structure and systems	Build up corporate culture (employees' culture)	Focus simultaneously on the hard (structures and systems) and the soft (corporate behavior and attitudes)
Process	Plan and establish	Experiment and evolve programs	Plan for spontaneity
Reward system	Motivate through financial incentives	Motivate through commitment, use pay as fair exchange	Use incentives to reinforce change but not to drive it
Use of consultants	Use consultants to analyze problems and shape solutions	Use consultants to support management in shaping its own solutions	Use consultants to empower employees

Source: Beer and Nohria, 2000, p. 137.

now understand that no matter how much market share they have, if they cannot reduce their costs, their organizations will not survive long enough to benefit from it. At the same time, some CEOs who made their mark by cutting costs and returning their organizations to profitability are asking, "What's next? I can't just continue to be against red ink. It's time to be *for* something."

Becoming the First Retrofits

Peter Senge and others (1999, p. 8) tell the story of talking with a group of managers on the front lines of leading-edge total quality management processes. One of the managers expressed his next challenges this way: "We've done all the easy things. In truth, things were so bad in many of our . . . facilities that it was enough just to give people a bit of authority to fix practices that many had known needed to be changed for a long time. Now we're up against much tougher problems and the rate of improvement is declining. Now we're up against problems where the real problem is us. We're pretty good at directing others to change, but not so great at changing ourselves."

We have to change several things—the way our senior management teams learn, the way we relate to our key constituencies, the overall tone we set for our organizations—and many of these changes begin with making subtle but important changes in ourselves. CEOs are, in essence, the "first retrofits" in a conscious change management program. There are a number of conscious steps health care managers can take to improve the environment for simultaneously managing change and cutting costs. The remainder of this chapter discusses several of them.

Creating the Right Culture and Structure

What is the right culture for today's and tomorrow's health care organization? We may not have all the answers, but some aspects seem clear.

A New Sense of Teamwork

The presence of teamwork in a health care organization is obvious to the patient and any outside observer. Some organizations have it, but most do not. When we discuss teamwork, we are referring to physicians working with physicians, physicians working with nurses and other clinicians, and clinicians and physicians working with administrative personnel. In the more advanced health care organizations, like Mayo and Dartmouth-Hitchcock, teamwork is ingrained in the culture. We believe this is one of the characteristics of the successful health care enterprise of the future.

Partnership with Physicians

The question of whether physicians are partners with hospitals or are the primary customers of hospitals remains unanswered in many organizations. One hospital CEO told us, "I think it is both. We are partners in some activities, and they are our customers in other respects. The Stark rules and private inurement make this a fuzzy and difficult area." We appreciate this point of view. However, we find it difficult to believe that in a future dominated by consumerism and technology, physicians and hospitals will be able to meet the needs of increasingly demanding consumers without a joint strategy and a relationship based on partnership. Hospitals working alone will not be able to do the job.

Consumers in many communities, perhaps most, do not differentiate between their physicians and the hospitals where they practice. Consumer research surveys have shown this over and over again. Medical malpractice suits also support this contention: when physicians err while performing medical procedures in the hospital, the hospital is almost always part of the resulting lawsuit. And the courts have generally upheld the principle that the two are inseparable.

Technological Sophistication

It is difficult to imagine health care leaders of the future who do not embrace the new information technologies, especially the Internet, as part of the way they run their practices or manage their departments. We have observed many physicians and administrators who have a fairly advanced knowledge of the uses of IT, and they have the best chance of becoming the health care leaders of the new century.

Robert Rowley, a family practice physician in Hayward, California, is an example. Rowley explains how and why he has incorporated IT into his practice:

> As a three-physician primary care practice in a heavily capitated environment, we face continuing challenges in our operational efficiency, growing patient volumes, slim margins, increased financial accountability, coordination of care, and demonstrating population-based medical outcomes. To accomplish this, we concluded that we had to develop our information technology capabilities. This was not a luxury.
>
> Our practice management system was the starting point. Data were available, we could generate reports, and we could set up patient reminder systems for mammography, immunizations and the like.
>
> Transcripts were the next thing to add. Linking dictated transcripts to demographic information on our patients was a huge step toward having an electronic medical record. With this, we could generate useful clinical reports and really begin to focus on population management.
>
> By adding high-speed Internet connectivity to all eight computers in the office, we were then able to verify health plan and payer eligibility through our IPA, Hill Physicians. We could submit claims electronically. We could connect into on-line formularies.
>
> We have been receiving 40 calls a day relative to prescription renewals. These calls are now linked to the patient's record, and this led to major changes in office procedures, and a streamlining of the processing of prescription renewals.
>
> The next step is Internet access for our patients so they can communicate with us on e-mail. We will then be able to share best practices among ourselves, and with patients. It will facilitate referrals to specialists [Rowley, 2000].

Steve McDermott, president and CEO of Hill Physicians Medical Group, the large northern California IPA that includes Rowley's group, says that at a meeting of a hundred physician leaders of the IPA, he asked Rowley to make this same presentation on how he and his colleagues were using technology in their practice. McDermott (2000) reports, "I asked how many were doing what Dr. Rowley's group is doing, and the response was none."

Is Rowley on the wrong track? We do not think so. Furthermore, he and his two partners are learning how to use many new information technologies, and they are doing it in a cost-effective manner. These are the kinds of physicians who possess the technological sophistication needed to become physician leaders in the new century.

A Higher Profile for Human Resources Issues

The demand for health care services is growing and will grow even faster as consumerism and technology further drive demand. This places additional strains on an industry that is labor intensive and already reeling from substantial labor shortages. One of the key challenges for health care organizations in the future will revolve around these human resources issues.

After years of worrying about downsizing, many hospital managers are reversing their focus and figuring out how to handle an expected surge in demand for both inpatient and outpatient services. For example, one large system in Minneapolis–Saint Paul reported a 19 percent increase in utilization in 1999. Outpatient diagnostic and surgical services are expected to continue the long-term growth trends that began in earnest in the early 1980s.

Burgeoning demand and constrained supply, especially the shortage of nurses and clinical support personnel, are forcing hospitals, medical groups, and integrated systems into different ways of operating. For example, nurses are increasingly playing a larger coordinating role, with greater use of licensed practical nurses and other personnel for many functions formerly performed by registered nurses.

Managers of health care systems may also find themselves more involved in the training of clinical personnel. This could include collaborating with other hospitals or medical groups in the region to support clinical training programs at local colleges and universities. Hospital staff and physician leaders may want to collaborate in establishing centralized pools of difficult-to-find clinical staff that can be shared among competing institutions.

At the same time that demand for health care services increases, reimbursement pressures will prevent the wholesale hiring of new staff. This will be a challenge for managers, who will need to figure out how to substitute IT and automation for people and how to staff more effectively.

New Linkages to Financial Analysts

Access to capital will continue to be a challenge for all types of health care organizations—hospitals, medical groups, and integrated systems. A key part of the answer is to maintain strong earnings and cash flow in order to demonstrate to the bond-rating agencies that debt service coverage ratios are more than adequate.

If the United States experiences a recession and a long-term drop in stock and bond prices, this would be a disaster for many hospitals that are already running in the red on operations and depending on returns on their investment portfolios for the cash flow necessary to sustain operations and invest in IT, new facilities, and medical technology. As one hospital CEO told us, "If an economic downturn and stock market bust were to happen, we would have to make ourselves available for acquisition. I didn't say sale, because I'm not sure anyone would pay anything for this hospital with its history of running in the red for the past few years."

The chief financial officers of not-for-profit hospitals are going to need all of the ingenuity they can muster to keep their organizations propped up financially. This will mean selling surplus assets, collaborating with other hospitals when possible, closing unprofitable services, and maximizing payment (without breaking the law) for services provided.

Finding the Right Leverage Points to Induce and Manage Change

What specific steps can be taken to anticipate and manage change? Based on observing what is working and not working as leading health care organizations try to prepare for consumerism, technology, and other change factors while also adjusting to scarce resources, we have ten modest proposals (summarized in Exhibit 13.1) for improving the odds.

**Exhibit 13.1. Ten Proposals for Adjusting
Management Approaches in Response to Changes
in Consumerism and Technology.**

1. Adopt a "learning persona" at the top.
2. Acknowledge discomfort and uncertainty.
3. Retool support systems.
4. Develop new linkages between early adapters.
5. Reduce management layers and insist on information crossover between departments.
6. Sit in the place of the consumer, then change seats.
7. Integrate overall strategy with IT strategy.
8. Initiate a knowledge acquisition and management plan.
9. Manage new initiatives as one portfolio.
10. Plan faster and replan more often.

Adopt a "Learning Persona" at the Top

In our view the average health care CEO and chief operating officer have to "get much more into the game" with respect to technological innovation, particularly in the IT area. To a lesser degree the same is true with developing a more in-depth understanding of consumerism and various market segments. Most senior health care managers need a self-taught crash course in new technology and marketing strategies, beginning with e-health care.

How are the Web sites of those using "best practices" organized to handle inquiries from patients with questions about cardiac problems? What are the best ways of integrating "bricks and clicks" initiatives into women's health programs? What are "zaplets," and how are they about to change e-mail? What are good information sources for deciding when to buy software and install it on the organization's network and when to contract with an outside vendor to have the software reside on the vendor's network? Who is strong in the business-to-physician segment of the e-health market, and what does this mean for a particular health care organization? These are examples of issues that health care leaders have to be conversant with.

Many senior managers in health care are not comfortable with these issues. Equally important, staffs know that their leaders do not know the answers. The first example CEOs and managers need to set is how to become aggressive learners. They have to embrace learning the new technologies. They have to create an environment where it is perfectly acceptable to look naive and uncomprehending but is totally unacceptable to be smug and uninterested.

A few months ago the two CEOs mentioned earlier as good examples of change leadership brought key board members, physicians, and managers from their two organizations together for a two-and-a-half-day learning and information-sharing session. This meeting was held in a unique setting that included elaborate writing boards, computer-based projections, and even music. More important, however, was that the CEOs were there, working through every exercise alongside their colleagues.

Acknowledge Discomfort and Uncertainty

These days, discomfort, uncertainty, and stress hang over most health care settings most of the time. Common sources of stress include physicians' income losses, nurses' problems in achieving new productivity targets, and managers' problems in increasing productivity in a very tight labor market. These and other immediate problems must be acknowledged and dealt with. However, pressing current problems cannot be used as an excuse not to deal with key change issues, such as consumerism and technology. Similarly, consumerism and technology cannot be used to delay addressing the other pressing problems.

Even after all is done that can be done, it is important to continue to acknowledge the residual uncertainty and stress—to acknowledge that the stress associated with change is being overlaid on an already high stress level. The two CEOs described at the beginning of the chapter make heavy use of humor to acknowledge uncertainty and defuse tension. Some of us can use humor to defuse stress; many of us cannot. Each of us has to find an approach that works for our personality and our situation (for example, a kind look or a show of energy).

Retool Support Systems

Senior managers need to ask themselves the following question: Do we have sufficient access to the right people, information sources, and other support systems around us to (1) be aggressive learners about consumerism and technology, (2) handle the added stress of new uncertainties piled on top of the old, and (3) manage the change? If not, they need to recognize this and retool their personal and organizational support systems.

Exhibit 13.2 is a suggested checklist for assessing the adequacy of support systems. The checklist can be applied at two levels in an organization: staff and senior management. For hospital systems it can also be applied for key partners, such as physicians.

Here are a few more important questions to address:

- *What do senior managers in the organization need in order to begin to address consumer marketing and service development seriously?* Consider these possibilities: teaching and discussion sessions on what is working in other industries where consumer-based marketing is "more mature"; a good source of either ongoing or occasional advice from outside the organization.
- *What does the organization need for aggressive learning and application of new technologies?* Consider these possibilities: a conference or primer on technology; some new periodicals to monitor; a source of trusted counsel, available on an as-needed basis.
- *Does staff or senior management need something more to help with stress?* Consider these possibilities: education sessions; more breaks; more discipline in taking family time and exercising.
- *What resources does the organization need for change management?*
- *What changes does the organization need to make with regard to its staff?*
- *What types of initiatives does staff need managerial permission to implement?*

Develop New Linkages Between Early Adapters

We have found that it is almost always a good idea to think in terms of and use market and attitudinal segments—not only consumer market segments but segments among employees, physicians, and other constituencies. Remember, people react to change in very different ways: some resist it strongly; others thrive on it.

These differences can be used as a tool to stimulate change. For example, getting early adapters in one part of the organization

**Exhibit 13.2. Checklist for Examining the Adequacy
of Support Systems.**

	Area of Concern			
Issue	*Consumer marketing*	*Technology learning and application*	*Stress management*	*Change management*
Ready, reliable sources of information				
Ready, trusted sources of counsel				
Effective ways to monitor progress				

together with early adapters in another department can stimulate innovation. The rest of the organization can be brought along later. Start, for example, with a few physicians (and their staffs) who are interested in experimenting with Internet-based consultation. Link them to the consumers who visit the organization's Web site asking about Internet-based consultation.

Link an early adapter program manager in oncology with the best and brightest in the IT department for experimental approaches to integrating in-house data with electronic data from peer organizations. Later, after the oncology experiment is a success, link a change-resisting manager in another department with the early adapter oncology manager.

Reduce Management Layers and Insist on Information Crossover Between Departments

Innovative, continuously learning organizations differ from static organizations in several ways. For example, innovative organizations usually have informal mechanisms for sharing information and trying out concepts that cross departmental lines. Numerous layers of management and rigid departmental boundaries are frequently the enemies of change, customer responsiveness, and productivity improvement. Consider reducing the number of layers of management—not just to cut costs but also to stimulate hands-on experiences that can lead to innovation. Also look for ways to consciously break down barriers between departments.

Figure 13.1 illustrates the relationship between these suggestions. Reducing layers of management is one approach to increasing the flow of information up and down the organization. Reducing departmental barriers is one means of increasing the flow of information across the organization. Linking early adapters is often a means of developing new flows of information up and down the organization, across the organization, and between the organization and the outside world (for example, with consumers). Another increasingly effective approach to stimulating communication that can often lead to innovation is Internet-based affinity groups (for example, groups in several health systems that are pursuing similar objectives and sharing results).

Sit in the Place of the Consumer, Then Change Seats

Senior managers often initiate change just by focusing on an issue and walking around their organization and observing. Try adopting the view of different customer segments—one day an elderly couple, one of whom has a heart problem, the next day a young couple expecting their first child, the next day a person with diabetes. Walk around, ask for reports and data, form impressions, and turn these impressions into tentative actions. Introduce these tentative actions to key managers in the relevant areas. When they resist, try to have them suggest constructive alternatives. Before acting, change seats. Consider the current situation and the tentative actions from the perspective of others, such as physicians and other employees working with the particular customer population involved.

Integrate Overall Strategy with Information Technology Strategy

Develop a strategy-level IT decision document summarizing the strategic implications, costs, and risks of different combinations of IT investments. Include an IT-based environmental assessment. For example, which physician practices are linked to which e-health business-to-business services? What are the projected changes in

Figure 13.1. Creating New Learning Paths in Mature Organizations.

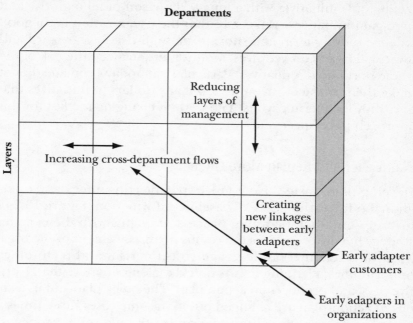

local health plans' IT positions and capabilities? Are e-health solutions threatening or strengthening local employee benefits and health plan brokers? This information can be factored into the overall strategy development process.

Initiate a Knowledge Acquisition and Management Plan

Meet as a senior management team and set goals for knowledge acquisition and management within and across departments or business units. Monitor progress and include results in managers' performance assessments. Consider establishing a small group to support and facilitate knowledge management across the organization and between your organization and others. Consider establishing a "resident experts" program, in which individuals become well versed in specific aspects of technology and then serve as resources for the rest of the organization.

Manage New Initiatives as One Portfolio

Do not make the mistake that so many have made in the past: selecting only initiatives with a long-term payoff or all high-risk and high-gain initiatives. Make sure that the organization has a good balance of long-term and short-term, high-risk–high-reward and low-risk–low-reward ventures. Monitor and manage the risk of the whole portfolio of initiatives. Particularly in today's climate, do not make the mistake of investing too many dollars in initiatives that have only long-term payoffs. The world is changing too fast for this approach to be successful.

Plan Faster and Replan More Often

Develop plans faster, using more specific consumer data, operational information, and IT baseline information. Figure 13.2 illustrates one such planning process. It begins with the existing strategy but also considers the results of an assessment of the organization's readiness to leverage consumerism and technology opportunities. Planning occurs quickly, taking no more than forty-five days, and produces an action plan. The quick plan and its associated action plan are changed often, in some cases three times a year. The informational foundation for the planning process—including information on legacy IT systems, consumer market research, and actions by other e-health players and trading communities—is updated on an ongoing basis.

Developing Clinical and Administrative Leadership

There is a growing recognition about the unique role of both physicians and professional administrators in managing complex health enterprises. The teaming of physicians and administrators is gaining ground, and we view this as a trend that is consistent with the needs of the new health care marketplace.

The next questions, then, are:

- How does a health care organization identify and develop both strong clinical and strong administrative leadership?
- What is the best way to move both clinical and administrative leaders in the direction of greater competence in consumer marketing and technology-based management?

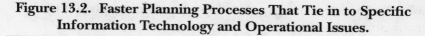

Figure 13.2. Faster Planning Processes That Tie in to Specific Information Technology and Operational Issues.

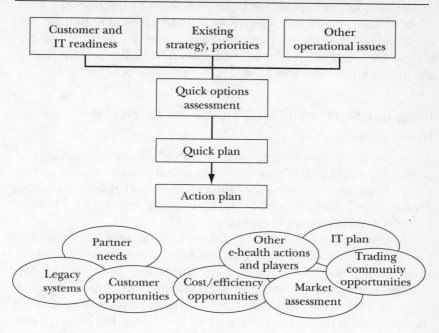

- What is the best way for clinical and administrative leaders to work together?

The following discussion presents lessons learned from our research.

Hiring Potential Team Players

The physician leader of a large clinic told us that when the clinic hires a new physician, it considers whether or not the newcomer will be a team player and have the potential to eventually become a leader of the organization: "If we see a big ego and the potential for trouble, we will not invite the candidate to join our organization. We can't afford to handle the train wrecks that these kinds of people cause. Also, we have to have a pool of younger physicians in order to assure our organization of a good supply of physician leadership on down the line."

In our view this approach is the exception rather than the rule. Most physicians are hired because of their clinical expertise and the needs of the organization. A young physician's long-term potential for leadership is often not considered. We believe that it should be a consideration.

Using Task Forces as a "Farm System" for Developing Future Managers

A number of major multispecialty clinics have large numbers of committees and task forces. Over the initial years of their careers, most physicians have the opportunity to serve on at least one committee. This is viewed as an important testing ground for identifying potential physician leaders.

In those organizations that do not have an extensive committee structure, existing physician leaders have to keep their eyes open for the physician leaders of the future and try to find opportunities to place these individuals in positions of responsibility in order to test them for potential leadership and administrative duties. As one physician leader of an organization that uses this approach told us, "It is a hit-or-miss proposition. So far, we have lucked out."

Choosing Physician Leaders from the Ranks of Highly Respected Clinicians

One consistent theme from our research into physician leadership is that physician leaders have to be recognized by their peers as highly respected clinicians. Why? One physician leader explained it this way: "My ability to lead and to have a following is based on how I am perceived as a practicing physician. This is by far the most important factor. If I don't have the respect of my colleagues for what I have accomplished, and continue to accomplish, in my medical specialty, they won't follow my leadership." Of course, this viewpoint is one reason why many physician leaders continue to practice medicine, usually on a part-time basis, and take after hours and weekend call. In our experience not all good clinicians make good administrative leaders; conversely, bad clinicians seldom make good physician administrators.

Using the Paired-Leadership Model

A growing number of large integrated systems form partnerships between physicians and administrators to manage service lines or clinical departments. This approach not only works well in most cases, but it helps identify individuals—both physicians and administrators—who have the potential to take on even more responsibilities.

Sending Physician Leaders for Additional Training in Business or Health Administration

Many large clinics and integrated systems encourage physicians to take courses in management and administration; others do not. The physician leader of one large multispecialty clinic told us that it would be the death knell for a physician's hopes of becoming involved in governance or management if the physician pursued an M.B.A. degree: "This would be viewed as being too aggressive." However, most physician-led organizations encourage physicians to take courses in management at local colleges or universities or to participate in courses in their professional association.

Conclusions: Management Challenges of the Future

The challenges of the future are fairly clear: cut costs, keep communication levels very high, anticipate salary hikes in a tight labor market, manage compliance risks, preserve morale, increase knowledge about opportunities created by changes in consumerism and technology, envision and pursue insistently the critical changes from the top down, nurture the organization's culture from the bottom up, and pursue the right administrative and physician leaders. No one ever said this would be easy.

Health care managers of the future will need a strong background in teamwork, IT, human resources, and finance. We expect to see increased use of physician-administrator teams, or partnerships, in many hospitals and integrated systems. We expect to see a radical increase in the demand for IT expertise among all leaders, but particularly in health plans.

Escalation in the demand for health care services will challenge many organizations. This will be a welcome relief from years of downsizing. However, improving quality of care, access, and service at the same time that financial resources are limited will be a daunting challenge.

There are serious questions about whether the management structures and teams of most health care organizations are positioned for the future. And, as we have said throughout this book, the changes in health care during the initial years of the twenty-first century will dwarf by comparison what has happened in the past decade, primarily because of the shift in emphasis to consumerism and technology. As suggested in the next chapter, there are similar questions concerning boards and governance structures.

Chapter Fourteen

Governance in Health Care

We have had the same governance structure for twenty years, and it isn't working like it used to. We need to reevaluate our governance model so that the decision-making process moves more quickly and the whole structure retains the confidence of physicians.
PHYSICIAN CEO OF A LARGE MULTISPECIALTY CLINIC IN THE MIDWEST

In many respects health care is unlike any other industry in the way it is governed and managed. A high proportion of all hospitals and multihospital systems are not-for-profit and are governed by community boards. Most medical groups are for-profit and governed by physicians. In integrated systems, where the hospital is almost always not-for-profit and physicians typically have their own entities (often for-profit), there are special challenges.

Despite the cumulative experience of several thousand boards of not-for-profit hospitals, multihospital systems, medical groups, and integrated health care organizations, there is still much to be learned about governance, particularly in an environment of more demanding consumers, different relationships between hospitals and physicians, increased competition, budget pressures, and rapid technological change.

Leadership and management are also critical in moving health care organizations forward in an era characterized by fundamental market shifts. Most health care organizations are concerned about developing strong physician leaders. Physicians have been key players in health care in the past, but their roles are likely to become even more critical in the future.

This chapter addresses several questions about health care governance, leadership, and structure:

- How have the traditional approaches to hospital governance changed over the past decade?
- What additional changes in hospital governance will be needed over the next five years?
- How are the governance models used in multispecialty clinics and integrated systems changing, and where is the governance of these types of organizations headed?
- What is the role of physician-led boards of governors?
- How will the most successful health care systems need to focus their organizational structure in the future?

This chapter addresses these and other issues regarding governance, leadership, and structure, with a focus on not-for-profit hospitals and both for-profit and not-for-profit medical groups and integrated systems. We begin with the area where there has been the most experience and where the governance practices are better developed—hospitals and multihospital systems.

Hospital and Health System Governance: Getting Away from Tradition

Don Arnwine, former president of VHA Inc., a board member of two hospitals, and a consultant to numerous hospital boards, says that over the past thirty years, the role of the typical hospital board has changed dramatically: "The role of board members, and the board as a whole, has expanded. It used to be that the hospital board would approve the annual budget, hire and fire the CEO, make decisions on major capital expenditures and bond issues, approve the recommendations of the medical director on medical staff privileges, and once every few years be involved in strategic planning. Of course, most boards expect their members to also be involved in fundraising." (All quotes and information from Arnwine in this chapter are taken from our interview with Arnwine, Apr. 2000).

Tough Times Revealing Flaws in Governance

Arnwine also told us, "Good times mask flaws and weakness. When things are going well, there is a lack of urgency in dealing with weaknesses or conflicts at the governance level." The belt tightening necessitated by decreasing reimbursement from both managed care and Medicare has brought out both the best and worst in boards. As Arnwine observed, "Bad times for hospitals bring out the best when the board reevaluates its direction, reaffirms the strategy of the organization, stands together, and steadfastly supports those charged with carrying out the mission of the hospital. It brings out the worst when the board becomes divided, political, and equivocal in its support of management."

Conflict at the Board Level: A Malignancy in the System

We have seen both the good and the bad—boards working smoothly with mutual respect among members and conflict among board members and between board members and management. Arnwine said, "When there is conflict in the boardroom between board members, or groups of board members, over direction, allocation of resources, or support of the CEO, it creates a destructive force that must be reconciled. The necessary flow of process, negotiation, decision making, and execution is either diverted or stifled. The inertia resulting from this type of situation can waste time and damage market positioning, and slow the development of necessary relationships to further the goals of the hospital."

CEOs' Assumption That They Cannot Fix Board Problems

"Many CEOs believe that they are not capable of dealing with many board problems; however, they must do it," Arnwine asserted. "In counseling with CEOs over these kinds of issues, I often am told by CEOs that they can change everything in the hospital but the board. But, over a period of time, many CEOs realize that they have to find ways to fix some of the board problems or move on."

How can a CEO, who is hired and fired by the board, be successful in changing the structure and direction of a governing board? Arnwine suggested several avenues. "One fairly simple approach," he explained, "is to suggest to an appropriate board member that he or she propose the creation of a process, or committee of the board, to evaluate the board's effectiveness. I have never heard of a hospital board turning down this kind of request coming from one of its own members."

This evaluation process might be followed by bringing in an outside facilitator to discuss how the board functions and how it might consider working in the future. These kinds of discussions are usually accompanied by an environmental and competitive assessment of where health care is headed in the community and what the hospital and board need to do to be successful.

In our experience this sort of honest appraisal will often lead to questions about the efficiency of the board's decision-making procedures, the size of the board, the need for additional expertise and diversity, and the opportunities for new thinking. For example, if the health care industry changes as we expect it will, it would be important to add one or two board members who work in e-commerce or who are highly knowledgeable about consumer marketing.

Dismantling of Past Restructuring Efforts

During the 1970s and 1980s, it was popular for hospitals to diversify into numerous activities, and attorneys usually advised that separate corporations, each with its own board, be established for each new business. Examples include networks of minor emergency centers, long-term care facilities, real estate ventures, a health plan, and wellness or rehabilitation programs.

Arnwine told us, "One CEO I know accepted a position with a prestigious organization and upon arrival found out that there were thirty-six different corporate entities, each with its own board. He and his management team were on several of these boards, but many involved community representatives." The CEO was responsible for coordinating the efforts and meetings of these boards; the management required to support this board structure took 30 percent of the CEO's time. Arnwine added, "It isn't just management time. It is the need to 'honor' the real or implied prerogatives of each of the different boards."

Arnwine described one hospital system where there were six boards with seventy different directors. There were eighteen monthly scheduled board or committee meetings, and several required the attendance of as many as seven administrators. However, as Arnwine explained, "After considerable discussion and appraisal by several of the boards, along with outside consultation, five of the boards were consolidated into a single governing board. The only separate board that remained was that of the philanthropic foundation."

Adoption of a Health Systems Perspective

For many hospital boards the challenge has been adjusting board structures and responsibilities as hospitals became part of larger systems or merged with one or more entities. The rapid rate of mergers and acquisitions in the hospital sector in the 1990s created radical changes for many hospital boards. For hospitals involved in a multihospital system, the focus of strategy, fiduciary responsibility, quality improvement, and overall governance is usually transferred to the system-level governing board. Hospital boards often serve in an advisory capacity and reflect the perspective of the local market and community needs.

Transition Planning

In some cases local governing boards are dominated by strong individuals who have been involved in governance of the hospital for twenty or thirty years. Arnwine said, "I have seen boards and hospitals continue to prosper in these kinds of situations, but over time, too much dependence on a single individual will wear thin and get a hospital in trouble." Arnwine advocates written board policies on terms of office and on the number of successive terms a board member or chair may serve.

Board Involvement in Day-to-Day Management

Every hospital board has one or two strong individuals, often leaders from the business and professional world. There is nothing wrong with this. However, it is not unusual for successful executives from other businesses to think that what worked for them in another industry is just what is needed for health care. This often leads to problems, particularly with the medical staff and the administrative team of the hospital.

Most hospital boards continue to grapple with the question of whether to get involved in operations or to limit their role to policy and strategy. Most CEOs prefer that boards set the general policies and that professional administrators and physicians manage day-to-day operations. But many board members, sometimes with the encouragement of management, cannot resist the temptation of involving themselves in operational details. However, neither boards nor individual board members should be involved in the day-to-day management of a hospital. Recognizing and honoring the distinctive roles of the administrative team, physician leaders, and board members will be especially critical as we move into the new health care marketplace.

A New Model of Governance

Although governing boards of not-for-profit organizations have their genesis in stewardship and fundraising, they have moved toward management oversight and fiduciary and community responsibility. Figure 14.1 depicts the evolution of governance in not-for-profit boards from the past to the future, showing what role governance will need to assume to succeed in a more dynamic marketplace.

In the future, strategic performance is the mandate. Writing in the *Harvard Business Review,* Barbara Taylor and her coauthors contend, "Nonprofit boards are often little more than a collection of high-powered people engaged in low-level activities. . . . A board's contribution is meant to be strategic, the joint product of talented people brought together to apply their knowledge and experience to the major challenges facing the institution" (Taylor, Chait, and Holland, 1996, p. 36). In this context a board needs to be in partnership with the organization's CEO, who should seek guidance and support from the board in refining this vision of the organization.

The Quest for Effective Governance

In the new health care marketplace, developing and sustaining effective governance will be even more important than in the past. Several elements are essential to achieving exceptional governance.

Optimal Board Size

In order to make effective decisions, boards need to be of manageable size and consist of the right mix of skills and talents. Boards of nine to fifteen members are usually adequate and can be re-

Figure 14.1. The Evolution of Governance in Not-for-Profit Boards.

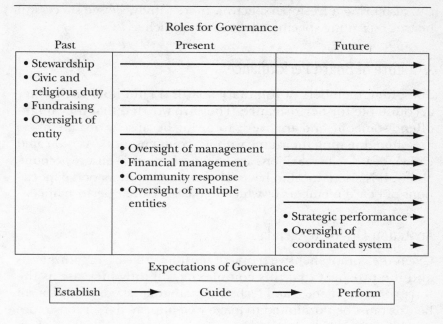

Roles for Governance

Past	Present	Future
• Stewardship • Civic and religious duty • Fundraising • Oversight of entity	• Oversight of management • Financial management • Community response • Oversight of multiple entities	• Strategic performance • Oversight of coordinated system

Expectations of Governance

Establish	→	Guide	→	Perform

sponsive and fast moving. As they have initially come together following a merger, many systems have started with larger boards. Over time these boards and management teams have found the postmerger structures to be unwieldy and unresponsive. Many multihospital systems continue to reduce their board size in an effort to become more focused and effective.

Board Composition

Barbara Taylor and her colleagues write that the board should be thought of as a constellation rather than a collection of stars (Taylor, Chait, and Holland, 1996). The parts need to support the whole with the skills and expertise they bring to the organization. Many hospital and health system boards have expanded the number of physicians in their governing structures to gain the perspective of this important stakeholder group. A smaller number of boards have also added the talents and unique perspectives of nursing executives. Involving individuals from outside the community, such as an administrator or physician from a noncompeting community, can also bring a fresh perspective. Increasingly, we see successful boards recruiting specific talent in areas such as IT.

A Culture of Board Performance

Too often, members of voluntary boards do not hold each other accountable for performance. They are worried that they might offend someone and are overly forgiving because board members are often donating their time without compensation. As indicated earlier, board self-evaluations are one mechanism to ensure accountability. It is also critical to have clear and well-understood expectations of board members by which to measure their performance.

An Action-Oriented Agenda

Given the comprehensive scope of most health care organizations and the prospect that this complexity will only increase as the forces of consumerism and technology are unleashed, not-for-profit boards must be positioned to make well-informed decisions more quickly than in the past. High-performance boards will insist on action-oriented agendas. Routine reporting is relegated to advance reports. Setting aside time on each agenda for education and strategy is also imperative for keeping the board focused on the "big picture."

Figure 14.2 illustrates a model board agenda in use by one of our clients. This agenda was developed to sharpen the focus of the meetings and keep the board attuned to the organization's mission and vision. No board members like to listen to routine reports or sit through long meetings. Our work with boards has revealed time and again that board members want to contribute to the organization in meaningful ways.

Tools for Measuring Performance

High-performance boards are equipped with tools they can use to quickly assess performance and evaluate key measures linked to their strategic plan. Major health care systems, such as Henry Ford

Figure 14.2. Model Board Agenda.

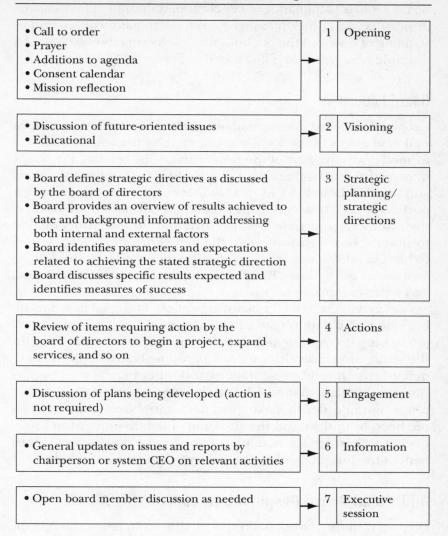

• Call to order • Prayer • Additions to agenda • Consent calendar • Mission reflection	1	Opening
• Discussion of future-oriented issues • Educational	2	Visioning
• Board defines strategic directives as discussed by the board of directors • Board provides an overview of results achieved to date and background information addressing both internal and external factors • Board identifies parameters and expectations related to achieving the stated strategic direction • Board discusses specific results expected and identifies measures of success	3	Strategic planning/ strategic directions
• Review of items requiring action by the board of directors to begin a project, expand services, and so on	4	Actions
• Discussion of plans being developed (action is not required)	5	Engagement
• General updates on issues and reports by chairperson or system CEO on relevant activities	6	Information
• Open board member discussion as needed	7	Executive session

Source: Avera Health System, Sioux Falls, South Dakota, May 2000.

Health System and Baylor Health Care, make extensive use of dashboard reports (summaries of key clinical, utilization, and financial indicators) and other measurement tools to gain a quick understanding of how well the organization is achieving its objectives. An example of such a tool is illustrated in Figure 14.3.

Board Education

Keeping the board informed about health care industry trends, as well as changes in the local market, enables trustees to make informed decisions. Part of the responsibility for keeping the board informed about local and national health care market conditions and trends falls to the CEO and management team. Dedicating a portion of each board meeting agenda for education can be effective. Retreats and new member orientation are also valuable forums for board education. At the same time, most boards need to budget additional funds to attend conferences such as those sponsored by the Estes Park Institute, the Governance Institute, and other organizations.

Related to the need for board education, a hospital board member who is also a university administrator told us, "It is part of my job to keep up with the trends in higher education, but I can't do the same thing in health care as a part-time board member. I am dependent on solid presentations and other educational opportunities. I realize that health care is entering into a new market phase, but in order to make good decisions, board members like me need to understand the situation. Take investment in information technology for example and how these dollars are likely to benefit the hospital and the community. This is complex stuff."

Additional Board Responsibilities: Looking Ahead

Dealing with the traditional responsibilities and issues will remain vital for boards in the future; however, the job is growing more complex, with new responsibilities and more significant decision making. Many new issues crowd the plate of most hospital and health system boards. These include dealing with potential mergers or acquisitions, helping the hospital interact with better-organized

Figure 14.3. Performance Measurement: Henry Ford Health System.

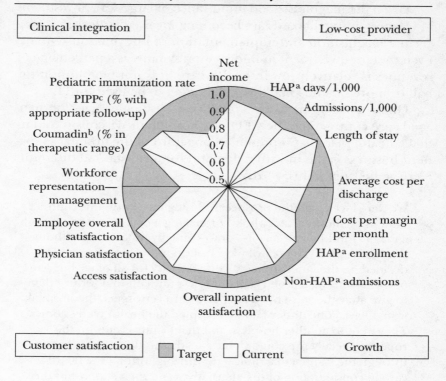

Note: HAP days and admissions are hospital days per 1000 members in health plan.

[a]Health Alliance Plan

[b]Prescription drug

[c]Internal Ford term

physician groups (including salaried physicians), and setting policies for managed care contracting.

Given the magnitude and importance of large-scale investment in IT, most hospital boards are becoming involved in decisions concerning acquisition and implementation of information systems. Even though investment in information systems as a percentage of revenues is relatively low in health care, it is not uncommon for half or more of a hospital's capital budget to be used for IT.

On the issue of the board's role in establishing policies for managed care contracting, the CEO of a hospital in Wisconsin told us that a health plan that represented one-third of the hospital's inpatient business came in with a demand for a substantial discount. Here is the story in his words:

> We were faced with the prospect of losing money on this contract (and in the hospital as a whole) or making a decision to go through a major—and I mean major—downsizing by proceeding without this health plan. The board was involved in this decision, and we decided on the latter strategy. This was scary for all of us, but one of the lessons we learned is that it is less difficult to downsize than to give away the store by cutting prices. In retrospect, the hospital would have gone under had we accepted the health plan's contract. They went to another hospital, and that facility is now on the ropes financially. We couldn't have made this decision and gone through the trauma of a radical downsizing without the board's careful consideration of the alternatives and their support of the final decision.

Additional examples of issues that make the typical hospital board member's job more complex and time consuming are discussed in the paragraphs that follow.

Purchase and Sale of Medical Groups

As mentioned earlier, for many hospitals that have acquired primary care practices, the results have been unsatisfactory from a financial perspective. Arnwine said, "When you employ primary care physicians and the hospital is losing an average of $100,000 a year on each doctor, the question of what you do almost always comes to the board or originates there." We know of a number of hospital boards that have forced management to confront this kind of difficult issue.

The primary care physicians (PCPs) who are employed by a hospital are often a valuable source of admissions to the hospital and referrals to the specialists on the medical staff. Therefore decisions about what to do (such as renegotiate contracts or terminate employed physicians) are tremendously important and potentially explosive. Board members often receive angry phone calls at home at night over matters like this.

In the 1980s and early 1990s, most hospital boards were not required to deal with these kinds of issues. The pressure of learning how to cope with managed care, the view that health care payment was moving toward capitation, the conventional wisdom that PCPs were the key to the future of most hospitals, and the belief that health plans wanted to contract with a single organization led to many of the original decisions to purchase physician practices, employ doctors, and form PHOs. Of course, many physician practices were purchased based on the notion that "if we don't do it, our competitors will." Managing the unwinding process is much more complex than the original decisions about whether to establish a primary care base, what to pay for physician practices, and how to integrate the practices into the hospital.

Conflicts Among Physicians Surfacing at the Board Level

Conflicts between PCPs and specialists, or between those in strong medical groups on one side and independent physicians and small groups on the other, often surface at the board level. Physicians' threats to "take their business elsewhere" often have serious implications for a hospital, and governing boards usually get involved.

For example, we worked with two hospitals and their combined medical staff of about two hundred physicians in analyzing the feasibility of starting a provider-owned health plan. The representation of PCPs and specialists on the governing board of the new entity turned out to be one of the most sensitive issues. After years of being beaten down (at least this was the perspective of many of the PCPs in this community), PCPs knew that they were key to the success of the health plan. They saw this as their chance to get back at the specialists, and they demanded disproportionate representation on the governing boards of the physician's organization and the PHO formed to provide services. Board members of the two hospitals ended up refereeing the dispute.

In other communities there are continuing conflicts surrounding larger medical groups, both single-specialty and multispecialty, and the special arrangements they often make with their hospital. Hospital board members typically end up being involved in decisions that allocate resources to various types of medical groups and independent physicians.

Joint Ventures with Medical Specialists

In the 1990s it was common to consider gain-sharing arrangements with specialists—for example, designating a hospital wing for cardiac, oncology, or orthopedic services—in order to develop centers of excellence and align financial incentives. Physicians could, for instance, share in the financial benefits if the center of excellence was profitable. These kinds of ventures always require board consideration and approval. Although federal rulings in 1999 made gain-sharing arrangements with physicians more difficult, there are still opportunities for physicians and hospitals to work together to create and expand centers of excellence. We believe these kinds of joint ventures make sense, and we expect to see more of them.

Hospital Boards of the Future: Conclusions

In the view of Donald E. L. Johnson (1999), former editor of *Modern Healthcare,* the performance and contributions of boards can be enhanced dramatically; we agree. We believe boards can increase their effectiveness in their most important areas of activity by clearly defining the role of the board vis-à-vis management, devoting more attention to strategy, providing more feedback from the community, asking more perceptive questions during board and committee meetings, and being open to opportunities for collaboration with other health care organizations and community agencies.

Perhaps one of the best ways to define high-performance governance is to explain what it is *not*. Experts who have reviewed the failed Allegheny Health, Education and Research Foundation (AHERF) point to several problems—brought about by ineffective governance—that led to this organization's downfall. Some of the key weaknesses of the AHERF governance system included the absence of board accountability, lack of board involvement in key policy formulations, and too little education and independent advice. Exhibit 14.1 presents a list of the weak points of the AHERF governance system—a list of pitfalls to avoid in order to help ensure effective governance.

Exhibit 14.1. Governance Pitfalls to Avoid: Lessons Learned from the AHERF Experience.

- Too little formal education for directors
- Board chair and CEO leadership that was too entrenched and strong for the circumstances
- Too few full board meetings
- Overreliance on the executive committee
- Too frequent delegation of decisions to the board chair and CEO
- Governance emphasizing civic honor, social activity, and fundraising more than fiduciary responsibility
- Too many reports, delivered too late, with too little time for full deliberation of issues
- Too little attention to alternative courses of action on proposals
- Inadequate board involvement in formulating corporate strategic plans and setting priorities
- Too many "off balance sheet" transactions without adequate explanation
- Too few internal audit functions
- Too little independent advice and attention to conflicts of interest
- Too little preparation for entry into nonhospital businesses or ventures

Source: Walker, 1999, p. 16.

Given the relatively short tenure of many hospital CEOs—around four years—it is important for the board and CEO to have a clear understanding of what is expected of them, what goals the organization has espoused, and how the board and management will work together.

Governance of Multispecialty Clinics and Integrated Systems

Based on our research, we believe the leaders of larger medical groups, both single-specialty and multispecialty, are taking governance more seriously. The physician leader of a three-hundred-physician multispecialty clinic told us, "We have had the same governance structure for twenty-five years, but we need to carefully examine how we make decisions and govern ourselves. Is this old structure still workable, or are there better models out there? With the increased strains on our group, we need a structure that engenders the confidence of our physicians."

This physician spoke from the experience of negotiating with a large PPM, suffering two years of losses in the health plan owned by the group, and dealing with a fractured relationship with a hospital that had been a longtime partner. The clinic board wavered but survived these pressures. However, how will it adapt to a future dominated by increasing IT investment pressures and the need to retain earnings and develop a capital base—a huge cultural shift for this group (and many others)?

The major challenges facing physician leaders, top administrators, and board chairpersons of multispecialty clinics and integrated systems as they attempt to design and implement a flexible yet enduring governance structure are shown in Exhibit 14.2. The paragraphs that follow discuss several of these elements of effective governance of physician-driven organizations.

Trust Building

We hear comments about the lack of trust more than any other criticism of various organizations and people in health care. Entire books have been written on this subject (see, for example, Annison and Wilford, 1998). Physicians do not trust each other and often do

Exhibit 14.2. Governance Challenges for Multispecialty Clinics and Integrated Systems.

- Building and maintaining trust among physicians and other participants
- Involving physicians in governance
- Ensuring limited turnover on the board and relatively long terms (from four to six years) for board members
- Using outside directors
- Compensating directors, either financially or with time off from other duties
- Identifying the potential for internal competition and eliminating it
- Maintaining credibility with physicians
- Focusing on policy and strategy without neglecting operational issues
- Avoiding inurement and Stark violations
- Guaranteeing equity in the compensation of physicians
- Focusing on the mission
- Introducing fairness and openness into the selection of board members
- Improving communication with physicians and clinical staff

not trust the CEO or administrative team. The CEO and board chair may not trust each other. As noted earlier, there are often gaps in trust between PCPs and specialists and between solo practitioners and physicians in larger medical groups.

How can organizations build and maintain trust? There are no easy answers, but a few fundamentals seem obvious: honor commitments, respect the views of others, be open and honest, and focus on what is best for the patient. And there is the old saying that we hear frequently among the leaders of integrated systems: Communicate, communicate, communicate. One former hospital CEO told us, "One of the best ways to build trust is to develop a few winners together. In this way physicians and administrators can learn that they can accomplish more together than going it alone."

Physicians' Role in Governance

George Lundberg (2000), M.D., former editor of the *Journal of the American Medical Association,* said, "The essence of professionalism is self-governance." Many physicians would agree, and this can be a source of problems in multispecialty clinics that are part of integrated systems. As Lundberg (2000) also indicated, physicians feel most comfortable when they play a role in the governance of the system as a whole, as well as in their own physician organization. In large integrated systems, this is often accomplished by limited representation on the overall system board of trustees and a physician-dominated board of governors. The Mayo Foundation and many other large systems use this approach. Figure 14.4 shows the relationships between the board of trustees and the physician boards of governors, and between the boards and the rest of the organization, in the Mayo Foundation.

Physician Board of Governors

The board of directors of a physician organization, often called the "board of governors" in integrated systems, typically meets more frequently than system boards and usually involves itself in day-to-day operations. This has been the pattern for years in many medical groups and is one of the reasons that physicians often have difficulty adjusting to their policy and strategy roles on a hospital or health system board.

Not every integrated system has a physician board of governors or believes that such a board is necessary. One physician leader told us, "Our primary goal is clinical integration and becoming more focused on patients. We want physicians to work more closely with administrators and develop strong clinical centers, such as oncology or cardiac services, within the overall system. If physicians retreat to a board of governors, we view this as a step backward."

A physician board of governors may not be desirable for all integrated systems. However, we believe that there are enough stresses on physicians that they should have their own organizational structure where they can consider special issues of direct importance to them. In many instances, the physician board of governors serves this purpose.

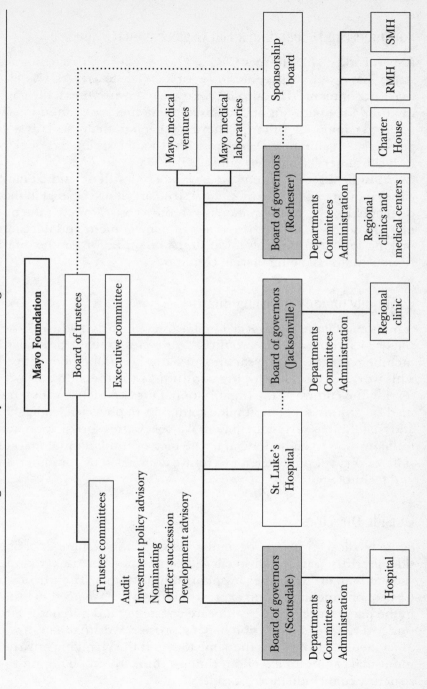

Figure 14.4. Mayo Foundation Organizational Structure.

Consumerism Demanding a Flat Organizational Structure

Robert Parker, M.D., former CEO of Carle Clinic in Urbana, Illinois, stated that health care is entering what he refers to as a "knowledge-rich environment." He said, "In this type of environment, the gaps in knowledge between physicians and patients are tremendously reduced compared with what they have been in the past. This suggests a flat organization where physicians can quickly interact directly with consumers" (interview, July 1999).

Most health care systems we have worked with or studied have either moved to a flat organizational structure or are headed in that direction. Part of the motivation is to reduce costs. However, the primary reason is to reduce the layers of management and decision making so that individuals lower in the organization can be more responsive to changing market conditions.

Continuity on the Governing Board

A number of large multispecialty clinics have boards made up of six physicians who rotate on two three-year cycles so that a new board member comes in each year and an older board member retires. This works well in developing continuity of leadership and preserving the culture of the organization. Our experience with large medical groups is that most value continuity of physician leadership and that this has served them well. We believe this sort of approach will continue to be beneficial in the face of fundamental market shifts of the type anticipated in a future dominated by consumerism and technology.

Outside Directors

Some medical groups are beginning to use a limited number of outside directors, usually individuals with strong business backgrounds, such as bankers or former hospital administrators. The physician CEO of one medical group expressed it this way: "We need to bring in the perspective of the health care consumer and purchaser into our governance and decision-making process. We are too ingrown. Most medical groups are the same way, and the changing environment makes this an excellent time to think about changing the structure to include more outsiders."

The physician leader of an orthopedic group that had two outside directors told us, "We gained a new perspective on many of the issues we faced. For example, when we discussed hiring a consultant to serve as interim executive director of the group, one of our board members had some valuable suggestions on how to set this up. Outside directors are also more objective and less emotional; this helps keep discussions on an even keel."

Compensation of Directors

One common issue is whether or not directors should be compensated for their time or, in the case of physicians who serve on the board, given a lighter patient load. As a general rule, we are not in favor of compensating inside directors of a medical group. However, whether this rule applies in a given case depends on the time commitment required of directors.

Some boards of medical groups meet for several hours a week, usually in the morning. As any board member will attest, time spent in meetings is only part of the obligation—there is also the time required to serve on committees and task forces and to talk with colleagues who have a special interest in matters before the board. In this type of situation, it seems fair to either pay physician board members a small amount or relieve them of a small portion of their patient care responsibilities. Our experience indicates that when the latter is done, many physician board members will appreciate the gesture but continue to carry a full load of patients.

An Equitable Selection Process

Many hospital boards are self-perpetuating; that is, a nominating committee of the board seeks out well-qualified prospects and presents recommendations to the full board. Potential governing board candidates are drawn from the ranks of foundation board members, nonboard committee members, professional acquaintances, and from other sources. In a medical group there are usually opportunities to observe physicians as they participate in committees and task forces. Most boards have nominating committees that develop lists of potential board members. When the time comes to put forward nominations, they have a basis for their recommendations.

Most large multispecialty clinics and integrated systems recognize that physicians who are invited to serve on the board of governors should be team players. Members of the board of governors also tend to be physicians who are highly respected by their peers for their clinical expertise, professionalism, and dealings with patients. Most medical groups have procedures for voting on new board members and approving the renewal of appointments of existing members. This election process introduces a measure of direct political accountability that differs from a self-perpetuating board. Except under unusual circumstances, this seems to work well and is perceived by physicians as being fair.

Distribution of the Results of Board Meetings

The intranets developed by most large medical groups provide an ideal vehicle for communicating with physicians. One large medical group posts a "sanitized" version of the minutes of its board meetings on the clinic's intranet within twelve hours of each meeting. A physician board member who advocated broadly distributing the minutes of board meetings said, "You would be surprised at the number of hits we get a month on the board minutes [on our intranet]. Physicians are interested." He added, "Furthermore, if a physician tells me that he didn't know about something important that the board was considering, I have a ready answer: look at the minutes on the intranet. What can they say?"

Conclusions

The ideal governance structure for multispecialty clinics and integrated systems has yet to be developed; it is a work in progress. However, we believe that applying the following principles will lead to the best long-term governance solution for most physician-driven organizations:

- Maintain a board of governors or a similar type of structure so that physicians have a voice.
- Create a mechanism that allows physician and hospital leaders to meet regularly to focus on issues of integration and cooperation. Many large integrated systems have such groups. The

group might include the team leaders—physicians and administrators—of the clinic and hospital.

- Let physicians know what they need to do to be considered for membership on the board of governors. Although very few will ask directly, it is important for those who might be interested to have an understanding of the path to board membership.
- Publish a version of the minutes of the board of governors' (or directors') meetings shortly after each meeting. Using an intranet facilitates this type of timely communication.
- Focus meetings of the board of governors on clinical coordination and on ways the organization can better meet the needs of customers.
- Acknowledge the distinctive roles of both the physician board of governors and the system board of trustees and recognize the way the two boards complement each other for the benefit of the entire organization and its customers.

Looking ahead, we see many opportunities to improve the governance of health care organizations. A focus on strategies for meeting the needs of the new health care marketplace will pay big dividends.

Chapter Fifteen

Health Care Marketing, Mass Customization, and Branding

The need to develop brand-name awareness hasn't been important in health care. But this is all changing very rapidly. As consumers are taking charge, they are increasingly favoring health care organizations with name recognition.

MARKETING DIRECTOR OF AN ACUTE-CARE HOSPITAL
IN NORTH CAROLINA, April 2000

This chapter focuses on health care marketing and how it will develop in the new health care marketplace. When we talk about marketing, we are referring to market research, market segmentation, advertising and public relations, distribution of products and services, communication with consumers, and branding. The proportion of health care resources invested in marketing is likely to increase dramatically in the years ahead, especially in a market where consumers play an increasingly important role. The past success of direct-to-consumer advertising and marketing of prescription drugs and a host of medical services (such as vision correction surgery and cosmetic surgery) has set the stage for exponential growth in the future.

This chapter focuses on four marketing-related questions:

- How will health care marketing change in the future?
- What will be the benefits versus the costs of the dollars spent on marketing?
- What advances can we expect in market segmentation?
- What will it take for health care organizations to establish brand names in their markets?

Health Care Marketing: Past, Present, and Future

With few exceptions over the past two decades, health care marketing has been a stop-and-start proposition. When times are tough, marketing is almost always one of the first departments (along with strategic planning) to be downsized. Like many industries, health care has a history of laying off marketing staffs and drastically cutting advertising budgets when things are not going well financially.

Marketing, Public Relations, and Fundraising in the 1980s

In the 1980s it was common for hospitals to combine marketing, public relations, and fundraising in a single department. In addition, responsibilities for strategic planning were often part of this department. Hospital marketing traditionally included market research and analysis, new product development, advertising, and distribution (taking services to the public). Market research usually included periodic telephone surveys of residents of the area, patient satisfaction surveys, focus groups with physicians (almost always viewed as the key customer group) and employers, and occasional meetings with representatives of health plans. Hospitals and state hospital associations generate huge amounts of data, so there have been ample opportunities to compare market share by DRG and to present other indicators of competition and market positioning.

Health Care Marketing in the 1990s

The thrust of health care marketing changed in the middle and late 1990s, when a number of larger and more sophisticated organizations shifted their focus to the consumer. In 1997, for example, the marketing manager of a large West Coast health plan told us, "My management wants me to know everything about every individual we serve. They instructed me to dig deeper and to stop dealing in generalities."

Of course, drug company advertising raised the level of spending in health care marketing, and marketing efforts by providers of an array of quality-of-life products and services followed. As any consumer can observe, there are huge amounts of advertising directed at potential customers for cosmetic surgery, vision correction surgery, teeth whitening, weight loss, and ultrafast heart scanning. The net result has been major increases in the amounts spent on health care marketing, both nationally and in local markets. Health care advertisements have become more common than political advertisements preceding an election.

Health Care Marketing in the Future

Spending on health care marketing and advertising can only increase. With national health care spending growing at $100 billion a year and various segments of the industry fighting for market share, marketing efforts will intensify. As consumerism continues to grow, as consumers pay a larger share of health care costs, and as the role of the more restrictive forms of managed care diminishes in importance, health care marketing is likely to explode.

Some of the money now spent on mass marketing—radio, television, magazine, and newspaper advertising—will be shifted to Web sites and other more direct marketing approaches. As marketers gain expertise in market segmentation, we expect increased use of direct mail, e-mail, and telephone solicitation. In much the same way that banks now encourage checking account customers to take out a home improvement loan or rent a safe-deposit box, collateral marketing—encouraging the purchaser of one product or service to purchase other products or services—will increase in health care.

In the meantime, without federal action to slow or stop it, we expect direct-to-consumer advertising by pharmaceutical companies to increase by 15 to 20 percent a year. The flow of new drugs will drive the need for more advertising, and we expect consumers to respond. To be convinced that drug company advertising has been effective, you need only ask your primary care physician how many patients come in each week to discuss a particular new drug and request a prescription. This has been one of the drivers of large increases in utilization of physician services in recent years.

Cost-Benefit Ratio of Health Care Marketing

One of the age-old dilemmas in marketing, especially in advertising, has been trying to measure the benefits against the costs. Will the ".com's" that spent $2 million for a thirty-second commercial during the Super Bowl get a return on their investment? It appears doubtful. However, we can be reasonably sure that these same companies or another group of firms will be back with cash in hand, ready to buy time, during the next Super Bowl and that the rates will be even higher. Having given this background, we present in the following paragraphs our opinions on the benefits versus the costs of marketing and advertising by pharmaceutical companies, hospitals, health plans, and medical groups.

Pharmaceutical Company Marketing

We suspect that most pharmaceutical companies have evidence that their advertising dollars have paid off in the sale of larger quantities of name brand prescription drugs. The fact that advertising directly to consumers has continued to increase dramatically is fairly good evidence that this is true. A representative of a pharmaceutical company denied this in a speech in Denver, saying, "It is the physician who writes the prescription, not the consumer. Our advertising is aimed at educating consumers." Needless to say, this statement is hard to believe.

Hospital Marketing

We know of a number of hospitals that have built up and downsized their marketing departments at least three separate times in the past decade. We also know from experience that most of the money spent by hospitals on marketing and advertising in the 1980s and early 1990s was largely ineffective. In an environment increasingly dominated by managed care, consumers exerted little or no influence over which hospital they used; physicians and health plans controlled hospital utilization. (Is it any wonder, then, that hospitals concluded physicians were their major customers?)

Hospital marketing efforts aimed at health plans and employers, however, were often subtle and highly effective. Hospitals typically advertised the geographical coverage of their physicians and outpatient facilities, their relative costs, the friendliness of their staff, the quality of their physicians, and their high-tech equipment and facilities. The existence of strong centers of excellence, especially in emergency medicine, obstetrics, oncology, and cardiac services, was important to ensuring that the hospital was included in a provider panel.

On the issue of centers of excellence, one hospital CEO told us, "We have one of the top two [obstetrics] programs in this market, and we intend to continue to market directly to consumers in order to create pressures on the health plans to include our hospital in their panel of providers." However, a hospital's boasting of strong centers of excellence is a catch-22: consumers who are sicker and more likely to need the services of a center of excellence in oncology or cardiology, for example, are more likely to sign up for the health plan. This is the very opposite of cherry picking by health plans, where they seek out the healthiest subscribers.

Based on experience in numerous communities, we believe that most hospitals have been effective in their public relations activities and have realized substantial returns on dollars spent for public relations. The development and use of strong volunteer organizations is part of the reason for this. The net result is strong community support for most hospitals, especially those in rural areas and smaller communities.

Health Plan Marketing

For health plans marketing and advertising have been a mixed blessing. Just when many health plans were on the verge of establishing solid reputations in their market areas, consumers were inundated with adverse publicity about HMOs. In addition, the highly publicized failures of some respected health plans, such as Harvard Pilgrim, further weakened the public's perception of HMOs. Many health plans have not yet recovered either their public image or their financial strength, and they probably will not.

There are several other factors that raise questions about the effectiveness of health plan marketing efforts. First, consolidation among health plans has left employers and employees confused because a large number of local plans have been absorbed by larger national health plans. Second, the constantly changing networks of physicians and the adverse publicity associated with these changes have further muddied the water. Third, the annual reports of membership growth and decline, as well as the mixed picture of profitability and losses, have confused almost everyone. Consumers do not want to sign up with a health plan that may go broke.

The most effective marketing by health plans goes unnoticed by the public. We are referring to efforts aimed at employers and benefits consultants, especially during enrollment periods, and presentations to employees of an organization once a health plan has been selected. Much of this marketing has taken the form of direct sales by the health plans' sales forces. Funds spent on marketing of this type appear to have paid off for most health plans.

None of this suggests that health plans will be well positioned to market directly to consumers in the kind of health care environment we anticipate. Health plans will need a major reprogramming of their marketing efforts and personnel in order to adjust to a consumer-dominated marketplace.

Medical Group Marketing

With the exception of cosmetic surgeons and ophthalmologists performing vision correction surgery, medical groups have traditionally devoted little or no effort to marketing their services and expertise. Some single-specialty groups, especially those in neurosciences, orthopedics, and cardiology, have learned how to effectively use public relations. For example, orthopedic surgeons compete for jobs as team physicians for college and professional sports teams; this leads to free publicity and generates self-referrals from patients, particularly younger individuals who are involved in exercise, fitness, and sports. Groups like the Steadman Hawkins Clinic in Vail, Colorado, have capitalized on their experience with skiers, high-profile athletes, and celebrities. Neurosurgeons have received free media coverage when their patients recover from strokes or brain tumors and are able to regain the ability to participate in athletic events, such as bike racing.

Many single-specialty physicians and groups have continued the tradition of marketing themselves to primary care physicians and other referral sources. However, this type of marketing is usually accomplished through participation in professional activities and on a one-on-one basis with a primary care physician. In our experience, this sort of low-key, professional marketing has paid off for many physicians and medical groups, and it is likely to continue in the future.

Marketing: Costs Versus Benefits

With the exception of pharmaceutical companies and health plans, spending on marketing by most health care organizations has historically represented a very small percentage of net revenues. Pharmaceutical advertising has obviously been a major success. However, we are not optimistic that health plans will be able to realize a reasonable return on their marketing and advertising investments in the future.

In our view most hospital marketing and advertising have been ineffective, but hospital public relations efforts have been valuable. We expect hospital marketing and advertising to change as hospital CEOs and marketers become more sophisticated and more focused on what they need to accomplish with their marketing dollars. Continued emphasis on public relations is a given, and we expect hospitals to continue to realize substantial benefits from these efforts.

We anticipate major increases in the marketing efforts of both single-specialty and multispecialty medical groups. As consumerism becomes more dominant, these types of medical groups will have a clearer picture of their target markets—consumers with certain economic and demographic characteristics (for example, women in certain age groups with above-average income). The success of single-specialty groups that have pursued quality-of-life products and services, such as cosmetic surgery, should be a source of encouragement to more traditional groups. We believe that strong medical groups have barely scratched the surface when it comes to effective marketing and realizable benefits.

Market Opportunities in Mass Customization

One of the outcomes of increased consumer power and choice is the inevitability of market segmentation. Look at any major retail industry, and you will see market segmentation at work. A client financial institution showed us its most recent market analysis, which identified over one hundred submarkets, ranging from the "pickups and gun racks" segment to the "kids and cul-de-sacs" group.

A number of individuals interviewed in the process of preparing this book cited market segmentation as a strategy that hospitals, medical groups, physician networks, integrated systems, and health plans need to learn—and learn fast. One physician leader said, "With the growth in consumerism, and consumers having more voice in their health care decisions, we have to be able to segment them by their economic and demographic characteristics and by their needs and wants."

KPMG Study of Consumerism

KPMG interviewed 321 individuals in seventy health care organizations and 1,812 consumers about the likely impact of consumer market segmentation in the future. Here is one of KPMG's findings (1998, p. 21): "Organizations will build competitive advantage by elevating market segmentation to a new art in all phases of its application—research, product design and development, advertising and promotion, branding and pricing. Leaders will efficiently convert that ability into everyday operations." The KPMG research notes that firms such as Levi's and Motorola, with their mass customization capabilities, have shown that narrow segmentation can be accomplished, and this concept can be successfully implemented by health care organizations.

"One Size Fits All": A Model That Misses the Mark

Historically, health care in the United States has evolved as a "one size fits all" service. With the advent of managed care, there have been attempts to segment the market into disease groupings—largely to facilitate disease management and contain costs. However, compared with other sectors of the economy, little has been done to recognize the unique needs of individuals and develop market-driven responses to those needs.

Health plans have sought to identify employer market segments. They have developed different strategies for large groups versus small groups and for firms that desire a rich benefits package versus those focusing on lower costs. Although this is clearly a form of market segmentation, it often misses the mark when it comes to the actual consumer. Small and medium-sized firms continue to select a "one size fits all" health plan design that fails to address the unique needs of the individuals who constitute their workforce.

A Perspective on Market Segmentation: The Senior Market

The elderly represent a market segment that is not well understood, even though this group spends more on health care than any other market segment. The sixty-five-plus age group is in reality a variety of distinct market segments, and these segments are undergoing rapid change.

As life expectancies increase, age sixty-five will not mark the beginning of the golden years but, rather, a continuation of middle age. The senior years will not start until age seventy-five or older. We have witnessed this trend in our own long-term care consulting practice. When we first started advising developers of senior housing fifteen years ago, we defined the target market as individuals sixty-five years old and older. Ten years later the threshold was typically seventy-five years of age. In the new millennium the vast majority of the elderly who are moving into senior housing that offers services such as congregate care and assisted living are in their early eighties.

Because the age band stretches over many decades and generations, it is misleading to lump seniors together in a single market segment. This would be the same as viewing college students in their early twenties and empty nesters in their late forties and early fifties (a twenty-five- to thirty-year spread) as a single segment. The life experiences of individuals who were eighty-five years old in 2000 are very different from those of individuals who were sixty-five in 2000. Many of the oldest Americans experienced World War I and the Great Depression during their formative years. Compare that with the most recent sixty-five-year-olds, who barely remember World War II, who relate more to the Korean conflict and the Cold War, and who grew up in the beginning of an era of economic prosperity.

Now look ahead a decade, to the time when the first baby boomer turns sixty-five. The experience of this generation has been one of upward mobility, geographical dispersion, higher education, more working women, and a booming economy and stock market. The Vietnam War and the tumultuous 1960s and 1970s shaped this generation. This segment has more income and spends it more freely than any preceding generation. It also has higher standards and expectations for all products and services, including health care. Those in health care who are not prepared for the baby boomers will reel under the impact of this large market segment.

Opportunities to Serve the More Affluent Consumer

Commercial banks have been seeking out wealthy individuals for years. Many large banks in metropolitan areas have private banking departments that focus on customers with high income and high net worth. Services are highly personalized; $50,000 loans for a vacation or new car are arranged with a single phone call, and the banker comes to the customer's home or business for the needed signature.

In a similar vein, one multispecialty group in the Southeast has created a "clinic within a clinic," called Corporate Health Services, where executives can go for a physical. Here is a description of the service: "A representative from Corporate Health Services escorts each incoming executive to a private waiting room, where there's access to business journals, a phone, and a fax machine. 'We see only one patient at a time,' says Marilyn Borrelli, a registered nurse and Corporate Health Services' coordinator. 'For patients who get fasting blood drawn, we offer coffee, juice, and a PowerBar. We also offer private showers, so an executive can change into his gym clothes for a stress test, shower, get back into his suit, and go to work'" (Kane, 1999, p. 128).

At the David Drew Clinic in Chevy Chase, Maryland, patients pay about $5,000 a year for diagnostic and preventive care. A doctor's visit lasts for hours, not minutes. Each patient receives an initial two-hour consultation, three physicals and additional consultations throughout the year, plus a roster of tests to detect diseases that routine exams may fail to identify (Kane, 1999).

In our view the growing affluent market in the United States, particularly among baby boomers, represents a huge untapped market opportunity for health care organizations that develop products and services to meet the very specific needs of small groups. These types of marketing efforts depend on sophisticated market research and require going well beyond what is typical today in terms of understanding customer needs and desires.

International Medicine: Another Example of Market Segmentation

A group of Philadelphia hospitals and other health care organizations have joined forces to promote Philadelphia as an international center for health care. Often labeled "the birthplace of American medicine," Philadelphia claims the largest concentration of health care providers in the country.

According to Philadelphia International Medicine (1999, p. 3), "More than 20 percent of physicians in America graduate from Philadelphia area medical schools or post-graduate medical education programs. Within a few miles of the city, there are more than 120 biotechnology and pharmaceutical companies, over 70 manufacturers of biomedical equipment and more than 60 biomedical research institutions." Raymond Uhlhorn, chairman of Philadelphia International Medicine, told us that in the few months since its inception, the consortium had attracted several million dollars in medical services provided by members to international sources. "However," he said, "this market is becoming more competitive and price sensitive, so it isn't going to get any easier" (interview, Jan. 2000).

Barriers to Market Segmentation

Information systems to help identify and understand distinct health care market segments have been woefully inadequate. Very few hospitals can tell you how much it actually costs to take care of a person with congestive heart failure or how these costs might vary by the age of the patient, the patient's socioeconomic status, or other pertinent factors. Health plans, the repository of claims data, are likewise often unable to articulate these key factors in anything but a vague, general way. This is quite a contrast to our financial services client who can identify one hundred different types of customers.

Databases for Market Segmentation

Where will health care marketers turn for help in developing and managing the databases needed for mass customization? Following is a summary of how databases for market segmentation have developed.

Geodemographic Systems

Jock Bickert is CEO of Looking Glass, a Denver-based market research and database firm. Discussing the evolution of databases for market segmentation, Bickert (1997, p. 367) says, "Until the late 1970s, efforts to segment consumers were generally limited to product-specific systems. For example, survey research would indicate that soft-drink buyers could be categorized into six groups. However, this system didn't travel well, meaning it was unable to explain and predict purchasing patterns in other products." According to Bickert, the development of geodemographic databases in the 1970s was the next step. "Some of the original research on cluster analysis showed that it was possible to aggregate people in various Census tracts and have consistency in such variables as income, ethnicity, education and occupation. The Claritas Corporation released the first geodemographics segmentation system called PRIZM (potential rating index for zip markets)" (interview, March 2000).

The Values and Lifestyles System

The values and lifestyles system (VALS) was developed by Stanford Research International. VALS had nine types. "Marketers hungry for a way to impose coherence on the complexity of consumer behavior embraced the VALS system. However, VALS proved to be a useful conceptual tool, but experienced limited applications" (Bickert, 1997, p. 368).

The Niches System

The niches system has three dimensions—needs, buying power, and spending patterns—derived from variables available in the Polk Company's eighty-million-name TotaList database. Needs consist of life-cycle stages, buying power is measured by wealth variables (such as income and type of dwelling), and spending patterns are gleaned from Polk's vast repository of auto and truck data. According to Bickert (1997), these three dimensions first produced 108 cells known as "SuperNiches." Through cluster analysis these were combined into twenty-six fairly homogeneous groups.

The DNA Demographic System

Metromail Corporation's household segmentation system is called the "DNA" demographic system. Part of this is a life-stage system, and part is made of behavioral data from a twenty-million-household behavioral database. Users can access one hundred highly homogeneous cells or twenty-five aggregated supercells in this system (Bickert, 1997).

The Cohorts System

A portion of the cohorts system is based on a database of close to forty million individuals who returned questionnaires that were packaged primarily with durable goods. The cohorts system includes demographic information (such as age, income, home ownership, and presence of children) and lifestyle factors—a combination of over seventy activities and interests (such as handicrafts, physical fitness, technology, investing, and motor sports) (Bickert, 1997).

The cohorts system has thirty-three unique segments, each of which is homogeneous with respect to the demographic and lifestyle variables but dissimilar to each of the other thirty-two segments. The main use of this system is to match the cohort database with characteristics of known customers or an organization and thus generate lists of individuals with the same characteristics. This, of course, facilitates targeted marketing.

Impact of the Internet on Market Segmentation Databases

Bickert (1997, p. 377) says, "The inevitable emergence of the Internet as a marketing medium will probably send the geodemographic systems to the dustbin. Geography, as a link between marketer and customer, will be meaningless." Of course, this has implications for health care. Bickert also believes that the Internet will make some household-based systems, like the VALS and niches systems, less relevant. "Even today," he observes, "the most desirable marketing unit is the individual, not the household. Since the household is the basic unit of most current databases, this will change" (p. 377).

Consumer Databases for Health Care

In terms of relevance to health care, Bickert believes that future databases on individuals will reflect lifestyle (including measures of health status) and the ability to pay for discretionary health services. He told us, "I would think that market segmentation for health care providers will become much more feasible in the future and will become the way most organizations do business." Summarizing his experience with market segmentation and the use of databases to support segmentation, Bickert said, "It doesn't do any good to segment the market unless you can do something about it" (interview, Mar. 3, 2000). This leads to a challenge for health care: figuring out how to reorganize the delivery of products and services to match the needs of various market segments.

Opportunities to Establish and Manage Brand Names

Here is the way one writer characterizes the importance of branding as a health care strategy: "The new healthcare consumer is well informed, technologically savvy and demands choices. So the old ways of attracting patients—location, word of mouth, a high ranking on the *U.S. News* 'Best Hospitals' list—are fading fast. Organizations will have to reach the new consumer through branding" (Serb, 1999).

What Is Branding?

Branding is more than a logo or slogan. Brand value is "strategic awareness plus perceived quality plus singular distinction" (Serb, 1999). The most powerful brands are known for superiority in a single area rather than for a general reputation for excellence (Serb, 1999). One marketing expert described the essence of a brand in this way: "A brand in fact is a relationship between an enterprise and its customers. A brand transcends logic: it's an emotional connection with our audience. It is both fragile and crucial to a company's ability to succeed" (Howgill, 1998, p. 33).

Creation and Management of a Brand

A *Harvard Business Review* article says, "In strong brands, brand equity is tied both to the actual quality of the product or service and to various intangible factors" (Keller, 2000, p. 148). The article goes on to describe the intangibles, which include the type of person who uses the brand, the type of personality the brand portrays, the feeling the brand tries to elicit from customers, and the relationship it seeks to build with its customers.

Branding in Financial Services: Lessons Learned

In another example from the financial services industry, an article in *The Economist* points out that branding attempts by financial firms are often rather dull. "Small wonder," the article comments, "that of the top 60 most valuable international brands, as calculated by Interbrand, a consultancy, only two—American Express (ranked 19th) and Citibank (25th)—are financial firms" ("Financial Brands," 1999). The article further indicates that there is much more to branding than putting up signs or advertising on television or in the newspapers. A brand is "the DNA of the firm": "It reflects, in other words, its culture. A good branding initiative builds on a firm's strength; but in marketing-speak, the firm must 'deliver on the promise'" ("Financial Brands," 1999).

Branding in Health Care: Not a New Strategy

The Mayo Clinic is a prime example of a health care organization with an internationally recognized brand. Large multispecialty groups have brands in their regional markets—Marshfield Clinic in Wisconsin, Scripps in southern California, Dartmouth-Hitchcock in Vermont and New Hampshire, and the Cleveland Clinic in the Midwest and Florida.

The impact of branding in health care has been partially reduced by managed care—a payment system that directs consumers
to specific physicians and hospitals. If branded providers, such as
well-known academic medical centers, have higher costs, many
health plans are unlikely to include them in their preferred provider panels, even if consumers want access to these prestigious
facilities. However, in an environment where the more restrictive
types of managed care plans are becoming less dominant and where
consumers are exercising more influence and footing more of the
bill, brand recognition takes on new meaning and will become an
imperative for many health care organizations.

Follow-Through

In any competitive health care market, there is an abundance of
billboard, newspaper, television, and radio advertisements, all trying to build an image, or brand, for a clinic, hospital system, health
plan, or specialized health care product or service. Are these efforts
successful? The answer depends on whether actual experience
matches the claims of the advertising. One industry observer notes,
"The brand can be polished and enhanced through advertising and
public relations. It can even be amplified. But it cannot be disguised
or covered up because no communications can permanently overcome the perceived dissonance between our actual experiences and
advertising messages that try to convince us that our experiences
are not valid" (Howgill, 1998, p. 39).

The dissonance between advertised claims and actual experience has been the biggest problem for health plans and hospitals.
Health plans advertise that they will take care of their customers
and eliminate all the hassles, yet patients experience diminished
choice, the need for referral authorizations, drug formularies, and
other cost containment features that many find distasteful. Hospitals advertise a caring environment, yet patients are frustrated
when no one answers when they push the nurse-call button. Consumers sense this dissonance, and thus attempts at branding an
organization as a caring place or a clinical service line as unique
usually do not take hold. If the dissonance is significant, it adds to
the public's cynicism about health care and makes it that much

harder to reach potential patients when a positive image and reality converge.

The Halo Effect

Long-established brands can provide enormous opportunities and are more resilient when it comes to an occasional negative perception. For example, the Mayo Clinic has capitalized on its brand name in establishing clinics in Arizona and Florida. We have seen hospitals and medical groups with strong reputations in a single area, such as cardiac services, capitalize on their reputation and brand for other clinical services. So for those pursuing a center-of-excellence strategy, the halo effect can be real.

Results-Based Branding

Scott MacStravic, a health care marketing consultant, says that basing a brand on the results achieved for customers is more powerful than other approaches. MacStravic (1999, p. 21) gives a few examples: "A fertility center in Los Angeles guarantees money back if its clients do not have babies. Cosmetic surgery and weight loss providers routinely show 'before and after' pictures to indicate the kinds of results they get. Outpatient—especially laparoscopic—surgery programs promise earlier recovery, and less scarring, discomfort, and time lost from normal activities than inpatient rivals." We anticipate that a consumer-dominated health care marketplace will respond well to these kinds of guarantees, and we expect to see much more of this over the initial years of the new millennium. Health care organizations that offer money-back guarantees will definitely be able to establish their brand name.

A Good Brand Turned Bad

Branding is a challenging strategy. If properly executed and delivered, it can be extremely effective. It can also turn on an organization if the brand is associated with a negative event. Columbia/HCA aggressively pursued a branding strategy during 1996 and 1997, but this approach deteriorated when the organization was accused of overbilling Medicare and other indiscretions. Columbia/HCA took its name off signs at its hospitals and changed the names of its local hospitals back to the names of their predecessor organizations. When consumer trust is betrayed, a branding strategy can come back to haunt an organization, which can be worse than if no brand had existed. Examples abound—the food poisoning issues of Jack-in-the-Box restaurants or a tainted hamburger at Burger King. It is clear that a bad event, even when confined to a single outlet, can taint an entire organization.

The Future of Branding Strategies in Health Care

Where is branding headed in health care? What should CEOs and marketers be doing to give their organizations brand name recognition in their markets? We believe that opportunities for achieving success in branding in health care are numerous. As noted earlier, the growth of managed care from the mid-1980s through the 1990s has somewhat weakened branding as a strategy and has contributed to health care being viewed as a commodity with price being the key differentiating factor. The focus of medical groups, hospitals, and integrated systems has been on developing primary care networks, improving their cost-effectiveness, and resisting pressures to discount their services. We believe that in the future establishing and nurturing a brand name will pay off for many health care organizations, large and small.

Conclusions

At the risk of offending some, it is our opinion that compared with other industries, most health care marketing has been primitive. Basic rules have been violated—lack of consistency in marketing efforts and messages, uneven delivery of products and services (thus not living up to promises), advertising directed at the wrong audiences, insufficient attention to market segmentation, superficial market research (millions of dollars wasted on poorly designed telephone interviews), and failure to capitalize on opportunities to develop and sustain a strong family of brand names. We are not talking about all health care organizations; there are a few notable success stories, including Mayo, the Cleveland Clinic, Ochsner in New Orleans, Johns Hopkins, and a number of regional systems and single-specialty medical groups.

The health care products and services that are sold directly to the public and paid for on an out-of-pocket basis are a model for the future. The pharmaceutical companies, which urge the consumer to make an appointment with a physician in order to request a specific name brand drug, have been successful. These kinds of marketing efforts are generally consistent over long periods of time, tell the consumer exactly what to do, and emphasize the positive results the customer can expect. And, for the most part, they deliver on their promise.

We expect a quantum leap in the number of dollars spent on marketing and in the cost-effectiveness of these efforts. In an industry that is growing at $100 billion a year and in which traditional providers such as hospitals are losing market share, the opportunities for carving out new product and service niches and building entire new businesses are immense. The success of such new or growing businesses will be based partly on more sophisticated marketing, including market segmentation, mass customization, and branding.

Part Four

The Future of Health Care

Essentials for Success in the New Consumer-Oriented Marketplace

It is not surprising that many boards and CEOs are confused about where health care is headed and what it will take to be successful. Many of us have been down a number of different paths, each of which promised to be "the answer." Now you are saying that we need to prepare for a new health care marketplace dominated by consumerism and technology. How do we get started?
CEO OF A MULTIHOSPITAL SYSTEM

The final two chapters deal with important issues: the characteristics of the health system of the future and the insights we can offer that will clarify the nature of the new health care marketplace.

Success Factors for the Future

The old arguments about whether or not vertical integration is the best strategy or whether hospitals and medical groups should "get back to basics" will become less relevant in the new health care marketplace. The key issue will be what health care organizations should do to position themselves for success in an era dominated by consumerism and technology. This is the subject of Chapter Sixteen.

Health Care Myths and Economic Realities

Chapter Seventeen concludes the book with our assessment of ten health care myths and ten economic realities. In a sense, our analysis of these myths and realities is another way of summarizing what the future is likely to bring and how major players might respond.

Successful Health Care Organizations of the Future

Should we proceed with our vertical integration strategy, or should we follow the advice of The Advisory Board and get back to basics? Our financial performance is of great concern to the board of our system. Even though we are in a solid financial position, we need to generate more cash flow for physical expansion and remodeling, and to acquire information systems and new technology. Can we pursue a vertical integration strategy and still meet our financial needs?
CEO OF A HOSPITAL-BASED INTEGRATED SYSTEM
IN THE ROCKY MOUNTAIN REGION, June 2000

These and similar questions are being asked by an increasing number of hospital and health system CEOs and board members and by the leaders of large multispecialty clinics. This issue forces us back to the drawing board to consider the characteristics of the successful health care system of the future.

We believe that, rather than arguing the merits of virtual integration versus ownership (of physician practices, a health plan, or other facilities) or of hospitals' sticking to "the basics" versus diversifying, the best approach to setting a direction for a hospital or group of physicians is to look closely at what the marketplace is likely to demand and value. Then we can define the characteristics that systems must develop to meet most or all of these marketplace needs. Considering the growth in consumerism and technology and the value-added criteria discussed in Part One, we believe there are at least fourteen fundamental characteristics that the successful health care system of the future will need to develop. These characteristics are listed in Exhibit 16.1.

There are other factors that could be on our list of key characteristics of the health system of the future. For example, we have not included cost cutting or improving an organization's financial position; however, better financial performance should follow from becoming a system that exhibits most of the fourteen characteristics. We could have discussed the development of a brand name, research and education, risk sharing with health plans, outcomes measurement, adaptability and flexibility, developing international markets, and being open to new partners or relationships. All of these success factors, and others, will be important, but we have

Exhibit 16.1. Fourteen Characteristics of the Health Care System of the Future.

1. Adoption of a sustainable set of core values that allow the health care system to adapt to changing conditions
2. Identification of market segments and development of programs that offer the best fit and profit potential (mass customization)
3. Development of centers of excellence
4. Establishment of leadership in IT and technological linkages with other organizations
5. Focus on the management of chronic diseases
6. Necessity of full geographical coverage of the marketplace
7. Encouragement of partnerships between hospitals and physicians
8. Cultivation of relationships among primary care physicians and specialists
9. Enhancement of performance and processes
10. Construction of well-designed facilities
11. Emphasis on prevention and wellness
12. Attention to providing superior service, convenience, and access
13. Integration of CAM into traditional medicine
14. Cultivation of outstanding management

focused on the fourteen we believe to be the most critical in a health care marketplace increasingly dominated by consumerism and technology.

These fourteen characteristics amount to strategies for success. A number of these strategies were discussed in earlier chapters dealing with hospitals, multihospital systems, and integrated health care organizations. However, the setting here is different, and the examples used here were not used earlier. Despite concern over duplication, we thought it was important to summarize what we consider to be the most critical overall strategies for the new health care marketplace.

Characteristic 1: Core Values

Over the past decade there has been considerable research showing that core values contribute the most to an organization's ability to adapt to and survive changing economic, technological, and market conditions. This is the thesis of Collins and Porras (1996) in "Building Your Company's Vision." A similar point of view is espoused by Arie de Geus (1997), formerly of the Royal Dutch/Shell Group, in an article in *Harvard Business Review.*

The Mayo Foundation

A number of health care organizations have been able to develop strong cultures and core values. The best example is the Mayo Foundation, established in 1919 and still going strong (it cannot keep up with the demand for its services). Mayo's most important core value, initially articulated by William J. Mayo, M.D., one of the Mayo brothers, and part of nearly every meeting today, is that the interests of the patient come first. A second core value is the importance of medical education, and a third relates to research. However, as important as they are, education and research do not detract from patient care and meeting the needs of patients.

While holding firmly to its core values, the Mayo Foundation has instituted several fundamental changes over the past two decades—forming new clinics in Jacksonville, Florida, and Scottsdale, Arizona, establishing regional systems in Minnesota, Wisconsin, and northern Iowa, and either acquiring or establishing hospitals in Rochester, Minnesota, Scottsdale, and Jacksonville. It has operated a medical school and graduate programs for years, and its research has led to many important medical discoveries. These major initiatives are all consistent with Mayo's core values and are important in terms of positioning the organization for the future. In looking ahead, Mayo's CEO, Michael Wood, M.D., said, "Although we don't know what the future will bring, we believe that our culture allows us to be in a position to deal with whatever curveballs are thrown our way" (interview, Dec. 1999). We agree with Wood in his assessment.

Other Multispecialty Clinics

We have worked with a number of large multispecialty clinics (smaller than the Mayo clinic) that serve regional markets and have strong cultures and core values. These include Marshfield in Wisconsin, Scott & White in central Texas, Dartmouth-Hitchcock in New Hampshire and Vermont, MeritCare in Fargo, North Dakota, and Park Nicollet in Minneapolis–Saint Paul. We expect many of these organizations to successfully adapt to a changing health care environment that emphasizes consumerism and technology.

Hospitals

We have also worked with many hospitals that have strong core values in terms of their commitments to the communities they serve. Many Catholic hospitals fall into this category. There are others as well, such as Franklin Memorial Hospital in Farmington, Maine, where community participation is part of the very essence of the organization (see Chapter Eight).

Core Values: Summary

In summary, to be a success story of the future, it is important to discover and develop core values and a company culture. We believe that the successful health care systems of the future will develop strong core values.

Characteristic 2: Market Segmentation and Program Development

We discuss the importance of market segmentation and mass customization in Chapter Fifteen. The health care system of the future will have the expertise and databases required to identify market segments (the frail elderly, Medicare patients, individuals with chronic diseases, women with children, families with high incomes or high net worth, baby boomers, working men, and so on), prioritize these market segments, and develop new programs and services for those segments that offer the greatest potential.

Highway to Health Provides an Example of Market Segmentation

Two entrepreneurs are building a company around providing health care for travelers. Angelo Masciantonio (1999, p. 94), one of the founders of Highway to Health, says, "I thought it would be extremely valuable if there were an easy way to access high-quality healthcare and coverage when you're traveling. I also thought about how the Internet could facilitate new physician-patient relationships."

Highway to Health's target market is people over the age of fifty who travel and who also have health plan coverage. If a member gets sick while traveling, the company contacts one of its physicians and makes an appointment for the traveler. The company says it is developing a network of physicians and hospitals in 350 top travel destinations worldwide (Masciantonio, 1999).

Internet Access Will Allow Greater Market Segmentation

One of the most important ways to segment the market over the next few years will be based on Internet access and usage. One hospital CEO told us that 60 percent of the consumers who use his hospital have access to the Internet and two-thirds of these individuals are active users. Of course, both of these proportions are expected to increase, as will the proportion of homes with high-speed Internet access. The CEO told us, "This is a critically important way of looking at the market. We are designing our whole patient flow process around consumer use of the Internet—from scheduling appointments to accessing their medical records—and we need to closely monitor those households that will prefer this approach. We will also use the Internet and e-mail to conduct real-time patient satisfaction surveys."

The "One Size Fits All" Model Will Not Work in the Future

What we visualize for the health system of the future is just the opposite of the "one size fits all" models of many health care organizations. An emphasis on market segmentation is consistent with the experience of other industries—airlines, financial services, retailers, automobile manufacturers and dealers, home builders, apparel manufacturers, and athletic and fitness clubs. It is difficult to think of examples of successful businesses that view their markets as homogeneous.

As we have pointed out, consumers are already demanding more choice in health services, and these expectations will only increase. Furthermore, consumers are becoming better educated about the alternatives. This means there are opportunities for health care organizations that can carefully identify consumer needs and find new products and services that satisfy those needs.

Market Segmentation Is Inevitable

Market segmentation is unavoidable for health care systems that want to position themselves for success in the future. However, the required investment in databases, research, and product development is not inconsequential. The sooner health systems establish the organizational structure and funding to begin this task, the better.

Characteristic 3: Centers of Excellence

Centers of excellence were introduced in our earlier discussion of hospital strategies, and we believe the health care system of the future will strive to create centers of excellence in order to distinguish itself in the market and provide top-quality care. Most health care systems already have one or two centers of excellence; in the future, health systems will add centers of excellence and strengthen those already in existence.

Reasons for a Focus on Centers of Excellence

Why should centers of excellence be one of the basic characteristics of the health care system of the future? Here are a few reasons:

- Consumers understand centers of excellence, and this understanding will become even more important in the marketplace of the future.
- Centers of excellence imply high quality of care and significant volume. Because of their size and nature, centers of excellence often facilitate monitoring quality and reporting the results to the public.
- It is possible to develop meaningful brand identification for centers of excellence.
- The "halo effect" of centers of excellence benefits other services. The best-known examples of this are in cardiac care, neurosciences, oncology, and neonatal care. In some markets a well-known emergency department can be a center of excellence and transmit the halo effect to the rest of the organization.
- Centers of excellence provide a perfect opportunity to develop partnerships with physicians. Centers of excellence cannot exist without physician involvement and commitment.

Centers of Excellence Versus "Focused Factories"

Centers of excellence are not much different from the "focused factories" advocated by Regina Herzlinger in *Market Driven Health Care* (1997). Herzlinger would prefer that these centers of excellence, or single-specialty centers, be outside the hospital or health system. However, we think they can perform well in, and benefit from being part of, a hospital or medical group. In fact, where health systems do not pursue this strategy, competitors of all types will fill the void.

Characteristic 4: Information Technology and Technological Linkages

Many hospitals, medical groups, health plans, and other health care organizations are approaching the rapid changes in technology as if they were a problem. For example, the *Wall Street Journal* ran a story with this headline: "Internet Medicine: Doctors Are Suddenly Swamped with Patients Who Think They Know a Lot More Than They Actually Do" (Jeffrey, 1998). Our conversations with literally hundreds of physicians lead us to a similar conclusion: the fact that consumers are arming themselves with medical information is perceived as a nuisance by many doctors.

There is no doubt that the health care system of the future will be a leader in technology, using Internet applications, intranet communication for staff and patients, Web sites, e-mail, voice recognition capabilities, telemedicine, telehealth, clinical information systems, EMRs, outcomes measurement, and cutting-edge medical technology.

What Is Technological Leadership?

We believe there will be two aspects to technological leadership: individuals with an entrepreneurial bent and access to the capital needed to acquire new technology. We expect that some of the entrepreneurial drive will come from physicians and that much of the capital will come from hospitals and multihospital systems. Internet companies (".com's") may also be a source of capital.

As we discussed in several chapters in Part Two, having the funds available to take a leadership position in technology poses serious challenges for many medical groups, hospitals, and health systems—even some of the largest and those offering the most comprehensive services. Perhaps this will lead to opportunities for companies that specialize in financing new medical technology, which could reduce the direct burden on the balance sheets of health care systems. Another alternative is increased collaboration with technology suppliers in the purchase and use of technology.

Technological Linkages

Technological linkages have tremendous potential for the health system of the future. By "technology linkages" we mean hospitals and medical groups linking with one another, over the Internet, over their own intranet, or through the careful design of Web sites. Telehealth, of course, will be a much more prominent form of technological linkage.

Information Technology and Technological Linkages: Summary

No matter how an organization gets the job done, it is difficult to envision a health care system of the future that is not developing a position of leadership in technology, especially IT. This includes the EMR and much, much more.

Characteristic 5: Disease Management

Growing evidence about disease management programs (which are introduced and discussed in Chapter Eleven) indicates that they are cost effective, that consumers like them, and that they are focused on individuals with more serious illnesses who are users of significant health care resources. With an estimated one hundred million Americans (over one-third of the population) suffering from one or more chronic illnesses, the potential market for disease management is huge.

Coordination of Care for Those with Chronic Diseases

There is a tremendous need for the coordination of care for those with chronic diseases, and disease management programs can partially or totally meet this need. We view this as an opportunity for local health care organizations. If health systems do not get involved, they will forfeit the field to pharmaceutical companies and the growing number of specialized disease management programs that operate nationally, usually funded by health plans or pharmaceutical companies.

Disease Management: A Way of Maintaining Control of the Local Health Care Market

Health systems of the future will not want to delegate disease management to outside organizations; disease management will be an integral part of the marketing efforts and care management services provided by local systems. The challenge, of course, is to figure out how to provide these services within the limits of reimbursement levels.

Dr. Kevin Fickenscher, senior vice president of CareInsite and a former executive with Catholic Healthcare West, told us: "I agree that local health care systems need to make sure that their customers have access to disease management services. However, I don't agree that local systems have the expertise or economies of scale to do this. They need to develop strategic alliances with disease management programs to ensure that these types of services are available locally" (interview, Sept. 1999).

Disease Management: Summary

It is difficult to envision a successful health care system of any size in the new health care marketplace that does not play a leading role in the management of the chronic diseases of consumers in the service area. For many organizations this represents a prime opportunity to increase market share.

Characteristic 6: Geographical Coverage

There is not a business we know of in which geographical coverage of the market is not important. In many parts of the country, health care providers have taken the approach that consumers will show up where the services are offered ("Build it, and they will come"). However, in other markets there is increasing emphasis on taking services to the consumer. An administrator of a large multispecialty clinic told us, "When people are very sick, they will come to the main clinic even if it means driving an hour or two. But, for the everyday ailments that afflict almost everyone, consumers want services to be convenient."

There are a number of ways that geographical coverage can be improved—for example, through outlying medical offices, outreach clinics, mobile services, technology (such as telemedicine and telehealth), and patient transportation. (Elements of convenience for consumers are discussed in Chapter Three.)

Regional Medical Offices

Regional medical offices are an especially popular and effective strategy for large integrated systems led by multispecialty clinics.

In a sense, this is similar to a branching network for a large banking system or grocery chain. Almost all large multispecialty clinics and integrated systems provide satellite medical offices or branches of some type throughout their primary service areas.

The Need for Consistency

One physician leader of a health care system that offered a network of medical offices had these observations: "I have seen a lack of consistency in these types of offices. Consumers don't know when they go from one office to another that they are all part of the same system. In the past, when health care was definitely local, this was OK. But in the future it will be more important to establish brand names and consistency from one center to another. Kaiser Permanente does a pretty good job in this and may be the model of the future."

Broader Scope of Services for Physician Offices

One interesting shift taking place in outlying physician offices is the addition of specialists on either a full- or part-time basis. Again, consumers are showing their support for specialty services and their appreciation for the convenience of satellite offices.

Outreach Clinics

There are many situations where physicians, medical groups, hospitals, and integrated systems have been active in providing outreach clinics to smaller communities, and consumers are very pleased with this. For example, in northwest Kansas, physicians travel to twenty different communities, some as much as a two-hour drive away, to provide services on either a weekly or monthly basis. The physicians who provide these outreach services are specialists in radiology, urology, general surgery, otolaryngology, ophthalmology, and cardiology. The benefits are happy patients in smaller communities and increased referrals to specialists at the regional center.

Mobile Services

Mobile CT scanners, MRIs, lithotripters, and cardiac catheterization labs have been around for years. These types of units represent one approach to reducing the cost of making technology available, particularly in small and medium-sized communities. They also enable smaller hospitals and medical groups to compete with larger regional or tertiary care centers that are trying to make inroads into their local market.

Technology

Two technological approaches that allow health systems to provide better geographical coverage are the Internet and telemedicine. Telehealth is becoming increasingly common and has many applications for the future. In many respects telehealth represents a new approach to disease management and home health care.

The expanded capacity of telephone and cable lines (through broadband technology) that run to homes, businesses, and health care facilities means that telemedicine should be less expensive and grow more rapidly than in the past, particularly in more sparsely populated areas of the country. With the much improved economics of telemedicine, this service will not be limited to a few facilities that have made the investment in two-way television; it will be used much more widely by all types of medical groups and hospitals.

Transportation Services

The importance of providing transportation, especially for the elderly, is something that health systems of the future will emphasize. Based on our experience, any community health care needs assessment will almost always identify transportation as an important need, especially for the elderly. One former hospital CEO told us of establishing a program for Native Americans who lived in the countryside surrounding the hospital: "We had this nice program, and we were pleased that we 'were doing the right thing.' However, the first day we opened the new facility, not a single patient showed up. We had neglected the importance of transportation; they had no way of getting to our facility."

Geographical Coverage: Summary

Geographical coverage is part of convenience, and as noted in Chapter Three, it is highly valued by consumers. We see this as one of the most important strategies of the health care system of the future.

Characteristic 7: Partnerships Between Hospitals and Physicians

Retreating to "the basics" or viewing hospitals as "doctors' work-shops" is the opposite of considering physicians as partners in meeting consumer needs. Partnerships with physicians characterize the successful integrated systems where physicians have taken leadership positions; in these systems the focus has shifted to the customers—consumers, employers, health plans, and government payers.

We believe that the concept of physicians as partners is fundamentally important for the successful health system of the future. This means that physicians and health system executives will find ways to work together in identifying market opportunities and in meeting consumer and payer needs through new programs, more focused clinical services, and other initiatives. The view of physicians as a hospital's best customers will not lead to the kind of partnership initiatives needed to be successful, especially in the new health care marketplace.

The "physician bonding" strategies of the old days were generally successful, but they will not usually be a key element of the health care system of the future. This does not mean that hospitals should not be considerate of physicians and their special needs; they should. However, the relationship will be based on seeing physicians as partners, not customers.

MeritCare uses terminology such as "executive partners" for physicians and administrators working as a team to head clinic service lines (such as cardiac care, oncology, and primary care). In MeritCare and many other large integrated systems (Mayo, Dartmouth-Hitchcock, and Scott & White, for example), physicians and administrators have been partnering for years—it works. (We have more to say about this characteristic of the successful health care system of the future in Chapter Seventeen.)

Characteristic 8: Relationships Among Primary Care Physicians and Specialists

In our research and consulting, we often work in local environments where primary care physicians and medical specialists are feuding and have lost respect for each other. However, when we work with more sophisticated organizations, this is not usually the case. We see mutual respect and admiration between the two groups. We know of many specialists who are appreciative of primary care doctors and vice versa. We also observe in many systems that nurses are not playing significant roles in management and decision making. By way of contrast, at the Mayo Clinic in Rochester, Minnesota, the top nurse executive has an office next to the CEO, and nurses serve on many key committees.

It is difficult to conceive of a health care system of the future where primary care physicians, specialists, nurses, and other clinicians are not coordinating their efforts and working smoothly as a team. There is no other way to meet consumer needs and successfully compete. What will it take for this to happen? The first step is viewing consumers, employers, and other payers as customers who have needs that can best be met by teams, or "microsystems of care," representing various medical specialties, including nurses. Some of the large integrated systems that have invested heavily in the development of care process models (often referred to as "clinical guidelines") have found that the process of developing guidelines brings various specialists and other health professionals together; this can be a way to take the first step.

In some markets health plans have driven a wedge between primary care physicians and specialists. The use of gatekeepers or the capitation of primary care networks are examples. The way financial incentives are structured—primary care physicians have an incentive to keep patients away from specialists—is another source of friction. The health system of the future will have to work hard to avoid situations where it is possible for health plans to split various medical specialties and divide physicians and hospitals.

Characteristic 9: Enhancement of Performance and Processes

We include in the category of process enhancement clinical as well as administrative processes. On the administrative side, one hospital CEO told us that he believes most health systems have already made substantial cuts in administrative costs and that there is little left in the way of potential to reduce expenses. We do not accept this point of view, especially for a future likely to be dominated by IT and automation. For most systems, however, clinical improvement represents the biggest potential payoff in terms of positioning the organization for the future. There are more dollars to be saved, and greater potential for improving both quality and cost-effectiveness, in clinical settings.

We do not view performance and process enhancement initiatives as "either-or" propositions. We think these kinds of initiatives are needed regardless of what the future brings. They make sense in both clinical and administrative areas under any scenario. We are concerned, however, that some hospitals, medical groups, and health systems are taking administrative process improvement to an extreme—investing in lowering costs and improving efficiency without adequate concern about positioning the organization for the future. We see the need for balance in the new health care marketplace.

Characteristic 10: Well-Designed Facilities

We worked with a Midwest medical group that wanted to build "the hospital of the future." Although this type of hospital was never clearly defined, it had these characteristics:

- Attractive design and modern construction
- Adequate parking and convenience
- Single-patient rooms
- Excellent lighting, heating, and air conditioning, attractive food service facilities, and other amenities
- State-of-the-art medical technology
- Extensive infrastructure for use of the Internet and information systems
- Excellent work flow for physicians and nurses

Many hospitals in the United States border on being obsolete and are badly in need of renovation or replacement. How much longer can these organizations maintain their accreditation, staffing, and market share without investing large sums of money in facilities and equipment?

J. Daniel Beckham (1999, p. 48), president of a strategic consulting company, says, "New facilities have provided one of the most effective avenues to new (or retained) market share. . . . A new highly visible facility usually speaks more loudly than any amount of advertising can about the environment of care the community can expect. And in smaller communities a new hospital can be a point of considerable civic pride." One health system CEO in New England told us something similar: "I think it is critical that we have one or more projects going on around here all the time. Not only do we need these upgrades, but it communicates to our employees, physicians, and patients that we are on the move."

The leaders of Dartmouth-Hitchcock credit their move from downtown Hanover to a large campus in nearby Lebanon, New Hampshire, with aiding in the clinical coordination of care and with fundamentally changing the organization. The physical proximity of the medical school, physicians, nurses, and administrators in the new building and the flow of patients were instrumental in achieving a restructuring of the enterprise.

An examination of the economic factors that make or break most health care systems shows that facility costs are not high on the list. For example, facility expenses are not in the same ballpark as labor and salary-related expenses in the hospital's overall cost structure. CEOs who have advocated investing in new facilities often report that the operating efficiencies more than make up for the added interest expense on debt incurred to modernize facilities.

Characteristic 11: Prevention and Wellness

Consumer research conducted over the past decade has shown that consumers place a high value on prevention and wellness. Our experience in conducting focus group interviews, especially with women, bears this out. Regardless of the health care topic being discussed, it almost always comes back to questions of prevention and wellness. This is what most women are vitally interested in, not just for themselves but for their families.

The frustration for most health systems is that there is little or no revenue to be generated from wellness and prevention. Money is made when people get sick. Capitated payment was supposed to change this, but capitation has stalled, and the future of this payment mechanism is in doubt. What will it take, then, for wellness and prevention to represent a viable market strategy for health systems?

It is quite possible that as consumers gain more control over how their health care dollars are spent, they will respond to programs that offer prevention as well as nonacute and acute care. The growth in use of personal trainers during the 1990s suggests that many consumers are willing to pay, out of their pockets, for services that help them improve their physical condition. (There are reported to be one hundred thousand personal trainers at work in this country.)

One of the challenges facing hospitals, medical groups, and other providers is how to offer prevention and wellness services on an economically feasible basis. Thus far, few employers or health plans have provided financial incentives for employees or plan members to take better care of themselves. One rural hospital offers employees of the largest employer in the area a 15 percent discount on health plan premiums if the employees are involved in some sort of wellness program—a hopeful sign. There are opportunities for innovative approaches that convert the desire for prevention and wellness into a viable business.

Characteristic 12: Superior Service, Convenience, and Access

No one in health care is satisfied with levels of service. The standards are not high in many organizations, and role models are few and far between. One physician leader of a large system told us that there are no easy solutions for improving service: "You just have to keep working at it, keep talking about it and educating new employees."

Another CEO believes that a major opportunity for improving service and access lies in the Internet. He said:

> When consumers schedule their appointments, we will e-mail them a confirmation that includes a map of how to get here, a code that gets them into the parking lot, and a picture and bio of the physician they will be seeing. When they drive into the parking lot, this will alert the office that they are on the property. In this way we can escort them directly to an examination room without a wait in the lobby. We won't give them a clipboard and ask them to provide a lot of information; this will either be done in advance or the data will be in the computer. When they finish their appointment, they

will be given key words for accessing information on the Internet about any physical problems they have. I will personally send them an e-mail that night thanking them for their business and inviting comments about the quality of service.

We devoted Chapter Three to consumers' need for service, convenience, and access. Suffice it to say that the health care system of the future must give a high priority to improving service, convenience, and access.

Characteristic 13: Complementary and Alternative Medicine

We believe that during the initial years of the new millennium, an increasing number of health care organizations will find ways to integrate their clinical services with those of CAM providers. It is already happening. Some physicians are partnering with providers of CAM, and some health plans (such as Kaiser Permanente in California) are offering limited CAM benefits.

One health system CEO observed, "We need to find new revenue sources. Don't be surprised if half of the new dollars are in areas that are not traditional to the services we presently offer." With a high proportion of consumers using both traditional medicine and CAM, the traditional and nontraditional worlds of health care are unlikely to continue to go in different directions. Consumers will drive the integration of CAM and traditional medicine. As discussed in Chapter Eleven, we anticipate many more medical groups will include CAM in the medical services they offer. We expect physicians and medical groups to seize this opportunity.

Characteristic 14: Outstanding Management

Outstanding management may be the most important factor of all. The commitment of the governing board, a strong CEO and management team, and exceptional physician leaders will be key to success in the health care system of the future.

Board Support

The CEO of a multihospital system told us, "Before I was asked to be CEO of this system, I was a consultant. I had seen a lot of different situations. However, I didn't realize the importance of one factor—board support of the CEO." He added, "We could not have accomplished the transformation of this system without board support every step of the way. The board had many opportunities to back down on certain initiatives, but they have stayed the course."

Recruitment and Retention of Top-Notch Health Care Managers

Why is it that some hospitals and health systems are able to attract and retain high-caliber CEOs and management teams? Although there are many factors at work (such as location, compensation, size and market position of the organization, and quality of the governing board), one factor seems to us to be at or near the top of the list—the opportunity to respond to challenges, meet needs in the market area, and build a superior system.

The chief operating officer of a hospital system had been on the job less than a year. He had come from a large hospital located eighty miles away in a large metropolitan area. Why did he make the move? In his words, he "got tired of working at a place where so much energy was devoted to moaning and groaning about unfair reimbursement of Medicare and managed care plans. There was a 'victim mentality' about the place, and it was depressing. It is like we have to accept the hand dealt to us and can't take the actions needed to gain control of our future."

Careful Allocation of Resources

Part of the formula for success of skilled health care managers is allocating financial resources, assigning accountability, and measuring performance. One physician leader noted that any successful organization should have rigorous criteria for return on investment for both proposed new ventures and current businesses. He said, "There also needs to be accountability for financial performance and no glossing over poor performance relative to budgets."

The CEO of a hospital system in the southeastern United States was well known among his staff for keeping a sharp eye on the numbers. The chief financial officer of the system told us, "Our CEO has the mentality of a controller. Furthermore, he strongly believes that every business unit should show a positive return on investment. He doesn't believe in subsidizing unprofitable operations."

Chapter Thirteen contains more detail on the characteristics of successful managers for the new health care marketplace, and Chapter Fourteen deals with governing boards. Strong governance, leadership, and management will definitely be needed in the health care system of the future.

Conclusions

Arguments about the merits of different types of vertical integration strategies and about whether hospitals should "get back to the basics" or become involved in a plethora of other activities do not address the questions most pertinent to the health care marketplace of the future. The key questions most health systems should ask themselves are these: Do we have, or can we develop, the core values needed for long-term survival in a dramatically changing health care marketplace? What will it take—including financial resources and management skills—for us to position ourselves to be successful in the future? Our suggestion is this: forget the old labels and arguments, and adopt the approaches that best meet the needs of customers today and in the future.

Some of the characteristics of the health system of the future will be similar to those of mature integrated systems—a strong culture and core values, physician and administrative teams, physicians and hospitals partnering to meet customer needs, elimination of friction between primary care physicians, nurses, and specialists, and excellent geographical coverage of the local market. Other characteristics, such as developing centers of excellence, partnering with CAM providers, improving facilities and services, acquiring technology, and focusing on market segmentation, are not the sole province of integrated systems. Organizations that want to maintain their own identities can take on many of these characteristics.

Health care is ready for a new type of organization that might be referred to as the *multidisciplinary clinical enterprise* of the future. The term *integrated system* is controversial and conjures up images of the failed PHOs and integration efforts of many hospitals and physicians in the middle to late 1990s. The other extreme is focused factories (single-specialty medical groups), which do not lead to clinical integration, do not usually help patients with multiple diagnoses, and definitely do not meet the needs of people who live in less populated areas. A new type of organization is needed—the consumer- and technology-focused multidisciplinary clinical enterprise.

Chapter Seventeen

Health Care Myths and Realities

The more I work in health care, the more I realize the extent of vested interests in maintaining the status quo. With a $1.3 trillion industry, lots of people and organizations aren't that interested in seeing massive change.
PHYSICIAN-ADMINISTRATOR OF A LARGE MULTISTATE
HEALTH PLAN, Summer 2000

We find there are many "vested interests" in understanding how the health care system works and where it is headed in the future. Many health plan executives, physicians, and hospital administrators become uneasy when the talk turns to the growing importance of consumerism and technology and what will be required to be successful in light of fundamental market shifts, both nationally and in local markets. Of course, among our objectives in writing this book is to challenge conventional thinking and to suggest other possibilities that may emerge.

This chapter presents our nominees for the ten most common myths and the ten key economic realities in health care relevant to the first five years of the new millennium. Having read this far, the reader may now ask, "So what does this all mean for the future of health care?" In a sense, our assessment of these myths and realities represents an answer to that question.

Health Care Myths

Our top ten health care myths are summarized in Exhibit 17.1 and discussed in the paragraphs that follow.

Myth 1: Physicians Are the Most Important Market for Hospitals

A key question for any health care organization is who are its customers. Are they health plans, consumers, employers, or physicians?

The conclusion for many hospitals is that "physicians are still our most important customers. Our success is directly tied to their practices and admission patterns. If we do whatever we can to make them successful, we will do well." Most hospitals, and especially their boards and CEOs, have been hurt emotionally and financially by physicians establishing enterprises that compete with the hospital. These include ambulatory surgery and imaging centers, rehabilitation facilities, cardiac services, and laboratories. Unfortunately, simply having excellent relationships with physicians—the hospital's "best customers"—does not necessarily slow the proliferation of these physician-owned, for-profit ventures.

Exhibit 17.1. Ten Health Care Myths, 2001–2005.

1. Physicians are the most important market for hospitals.
2. "Focused factories" are the best way to deliver medical services.
3. Private sector health plans are more efficient than Medicare.
4. Vertical integration is a failed strategy.
5. Without capitation there is little hope of controlling costs.
6. The quality of care provided under managed care, particularly HMOs, is substandard.
7. Health care is a commodity, with price being the most important consideration.
8. There is a shortage of primary care physicians.
9. Focusing on "the basics" is sufficient.
10. The health care industry is in decline and disa

One of the differentiating factors between hospitals and true integrated systems is their respective views about the role of physicians. In the more advanced integrated systems, physicians either drive the organization or are partners with the administration and board; employers, health plans, and consumers are the customers. There is a big difference between being a partner in a business and being a customer.

If physicians are the primary customers, what about the movement toward consumerism and greater empowerment of consumers? Are consumers, then, competing with physicians as the best customers of hospitals? It will be difficult, if not impossible, for a hospital to meet the needs of consumers if physicians are not clearly seen as partners in the effort.

In the future, consumers will have more choice, not less. There will be plenty of hospitals and medical groups seeking their business, and geographical advantage will not mean as much as it has in the past. In other words, neither physicians nor hospitals can count on retaining their base of patients because of their locational advantage. Telemedicine, prescriptions over the Internet, telehealth, outside disease management programs, patients controlling their own medical records, prestigious tertiary care centers and medical groups vying for business in larger and larger service areas—these are the realities of the new health care marketplace.

We believe that a better alternative is for physicians and hospitals in a local market to sit down together and jointly develop strategies for the future. As we discuss in Chapter Seven, this might lead to the development of a new type of PHO. Some key questions physicians and hospitals could jointly address are the following:

- How can we do a better job of meeting the needs of the customers—purchasing coalitions, health plans, employers, and consumers—in our market?
- What can we do to gain competitive advantage and differentiate ourselves from the host of new physician and hospital competitors?
- How can we make sure we have the capital needed to develop the information systems, new programs, and other initiatives we need to be successful?

Myth 2: "Focused Factories" Are the Best Way to Deliver Medical Services

The thesis of Regina Herzlinger's popular 1997 book *Market Driven Health Care* is that "focused factories" (medical service firms that focus on a single disease) are the best way to deliver medical services. She makes compelling arguments about the higher levels of service and operating efficiencies possible in focused factories. In Herzlinger's view a substantial portion of all health care services would be best delivered in focused factories, such as specialty clinics for hernia repair, cosmetic surgery, or outpatient orthopedics and organizations like MedCath, a PPM that manages all heart services from routine checkups to open-heart surgery and inpatient hospitalization.

Herzlinger makes several interesting points and is an excellent speaker and advocate of her central theme. Nonetheless, we find her views about the way health care should be organized to be unrealistic. This is not to say that focused factories in cardiac services, orthopedics, or pediatrics do not make sense in certain markets. In our view, however, the kinds of solutions she advocates are applicable to less than 10 percent of all health care services.

Herzlinger suggests an approach that, if enacted, would be devastating to many community hospitals, primary care physician practices, multispecialty groups, and residents of areas without a large population base, where only a limited number of focused factories may make economic sense. Many rural hospitals, fighting for their survival, are already concerned about patients leaving for larger and more sophisticated medical centers (for example, patients in southern Maine or New Hampshire leaving to receive care in Boston). Herzlinger's remedy for the U.S. health care system also gives insufficient attention to the fact that a number of medical problems do not fall within the purview of a focused factory. For example, many elderly patients require treatment for multiple ailments.

For Herzlinger to argue that focused factories are superior to integrated health care systems, such as Marshfield in Wisconsin, Scott & White in Texas, the Cleveland Clinic in Ohio, or Carle in Illinois, is to miss the point. (At the same time that Herzlinger speaks disparagingly of large integrated systems, she is an advocate of the Mayo Foundation. In our view the multispecialty Mayo Clinic is a prime example of a large integrated system.) We believe that the potential to improve the performance of the U.S. health care system lies in coordination of care, seamless delivery of services, clinical integration, and measurement of outcomes. Focused factories can contribute to the solution but are far from the complete answer.

Myth 3: Private Sector Health Plans Are More Efficient Than Medicare

Richard Huber (1999), former chairman and CEO of Aetna U.S. Healthcare, asked this question: "How many business leaders worried about health costs are willing to test the assertion that a government monopoly (the same people who brought you $600 toilet seats) would add less overhead than a private system where hundreds of health plans compete for their business?" Huber's assertion that the present fragmented health care system has less overhead than a single-payer system is accepted by many; however, it is a myth of vast proportions. One of the factors leading to the defeat of the Clinton health care reform proposal was opponents' success in labeling it a "government takeover of health care," with the implication of gross inefficiencies. The fact is that government-run programs like Medicare operate with far less overhead than many private health plans, even when allowances are made for differences in the services they provide.

The administrative overhead associated with most managed care plans is high. This overhead has several components: health plan administration (around 9 to 12 percent for the best-managed plans, but often more), expenses incurred by physicians for maintaining a network (such as an IPA or PHO) to contract with health plans, additional employees in physician offices, and the costs to employers of administering a variety of plans for the benefit of employees. If you included the additional administrative burden for consumers (time spent waiting on the phone or going through a primary care gatekeeper), the total overhead associated with the managed care model would easily exceed 25 percent.

An open letter from fourteen nationally known health care leaders to Congress and the executive branch, urging more financing for staffing of the Health Care Financing Administration (HCFA), said, "When HCFA was created in 1977, Medicare spending totaled $21.5 billion, the number of beneficiaries served was twenty-six million, and the agency had a staff of about 4,000 full-time equivalent workers. By 1997 Medicare spending had increased almost tenfold to $207 billion, the number of beneficiaries served had grown to thirty-nine million, but the agency's workforce was actually smaller than it had been two decades earlier" (Butler and others, 1999, p. 9). Concerning the administrative overhead associated with Medicare, Donna Shalala, secretary of health and human services, said, "People just can't get the stereotype of big bureaucracy out of their heads. And the idea that Medicare's administrative expenses are 3 or 4 percent while the private sector spends 12 percent just doesn't register with many people, particularly those who see healthcare as a business" (Shalala and Reinhardt, 1999, p. 50).

Today's managed care systems do offer choices and perform services that Medicare does not. However, they are drastically more expensive, and there are other alternatives. For example, the administrative expenses associated with running the Buyer's Health Care Action Group (BHCAG) in Minnesota are around 10 percent. Consumers have decision-making power over which "care system" they want. This simplifies the task of employers' human resources departments. If consumers think the administrative hassles of their care system are too great, they can easily switch to one of the other fourteen alternatives.

Of course, simplifying the health care system is one of the primary goals of those who advocate the single-payer system. We believe that those who prefer alternatives to a single-payer model (including the authors of this book) share the burden of proof as far as finding ways to reduce the overhead and complexity associated with the present U.S. health care system.

IT offers an incredible opportunity to lower costs in the health care system. In doing so, it will be necessary to make drastic changes to today's managed care plans. Information technology that exists today—and is already used to cut costs in other industries—is capable of dramatically reducing costs in health care in many ways:

- Tracking and verifying consumers' health plan information, including eligibility, plan types, and plan reimbursement characteristics

- Tracking and managing referrals, precertifications, postcertifications, and second opinions
- Analyzing the effectiveness of precertifications and other approaches to managed care and designing better, faster, and cheaper options
- Identifying physicians, facilities, and other care providers with an unusually high error rate, cost of care, or number of customer complaints
- Processing payments to providers more accurately, quickly, and cheaply
- Facilitating more customer choice and less administrative intervention between customers and their care

Myth 4: Vertical Integration Is a Failed Strategy

The poor financial performance and "disintegration" of many "integrated" systems provide the skeptics and naysayers with plenty of ammunition for the argument that vertical integration is a failed strategy. As a result, many governing boards and physician leaders of hospital-driven integrated systems have lost confidence in vertical integration. However, our continuing research into the performance of vertically integrated systems paints a different picture. We believe that with the right leadership (with physicians almost always playing a key role, usually as partners with professional administrators), well-designed governance and management structures, and in the right markets, vertically integrated systems are capable of delivering high levels of quality and service and earning adequate financial returns.

We are especially optimistic about integrated systems led by large multispecialty clinics. Examples include Mayo, Marshfield, Fallon, MeritCare, Cleveland Clinic, Henry Ford, Dartmouth-Hitchcock, and Scott & White. Physician leadership is a key ingredient for success in vertical integration, and these types of clinics have strong physician leaders and internal structures (for example, physician-led committees) that ensure a future supply of leaders. Furthermore, these leaders have many years of experience in working together. Critics of integrated health care who fail to differentiate between large hospital systems that are attempting to become integrated and those organizations led by strong physician groups (such as those just listed) confuse the issue, misleading many hospital governing boards and doing a disservice to a promising alternative form of health care delivery.

Many of the clinic-led systems can provide reams of customer surveys, and plenty of hard data based on utilization and growth in patient visits, showing that large numbers of consumers prefer a coordinated, seamless system of care. Our research indicates that these systems are typically growing and increasing their share of the markets they serve. One of the major problems for several of these organizations is that they cannot keep up with the growing demand for their services. At the same time, the leaders of these types of more advanced integrated systems would be the first to acknowledge that there are tremendous opportunities for improving quality of care, coordination, service, and cost-effectiveness. They are often frustrated at how long it takes to improve health care delivery, even when the system controls all or most of the elements of production.

One conclusion we draw is that what is important and enduring is what a health care system does. Does it, for example, promote cooperation and partnership between physicians and other health care managers in identifying and meeting the needs of customers in a faster, better, and cheaper way? What is less important is what legal form a health care system adopts. Whether the health plan, hospital, and physicians are in one organization or three is significant only to the degree that it affects performance. And it is not clear that the optimum organizational structure is the same in every situation.

A second conclusion is that it is premature to judge vertical integration a failure. It has taken Henry Ford Health System, Mayo, Marshfield, Scott & White, and many of the other physician-led systems a long time to get where they are today. Hospitals and multi-hospital systems that began pursuing vertical integration in the early 1990s have not been at it long enough for anyone to conclude whether it makes sense in their specific markets. Patience and a desire to keep innovating are the keys here. For some situations these systems still offer by far the most attractive business model.

Myth 5: Without Capitation There Is Little Hope of Controlling Costs

Paying medical groups and hospitals a fixed amount per member per month certainly continues to be one option for controlling costs. Capitation aligns financial incentives in the sense that there are motivations to avoid the overdiagnosis and overtreatment of patients. Under capitation there are strong incentives for physicians to develop clinical guidelines, telephone triage, and other initiatives to serve patients economically.

By contrast, the predominant fee-for-service system of payment, whether through a PPO or old-fashioned indemnity insurance, does not appropriately align financial incentives. There are strong incentives for physicians and hospitals to provide more services and thus maximize their revenues, and there is plenty of evidence that this is exactly what has happened over the past twenty years. And with the lack of growth in capitation, unexplained clinical variation continues to be a serious problem for the U.S. health care system.

However, there are other, promising approaches that may emerge in a system that gives the consumer an incentive to control costs, such as vouchers, provider-sponsored health plans, defined contributions, and disease management for chronic illnesses.

Vouchers

Voucher-type approaches appear to have potential. The pioneering work of BHCAG, with its voucherlike Choice Plus plan, is an example. BHCAG does an excellent job of providing physicians and hospitals with incentives to improve quality and service and reduce costs. Furthermore, employees and their families have the responsibility of making the trade-offs among quality, service, and cost and then deciding which of a number of available care systems to select. All of this is accomplished with self-insured employers who are at risk financially for the results of the system—and with a minimum of fuss and muss.

Provider-Sponsored Health Plans

Provider-sponsored health plans can align incentives and promote innovation. Owning a health plan is another way for a health care system or network of physicians and hospitals to align financial incentives. Despite the skepticism about provider-owned health plans, there are numerous examples of medical groups and integrated systems that own their own health plans (such as Scott & White Health Plan, Geisinger Health Plan, Marshfield's Security Health Plan, and Carle's Health Alliance Medical Plan). Under these models there are financial incentives to make the health plan work. To succeed, there has to be a cooperative effort between physicians and hospitals, which also own all or part of the health plan, to control the medical loss ratio and overhead. In other words, the goals of the health plan, medical group, and hospital are in harmony.

As noted in earlier chapters, we also recognize that this strategy has been falling out of favor and that more provider organizations are discontinuing health plans than are establishing new ones. This is unfortunate, but it is the reality of the early years of the twenty-first century.

Defined Contributions

Defined contributions, as opposed to defined benefits, can stimulate the development of new health plan options. Any of the existing or proposed approaches that use defined contributions rather than such defined benefits as paying everything that falls within the benefits definition should help align financial incentives. The consumer will be motivated to limit out-of-pocket spending that exceeds the amount of the defined contribution and is more likely to select providers with a track record of delivering high quality at reasonable costs.

Disease Management for Chronic Illnesses

Programs that focus on chronic diseases can coexist with many different payment models and still cut costs. We are encouraged by new thinking about how to organize health plans and provider groups based on serving the needs of those with chronic diseases. As we discussed in Chapter Twelve, new pricing approaches are being considered that offer consumers with chronic illnesses incentives to be served by small but select panels of physicians. It appears to us that this focus offers an opportunity to better align incentives and control costs while better serving the needs of those who most need health care.

A growing number of large health care systems are blending their clinical guidelines into disease management programs. For example, MeritCare has taken its clinical guideline on the treatment of diabetes a step further and made it available to physicians, nurses, and patients to improve day-to-day care. MeritCare is moving ahead with a similar program for congestive heart failure.

Capitation and Cost Control: Summary

The fact that payment models other than capitation will work is encouraging. It means that the inherent difficulties of implementing capitation (such as a small population base, lack of organized provider groups, and insufficient capital by medical groups that accept risk) do not doom efforts to align the financial incentives among employers, employees, consumers, physicians, and hospitals.

Myth 6: The Quality of Care Provided Under Managed Care, Particularly HMOs, Is Substandard

Many consumers and physicians believe the quality of care provided under managed care is substandard. This is partly due to the suspicion that managed care plans—at least those that pay providers on a salary or capitated basis—withhold care. However, there is plenty of objective evidence indicating that the quality of care offered by HMOs is at least as good as that offered by indemnity health plans, which pay physicians on a fee-for-service basis (thereby creating an incentive to perform more tests and procedures). Furthermore, the abuses of overtreatment—inappropriate and unnecessary care—inherent in the fee-for-service payment system for so many years, have become increasingly obvious when compared with what can be accomplished with capitation and managed care. There is a strong need for consumers to have more information and better distinguish between those HMOs that are doing a good job of facilitating good care at a reasonable cost and those that are not.

The Experience of One Large Health Plan

UnitedHealth Group, the nation's third largest HMO (with thirteen million members), says that its relationship with physicians has begun to improve the quality of care: "The contention, which defies the popular perception of HMOs as caring more about cost than quality, rests on an extensive evaluation of the performance of more than 42,000 doctors in 17 states, all participants in one or another UnitedHealth plan. The evaluation shows that those physicians are doing a better job of executing the fundamentals of medicine than when UnitedHealth conducted its first evaluation back in 1997" (Burton, 1999). The most recent information prepared by UnitedHealth shows improvement in a wide range of commonly accepted clinical measures, such as treatment of diabetes, use of mammograms, and use of beta-blockers for heart attack victims: "The clinical-performance measures that were evaluated are things doctors widely agree to be beneficial for patients" (Burton, 1999).

Quality Issues and Financial Incentives

On a broader basis Whitelaw and Warden (1999, p. 140) of the Henry Ford Health System note, "Current attacks on quality under managed care overlook quality problems throughout health care. Our attention should be focused on the quality and appropriateness of health care, which are often unrelated to current changes in financial incentive." There is little disagreement over the proposition that there is plenty of room for improvement in health care quality. However, the assertion that managed care plans provide poorer quality is, in most cases, simply not true. The evidence does not support this point of view.

Myth 7: Health Care Is a Commodity, with Price Being the Most Important Consideration

Many hospital CEOs, physician leaders, and individuals running integrated systems are deeply concerned because they perceive that their customers—employers, government payers, and consumers—only care about price. One physician told us, "I wish I could believe you that employers in our area purchase health care based on value added; all the evidence I see indicates that unit prices are 90 percent of the ball game." While we acknowledge the growing body of evidence suggesting that price is important (for example, the switch of BHCAG employees and their families from higher-priced care centers to those that are cheaper), we would have to consider health care an undifferentiated commodity in order to accept this viewpoint.

We find it difficult to think of any large industry where there are more opportunities for product differentiation than there are in health care. As we discuss in Chapter Five, the opportunities for innovation are unlimited. To equate health care with a commodity like agricultural products or raw materials (such as iron ore, wood, cement, or gravel) misses the mark, especially in an era where consumers are playing a bigger role.

In our view the problem is that those health care providers offering more added value to employers and consumers have not been able to demonstrate this to their customers. For years we have heard the excuse that data are not available to measure clinical outcomes. However, we are aware of the increasing number of both large and small health care organizations that systematically measure patient satisfaction with physicians and their offices (one important contributor to outcomes). Of course, with a shift toward consumer decision making, there will be tremendous opportunities to demonstrate value to the direct beneficiaries of health care services.

Myth 8: There Is a Shortage of Primary Care Physicians

We are continually surprised at reports we receive from various metropolitan areas, and at information we come across in our research and consulting, about physician supply and demand. In the early 1990s, at the time of the Clinton health care proposal, there was serious concern about a shortage of primary care physicians, especially in family practice, general internal medicine, pediatrics, obstetrics, and gynecology. A number of states and the federal government put pressure on medical schools to produce more primary care physicians. At the same time, it was agreed that it would take many years for the supply of primary care physicians to grow to the point where it was meeting the demand. One of the drivers, of course, was the growth of managed care, and the anticipated need for primary care physicians to serve as gatekeepers, or coordinators of care.

However, the reality of the early part of the new century is that in many parts of the country there is a more than adequate supply of primary care physicians but a serious shortage of certain types of specialists and subspecialists. For example, in Minneapolis–Saint

Paul, an area generally considered to have a serious oversupply of physicians, it is difficult to find a sufficient number of cardiologists, gastroenterologists, and otolaryngologists. One physician leader told us, "There are a number of medical schools and training programs in this area, and they produce quite a number of primary care physicians. However, the number of new specialists produced each year is a handful. Those new physicians who come out in these specialties can pretty much go where they want." This is also true in central Illinois; a physician associated with Carle Clinic told us that many specialists are in short supply and that there is an abundance of primary care physicians.

Physician supply and demand is increasingly becoming a regional issue, and it is impossible to generalize about shortages or surpluses. With few exceptions, however, the much publicized shortage of primary care physicians has not developed. And, even more surprising, we are seeing shortages of specialists in many parts of the country. This is a far cry from what was anticipated just a few short years ago.

Myth 9: Focusing on "the Basics" Is Sufficient

The importance of "getting back to the basics" is espoused by many hospital and health system CEOs and physician leaders, in part because of disappointing experiences with integration strategies (such as forming a PHO, owning a health plan, or acquiring primary care practices), mergers that are not working as expected, or (for physicians) being acquired by a PPM. The attitude is often expressed this way: "We have tried to anticipate the future, and look where it has put us. We weren't doing well financially, and then we got hammered by the BBA. We need to focus our efforts on performance improvement and get our operations back where they should be." Individuals holding this view often cite the experience of AHERF in Pennsylvania and the continued downgrading of hospital debt by rating agencies.

The physician leader of a large West Coast health system told us, "Any organization that doesn't perform well in its core businesses will not have the financial resources or management skills to experiment with new strategies." We agree with this physician's viewpoint. However, we are concerned that too much attention is being given to a "back to the basics" approach and insufficient attention to the future. Compared with what it has been in the past, health care is shaping up as a totally different industry, with new players, new rules, and new ways of keeping score. Although it may help to generate a strong bottom line in the short term (which obviously is important), going "back to the basics" does not adequately reposition an organization to handle fundamental market and technological shifts of the magnitude expected over the next few years.

Here are several "nontraditional" initiatives that need serious consideration:

- Investing in databases on consumers and in market research to determine their health care needs
- Identifying new products and services for groups of consumers who have their own money to spend on the health care services they want
- Either investing in a sophisticated management information system—what Bill Gates (1999) calls a "central nervous system" for the organization—or joining with another organization that offers this capability
- Learning how to better manage individuals with chronic diseases, who represent about one-third of all potential customers in any given service area, before outside organizations take over the management of these populations
- Identifying new ways to work with individuals and organizations that offer CAM
- Finding collaborative ways to work with competitors in providing certain types of community services

We are not suggesting that health care executives ignore the importance of strong day-to-day management. In the Middle Ages there was a saying that bad money drives out good money. In the same way, we all know that short-term pressures drive out long-term planning. To the extent that focusing on the current situation does not leave time for strategic planning, innovation, and looking outside the walls toward consumers and the rapidly changing health care environment, we think that a "back to the basics" approach may backfire. Health care systems need a balanced approach—

sufficient attention to day-to-day management without ignoring the need to begin to transform the organization for the future.

Myth 10: The Health Care Industry Is in Decline and Disarray

We often hear about the large numbers of discouraged, disillusioned, and depressed people in health care. Many individuals who leave their health care jobs are searching in other industries for work and professional satisfaction. Surveys show that two-thirds or more of all physicians are unhappy with managed care. Following the PPM debacle, which included several bankruptcies and the sudden shrinking of MedPartners, many investors (and those who advise investors) are disillusioned with health care. Hospital boards and administrators are panicked about the impact of the BBA and their ability to continue to finance what they need in the way of improvements to the physical plant, medical technology, and information systems. Employers are increasingly concerned about rising health care costs but are afraid to rock the boat for fear of losing valued employees or upsetting labor unions. Many consumers are not impressed with the level of service they receive from health plans and health care providers. On and on it goes.

One large integrated system has "joy" as part of its culture and core values. The CEO told us, "This is a difficult one. When you have just gone through a layoff, there isn't much to be happy about. While this is a good place to work, I can't really say that people here are joyful." That a large number of key health care professionals and staff have lost their enthusiasm—are just plain discouraged—is not a myth. The myth consists in the fact that perceptions about the health care system today do not match the reality of where health care is headed over the next five years.

Consider, for example, the following points:

- Health care spending is conservatively projected to increase at an annual rate of more than $100 billion during the first few years of the new century. This is on top of a base of $1.3 trillion in 2000.
- The aging of the population and improvements in longevity and quality of life for the elderly will be growing drivers of demand for health services.

- The annual rate of advances in medical technology is at an all-time high, and many new products promise better clinical outcomes with less patient discomfort and suffering.
- Many new prescription drugs promise relief from chronic conditions, and with fewer side effects.
- IT promises to make great gains in the areas of the EMR, information on clinical outcomes, and automation of processes and to allow reductions in inappropriate care, including a reduction in the number of unnecessary deaths.
- There will be major improvements in the models of organization in health care, with physicians likely to play increasingly important leadership roles.
- Consumers will be better educated and more interested in participating in their own care.

In our view these points do not add up to an industry in trouble. Instead, they suggest a rapidly growing and dynamic industry with a tremendously important role to play in society. A minority of those working in health care, but a rapidly growing group, are excited about the future of medicine.

Physicians, nurses, and staff at the Mayo Clinic in Rochester, Minnesota, are not discouraged about the future. They are concerned about how to keep up with the demand for their services. Mayo and a number of other large integrated systems led by physicians and multispecialty clinics are facing the future optimistically. They feel good about the results they are achieving and are excited about the opportunities to do more for their patients. At Mayo and many other successful health care systems, the focus is on the patient. All other matters are of secondary importance. Perhaps this is the key to regaining an optimistic view of the future for most of those in health care.

Economic Realities for Health Care

Our list of the top economic realities that we believe will affect health care in the twenty-first century are summarized in Exhibit 17.2 and described in the paragraphs that follow.

Exhibit 17.2. Ten Economic Realities, 2001–2005.

1. The combination of more demanding consumers and technology will affect every hospital, medical group, and health plan.

2. Investor-owned hospitals, health plans, and medical groups will continue to produce disappointing financial results.

3. It is time for physicians' expectations to become more reasonable.

4. Hospitals' share of total health care spending will continue to decline.

5. Modifying the BBA will not, by itself, save hospitals.

6. There are opportunities, and a critical need, to focus on reducing clinical variation.

7. Health care consolidation will create opportunities to develop niche markets.

8. Many of the growth opportunities in health care will be based on the Internet, advances in medical technology, and new drugs.

9. Health care will increasingly involve quality of life.

10. Health care will experience a fundamental market shift during the first five years of the new millennium.

Reality 1: The Combination of More Demanding Consumers and Technology Will Affect Every Hospital, Medical Group, and Health Plan

The growth of consumerism and the development of technology will affect every hospital, medical group, and health plan. To think otherwise is unrealistic. We acknowledge that it is impossible to predict or visualize much more than the general parameters of the future impact of consumerism and technology; that is why we have considered several scenarios. One thing, however, is clear: a fundamental market shift is inevitable.

The Health Care Advisory Board (1999, p. viii) says that many hospital CEOs are concerned about how far the consumer impulse will go and worry that service levels at their institutions may not measure up to future market demands: "For most hospitals, these worries appear misplaced. The Advisory Board believes that the up-tick in consumerism is unlikely to revolutionize hospital economics for the foreseeable future. Physicians, not consumers, will continue to be the ultimate arbiters of hospital selection, while the minority of patients who elect to choose hospitals themselves are likely to base their decisions on clinical reputation rather than service excellence." We take a contrary view. The increase in consumerism in health care would be more accurately characterized as an *explosion* than an up-tick. Hospital CEOs *should* be worried about service excellence and the clinical reputations of their organizations.

Our viewpoint is supported by a survey of 321 health care exec-utives conducted by KPMG (1998, p. 4). On a scale from 1 to 5, with 5 being complete agreement and 1 being disagreement, KPMG found very high agreement with these two statements: "Health care organizations will develop new products, offer more choice, and pro-vide service enhancements to respond directly to consumer pref-erences" (the mean score of agreement was 4.69) and "Health care organizations will increasingly invest in feedback mechanisms to assure they are 'in touch' with consumer needs and meeting their expectations" (the mean score of agreement was 4.76).

In our view the changes are already arriving on the scene. The likely response of many hospitals, medical groups, and health plans will lead to tremendous improvements in the health of con-sumers and to greater satisfaction on the part of many physicians and leaders of health care provider organizations. We are opti-mistic in this area.

Reality 2: Investor-Owned Hospitals, Health Plans, and Medical Groups Will Continue to Produce Disappointing Financial Results

The track record of for-profit hospital systems and PPMs does noth-ing to instill confidence that investor ownership makes sense for most hospitals and medical groups. Investor-owned organizations have yet to prove they can bring more added value and better man-agement to hospitals and physician practices. A large part of the problem is meeting Wall Street expectations for ever-increasing revenues and earnings, which affect the market value of most stocks. We have already seen the troubles experienced by Columbia/HCA, PhyCor, and many other publicly owned PPMs in trying to live up to investors' expectations.

For most hospitals, medical groups, and health plans, there are too many external variables affecting operations to make revenues and earnings predictable year in and year out. For health plans there is the historical underwriting cycle of three good years followed by three poor ones. Hospitals that push hard to increase earnings run the risk of violating fraud and abuse laws and being reported for lack of compliance with Medicare rules. For most medical groups, outside pressures on billing rates and the coming and going of key physicians make predictability difficult.

In the present U.S. health care system, community not-for-profit hospitals are at financial risk for their performance. If they experience a succession of good years, they have the opportunity to accumulate cash and reserves that can be used for new technology, rehabilitation of older facilities, and expansion. When the inevitable poor years hit, they have to find ways to reduce operating expenses or draw down reserves. But this is a community decision as reflected by the hospital board.

Physicians in medical groups are also responsible for their financial performance. If earnings are down, bonuses and other cash distributions are eliminated; there may even be salary cuts and layoffs. In good times physicians can increase their take-home pay or set aside reserves (which is not done often, but we are encouraged to see a tiny trend developing in this direction).

Some health plans are part of much larger insurance companies, like Aetna U.S. Healthcare and CIGNA, and are able to weather the wide fluctuations in earnings inherent in health care. The more focused health plans have incentives to merge with stronger plans, improve market positioning, gain more leverage over providers, and increase financial reserves. These types of organizations need access to outside equity capital. However, shareholders should expect large fluctuations in share price.

Reality 3: It Is Time for Physicians' Expectations to Become More Reasonable

When we say physicians' expectations need to become more reasonable, we are talking primarily about physicians' expectations regarding earnings potential, practice styles, and independence. Although not true for every physician, for many the practice styles they had planned to develop and the income they had hoped to earn from a career in medicine are unlikely to materialize. The result will be many unhappy, disillusioned, and depressed physicians. We are already seeing this happen in many markets.

Here is the way the situation was described to us by the physician leader of an integrated system comprising over seven hundred physicians: "The morale of our physicians has been declining for several years. They feel undervalued. Many physicians went into medical practice for the intellectual challenges, the opportunity to be of service, and financial security. They don't have the options they had at one time; the grass is *not* greener on the other side of the fence. So they feel like they are stuck in a bad situation." This physician said that the key is managing physicians' expectations and that this begins with a recognition that expectations have to change: "Physicians are not going to make the kind of money they have in the past, and they are not going to enjoy the independence in clinical decision making that they have experienced or hoped to experience."

We observed the clash between expectations and economic reality in working with a professional society of five thousand board-certified plastic surgeons. Many plastic surgeons prefer reconstructive surgery, but reimbursement is relatively poor. The money is in cosmetic surgery, but this is less challenging and not as professionally rewarding.

Economic reality 3 may seem unduly pessimistic considering our overall assessment of the rapid growth and changing nature of the new health care marketplace. However, we anticipate increased competition for physicians coming from many directions—CAM providers, physician's assistants, nurse practitioners, and consumers themselves (for example, through increased use of the Internet and self-care). The ability of consumers to obtain prescriptions over the Internet is an increasing source of competition. Personal trainers may even be competitors for some primary care physicians.

We also anticipate more recognition of the top-performing physicians and medical groups by health plans and other payers. Payment methods are likely to reward those physicians who have a demonstrable track record of producing both the best clinical outcomes and the highest proportion of satisfied patients. Physicians who are unable to enter these elite medical groups are the ones most likely to earn less than they expected.

Reality 4: Hospitals' Share of Total Health Care Spending Will Continue to Decline

Hospitals' share of health care spending has dropped from 40 percent in 1980 to 32 percent in 2000, and it is likely to drop to below 28 percent by 2005. Of course, these percentages represent a smaller share of a rapidly expanding market, so the news is not all bad.

We are concerned about the future of many small hospitals serving a high proportion of older residents. The cumulative effect of new drugs will be to keep people out of hospitals. Given that most prescription drugs are consumed by those on Medicare, hospitals with a high proportion of Medicare patients are likely to lose proportionately more patients. This can make a significant difference when many hospitals are operating with little or no margin.

One physician leader with experience in rural areas told us, "Many rural hospitals have become community care centers. The primary care physicians' offices are right in the hospital, and a long-term care facility is physically attached. These organizations often provide home health and work closely with county health departments." He added, "In many respects these smaller organizations represent a model for the future."

We agree. However, smaller hospitals will need to move even more aggressively to develop new roles in their service areas—be it the role of safety net, integrator of care, outpatient services provider, or community health care center. The inpatient business will continue to decline; there is not much question about that.

Reality 5: Modifying the Balanced Budget Act of 1997 Will Not, by Itself, Save Hospitals

The comments of many hospital CEOs and others representing the hospital industry make it seem as though relief from the payment limitations of the BBA would be sufficient to secure the financial future of hospitals, especially academic medical centers and rehabilitation facilities. Although we agree that additional relief beyond that granted in 1999 is warranted, we believe there is much more to the issue of the future financial viability of hospitals.

Hospitals brought on their own problems. Many of the health care policy experts we interviewed in connection with this book believe that hospitals brought their financial woes on themselves by acquiring money-losing physician practices, making low-cost deals with managed care plans, starting their own health plans, pouring money into poorly conceived information systems, and investing in ventures with little or no chance of offering a reasonable return on investment. One Washington-based policy expert put it this way: "Since Medicare has been one of the best payers for several years, hospitals expect the government to continue to bail them out from the bad decisions they have made across the board. While there will undoubtedly be some relief, we aren't very sympathetic."

The solution for hospital economic viability is multifaceted. The economic realities facing hospitals have both revenue and expense implications; in most cases expanding the revenue side has the greatest potential for long-term financial benefits. In many cases the potential for reducing costs, other than by cutting out entire departments and outreach services, is minimal. As one CEO put it, "If our only strategy is to cut costs, we will disappear."

We were impressed that Scripps Health in San Diego was able to terminate over 100 managed care contracts in mid-1999 and renegotiate almost all of them by the end of the year. The benefit to the hospital system was that the proportion of revenues from capitated contracts (most of which were unprofitable) dropped from 28 percent in 1997 to three to four percent.

With the health care market growing at the rate of $100 billion a year, it appears to us that revenue-generating opportunities, including the strategy of renegotiating unfavorable contracts, are the order of the day. Of course, there are also significant prospects in outpatient services and in providing services that improve the quality of life for persons living in the local market.

Reality 6: There Are Opportunities, and a Critical Need, to Focus on Reducing Clinical Variation

We have previously referred to the Dartmouth studies of clinical variation in small geographical areas (Dartmouth Medical School, 1999) and the comments of many in health care about the tremendous amount of clinical variation that continues to plague the U.S. health care system. The best estimates indicate that inappropriate and unnecessary care accounts for one-quarter to one-third of all health care spending.

Most physician leaders believe that there are substantial opportunities to reduce clinical variation. The ability of the health care system to successfully attack clinical variation will be facilitated by improvements in clinical information systems leading to better and more accessible databases and by changing financial incentives from payers. For example, as noted earlier, we expect major efforts to focus on those individuals who are heavy users of the health care system—those with chronic diseases and serious illnesses and a few others who are simply taking advantage of the system. Unfortunately, some of the individuals in the latter group are encouraged by their physicians.

Coordination of care is part of the answer to the problem of clinical variation. Differences in the training of physicians are a major cause of clinical variation. A number of large organizations are attacking this issue by establishing their own in-house "universities," or physician-training programs.

Reality 7: Health Care Consolidation Will Create Opportunities to Develop Niche Markets

Although hospital consolidation slowed in 1998 and 1999, we expect to see continued consolidation in the new century. It is not unreasonable to expect half a dozen major health plans to emerge, with two or three of them dominating individual markets. Despite impressive consolidation during the 1990s, medical groups and physician practices are still fragmented, and consolidation will continue.

Along with hospital, health plan, and physician consolidation, there will be opportunities for niche players. We saw it in banking in the 1980s and 1990s. As large national and international banking organizations acquired statewide and smaller banking organizations, there were numerous opportunities for the formation of new banks that focused on specific types of services and market segments (for example, private banking for wealthy individuals, children's banks, women's banks, and now Internet-only banks).

With the consolidation in health care, we are likely to see more specialty hospitals and strong single-specialty medical groups serving specific market areas. This is not necessarily in the best interests of acute care hospitals and integrated systems, but we expect consumers to support many of these specialized facilities and clinics. As noted earlier, we disagree with Herzlinger that this is the way that health care must go to satisfy consumers. At the same time, we acknowledge the existence of specific opportunities.

Reality 8: Many of the Growth Opportunities in Health Care Will Be Based on the Internet, Advances in Medical Technology, and New Drugs

The factors driving growth in health care spending are numerous and fundamental: aging of the population, growth in drugs and medical technology, failure of managed care and other programs to stem the long-term growth in costs, the complexity of the system leading to frustration and high administrative expenses, and the structure of the health care system (for example, first-dollar coverage shielding employees from the total costs and consumer demand for more and more health care services).

Where will the best growth opportunities be? The obvious choices are outpatient diagnostic services and surgery, long-term care (assisted living, congregate care, nursing home care), telehealth, medical groups, discretionary services (such as cosmetic surgery), new drugs, and health information and education.

For some health care organizations, international markets represent a new and exciting opportunity, especially when the worldwide economy is strong. Kevin Fickenscher, M.D., senior vice president of CareInsite and former leader of health systems in California and Wisconsin, believes that the international health care market will become enormous. "This could eventually overshadow the U.S. market, where 6 percent of the world population lives," he said (interview, July 1999).

Fickenscher's point is that international health care could become more than just a marginal business for a few prestigious organizations. The worldwide market goes beyond just a few organizations and may be open for many medical groups and health systems that, without the Internet, would never have considered such a possibility. Perhaps the sister city program involving many U.S. and overseas communities could be a model.

Reality 9: Health Care Will Increasingly Involve Quality of Life

Yes, health care continues to be concerned about healing those who are sick. But several of the growth segments of health care are prevention, CAM, and medical services, procedures, and products that improve consumers' quality of life.

Several months ago one of the authors asked a nursing home executive how she coped with the often discouraging situations she and her staff encounter with the types of frail elderly persons they care for. Her response: "We don't find it discouraging. We are in the business of improving the quality of life for our patients. We realize that they can't do what they used to do. We don't focus on their limitations; we focus on helping them live the most fruitful, rewarding, and enjoyable lives they can at this point in time."

But long-term care is not the only segment of health care where quality-of-life factors are becoming increasingly important. Here are several others:

- Orthopedic surgery to replace hips and knees, alleviating pain and increasing mobility
- Cosmetic surgery to improve personal appearance
- Laser eye surgery to improve vision and hearing aids to improve hearing
- New drugs—most notably Viagra—chiefly marketed to those concerned about the quality of their sex lives
- Ultra-high-speed cardiac scanning to provide consumers with a sense of well-being by reassuring them that they do not have heart problems

Calvary Hospital in the Bronx, a hospital that caters to the dying, offers another example of quality of life winning out over saving money:

To die at Calvary is a tender affair. Patients are handed a rose upon arrival. They stay in one of the hospital's 200 private rooms, are given physical therapy until the end, and get free televisions with VCRs. They are offered copious emotional support; priests, nuns, a rabbi and a psychiatrist work to alleviate their terror and distress. They can order omelets for breakfast, sizzling steaks or lobster tails for dinner. Two nights a week, a cart stocked with wine and liquor, including bottles of Johnnie Walker's Black Label and Harveys Bristol Cream, makes the rounds.

Extravagant? Not so, says Kathleen Foley, a cancer and pain specialist at New York's Memorial Sloan-Kettering hospital, which frequently refers patients to Calvary. "Why should quality of life for someone who will live a day be different than quality of living for someone who may live much longer?" [Lagnado, 2000, p. A1].

The article on Calvary Hospital from which this quote is taken focuses on the fact that Calvary has been successful in appealing to the New York legislature for special relief so that it can continue to offer what HMOs and other payers consider to be unduly expensive care for dying patients. This is another example of quality of life being recognized as important by both lawmakers and the public.

The ramifications of this dramatic shift are several. First, the trend toward health care for quality-of-life improvement is a major factor driving up revenues for providers and costs for payers and consumers. Second, as it becomes harder to separate medical necessity from quality of life, the development of public policy on the growing number of uninsured individuals and on what medical benefits to include in Medicare will become more complex. Third, as consumers pay an increasing share of their health care costs, they will become more demanding with regard to the level of service they receive from providers and the quality of the experience of visiting a provider's office or facility.

We believe many health care services and products need to be viewed more accurately; they need to be seen as what they really are—efforts to improve quality of life. This is one reason why the relatively high health care spending in the United States compared with other developed countries has not led to improvements in most of the standard measures of health status (such as infant mortality and longevity rates).

One of the age-old debates in the United States is whether health care is a right or a privilege. Those who most vigorously advocate universal coverage, a payment source for all Americans, often argue that basic health care is a right. Although we are strong advocates of moving toward universal coverage, we believe that those who argue that access to health care is a privilege have the stronger argument, especially in a country where a growing share of health care spending is for quality-of-life improvements, and not for "pure" medical necessity.

Reality 10: Health Care Will Experience a Fundamental Market Shift During the First Five Years of the New Millennium

Paradigm shifts in an industry almost always arise from external factors and are not usually seen or accepted by those inside an industry until it is too late. How, then, can we say with any credibility that we expect a fundamental market shift coming in health care?

As we indicated in earlier chapters, we disagree with many in health care that the industry has been dynamic and in a constant state of flux. We view health care as having fallen into predictable patterns, with managed care taking on the characteristics of a stagnant industry. Yes, there is the BBA and its negative financial impact, especially on hospitals, rehabilitation providers, research and teaching organizations, and home health. Managed care will feel pressure on two fronts—on the one hand, employers and consumers trying to control spending, on the other, physicians and hospitals negotiating hard to protect their revenues—and this will lead to increasing pressure on providers.

The combination of increased consumer involvement and personal responsibility and increased use of technology are interrelated. This connection is manifested, for example, in pharmaceutical companies marketing new drugs directly to consumers and consumers using the Internet to become better educated about treatment options. Although many individuals we interviewed scoffed at possible changes in the payment system as drastic as those we anticipate— employers moving toward defined contributions, increased interest in MSAs and vouchers, significant reductions in the number of the uninsured, or tax reform providing incentives for individual insurance—we believe there is a reasonable chance that many such changes will be in process by 2005. Going back five years, who would have predicted the impact of the Internet? Who would have anticipated the early completion of the Human Genome Project and the competing private sector efforts? Who would have thought that managed care would saturate the market and face increasingly disgruntled consumers and alienated physicians?

In looking ahead, we can detect only the faintest outlines of what health care will be like in 2005. What we can see suggests that physicians, hospitals, and other health care organizations have the opportunity to find new ways of positioning themselves in their markets through dramatic improvements in service, convenience, quality of care, and cost-effectiveness.

Conclusions: The Positive Factors Outweigh the Negative

Many in health care have become negative. This is true of hospital trustees and managers, physicians, health plan executives, and the human resources representatives of large employers. The CEO of a hospital in Nevada referred to a certain "crankiness" that permeates the organization, including physicians on the medical staff and board members.

It is refreshing to hear someone who is positive about the future of health care, an industry that is expected to grow rapidly over the next few years. Such voices are rare but much appreciated. Yes, health care dollars will be spent differently than in the past, and consumers will become more demanding. However, for many in health care the dramatic changes anticipated over the first five years of the new millennium are challenging and exciting—we agree with those who hold this viewpoint. So go for it!

Appendix: Planning for the New Health Care Marketplace

Certainly the technology matters, but getting the business strategy right matters even more.
"Business and the Internet," *The Economist,*
June 1999

Hospital earnings have been wiped out by the BBA. Investment in Y2K remedies have far exceeded projections. Physicians and medical groups have been looking for new capital partners after dropping out of PPMs. Hospitals have divested themselves of primary care groups or have restructured their contracts with physicians. Bond ratings for large hospital systems have been downgraded. Employers have been asked to absorb huge increases in health plan premiums, and a growing number of small and medium-sized firms are dropping health insurance coverage for their employees. Medicaid and Medicare payments are inadequate to cover direct costs of care. It is no wonder that many hospital board members and CEOs, physician leaders, and other executives in health care are focused on short-term survival.

John Cochrane (1999, p. 1), former editor of *Integrated Health-care Report,* writes, "Hospital administrators are on the brink of revolt. . . . This summer, the healthcare industry reached a new low. Carnage is everywhere, when in the rest of the economy unemployment is at an all-time low and America is booming. What is happening?" Alden Solovy, editor of *Hospitals & Health Networks,* agrees and believes that health care executives are fed up with "the future." "After all," Solovy (1999) says, "we've been working in the future for 25 years." He cites DRGs, the Resource-Based Relative Value Scale, risk contracting, total quality management, and patient-focused care.

Much energy and money have gone into the management techniques and organizational models that were supposed to solve many of health care's problems, and the results have been unimpressive. Furthermore, many in health care freely admit that they do not know what the future is likely to bring in the way of change. As one CEO told us, "We have been burned many times by those who told us that this or that was going to happen and we had better get ready." He was referring to PHOs, provider-sponsored health plans, continuous quality improvement, and capitated payment.

Despite short-term pressures—and they are immense—*there has never been a time in health care when the development of strategy has been more important.* We agree with Arie P. de Geus (1988, p. 3), who observes, "Once in a crisis, everyone in the organization feels the pain. The need for change is clear. The problem is that you usually have little time and few options. The deeper into the crisis you are, the fewer options remain. Crisis management, by necessity, becomes autocratic management. The positive characteristic of a crisis is that the decisions are quick. The other side of that coin is that the implementation is rarely good; many companies fail to survive." He concludes that "[t]he challenge, therefore, is to recognize and react to environmental change before the pain of a crisis." This is what we are urging in this book, and especially in this Appendix.

Our experience in strategy consulting—the authors have directed or participated in more than one hundred such assignments for entities in a variety of industries—is that the strategy process is especially valuable for not-for-profit organizations (such as health care, quasi-government, or religious entities), whose direction is often fragmented. Furthermore, the development of strategy is especially valuable where there is confusion about the roles of various participants (such as board members or managers) and a lack of alignment of financial incentives—which generally characterizes health care.

This Appendix focuses on strategy development and implementation under conditions of uncertainty, with an emphasis on the impact of consumerism and technology—that is, an emphasis on scenarios 3 and 4 (see Chapter One for an explanation of these scenarios). We have taken more of a how-to approach in the Appendix, dealing with the nuts and bolts of developing a strategy. We address the following questions:

- What is the appropriate level of effort for visioning and strategy?
- What should be the steps in a strategy process designed for the new millennium? What kinds of information and analysis should be included to reflect the changing environment dominated by consumerism and technology?
- What are the strategic issues for hospitals, medical groups, integrated systems, and health plans?
- When the strategy process has been completed, how do you know that it has been worth the effort? How can the CEO and board discern whether or not the development of strategy has been successful?

Strategy Development: Appropriate Level of Effort

In health care the development of strategy can range from a half-day retreat (usually including a social hour and a nice dinner) to a six-month intensive effort involving a number of task forces. It is common for hospital boards to have Friday night and Saturday retreats, with some staff preparation and professional facilitation. Smaller medical groups and physician organizations (such as IPAs or PHOs) typically schedule evening retreats, often with little or no preparation. Our experience indicates that the number of half-day retreats is increasing but that the in-depth, intensive efforts have mostly disappeared. However, it is important to strike an appropriate balance between the "quick and dirty" versus more in-depth planning.

A Vision Is Not a Strategy

It is common for a visioning process—"Who are we, and what are we trying to accomplish?"—to be viewed as strategy development. Retreats asking these questions focus on revisiting and refining mission and vision statements. In our view they are generally "feel good" sessions without much lasting value other than the fellowship that occurs during the breaks and after the meeting. We are not suggesting that it is unimportant to discuss the organization's vision, mission, and core values. However, this should not be confused with the essence of developing a strategy. (We discuss how visioning fits into the picture in more detail later in the Appendix.)

Preparation Is Important

A strategy retreat without significant preparation—"It's that time of year again. We need to spend Saturday morning planning for the coming year. Anyone have any suggestions on what should be on the agenda?"—is probably not worth the effort. We do not have high expectations for what will result from this sort of get-together.

Benefits of Midlevel Efforts Usually Exceed the Costs

We believe that most health care organizations can gain significant value from a midlevel effort—a limited assessment of the environment (especially the growing impact of consumers and technology), a brief review of internal business operations, a look ahead at finances, and agreement on directions for the future. This may involve three or four meetings of the management team, a limited amount of staff work, and a board session and might be carried out over a one- to two-month period.

Like many things in life, a health care organization gets out of strategy development what it puts into it. In our view the investment of staff resources, management, board, physician time, and out-of-pocket expenses for a facilitator or for renting a meeting place will produce benefits that far exceed costs. At a time when health care is facing the strong possibility of a shift to a consumer- and technology-driven marketplace, *this type of strategizing represents an investment with potentially high returns.*

The Strategy Process in Health Care

This part of the Appendix reviews the typical steps we use in developing strategy for a health care organization, with an emphasis on how to consider the twin forces of consumers and technology. The key steps in the strategy process are summarized in Exhibit A.1. In the pages that follow, each step in the process is briefly described, with shortcuts and tips on how to make strategy development move smoothly. We include a checklist of factors to consider in evaluating the external environment and a focus group interview guide.

Step 1: Core Values, Visioning, and Mission Statements

Jim Collins and Jerry Porras, coauthors of the best-selling book *Built to Last: Successful Habits of Visionary Companies,* say a well-conceived vision consists of two major components: a core ideology and an envisioned future. The core ideology defines what an organization stands for and why it exists. The envisioned future is what an organization aspires to become or achieve—something that requires significant progress and change to attain (Collins and Porras, 1996).

Core Values: An Issue Often Overlooked

In reflecting on the changes in direction that have marked many health care organizations over the past two decades, it is evident that insufficient attention has been given to core values. As Collins

---

Exhibit A.1. Key Steps in the Strategy Process.

1. Core values, visioning, and mission statements
2. Environmental, consumerism, and technology assessment
3. Market analysis, including market segmentation and competitive assessment
4. Internal business assessment
5. Development of a financial model
6. Identification of key issues and opportunities
7. Development of a list of strategic initiatives
8. Prioritization of strategies
9. "What if" scenarios
10. Finalization of strategies
11. Presentations and stakeholder buy-in
12. Implementation

---

and Porras explain, "Core ideology provides the glue that holds an organization together as it grows, decentralizes, diversifies, expands globally, and develops workplace diversity. Core values are the essential and enduring tenets of an organization" (1996, p. 66). Collins and Porras say their research shows that successful organizations do not create or establish core ideology but, rather, that they discover core ideology: "Do not ask, What core values should we hold? Ask instead, What core values do we truly and passionately hold?" (p. 71).

Core Values: Examples

The Health Care Advisory Board is a highly regarded research and educational organization serving the health care industry. Here is a statement of its core values: "*Our corporate privilege is to serve as modest scribe to the remarkable advance of great ideas in health care.* The revolutions in our time are of the mind, the triumph of sound and inspired ideas. . . . Good ideas triumph. *Ours is the task to find them*" (Health Care Advisory Board, Nursing Executive Center, 1999, p. 9, emphasis added).

The board and management team of a Catholic hospital in New England thinks it is important to understand what the founders had in mind when they established the organization in the mid-1880s. The CEO told us, "Our efforts to better understand the vision of our founders have led us into some surprising new initiatives that might stretch the definition of health care. For example, we are taking the lead in helping settle refugees from Kosovo and several African countries who want to come to our area. We are actively involved in redeveloping housing in some of the older parts of our city."

Many health care organizations focus on what they would like to become. We often observe a sameness and much wishful thinking in vision and mission statements of hospitals, health systems, and large medical groups. For example, it is popular to talk about "meeting the health care needs of the community," but examples of really doing this are few and far between. (We describe one success story—that of Franklin Community Health Network in Maine—in Chapter Eight.) Exhibit A.2 shows the vision and mission statements of several large health care organizations. There are substantial differences between the examples shown in Exhibit A.2, which is understandable given the origins of each organization.

Exhibit A.2. Examples of Vision and Mission Statements of Health Care Organizations.

Lovelace Health Systems

The vision of Lovelace Health Systems is "to be recognized as the best health care system in the Southwest." (Lovelace Health Systems is based in Albuquerque, New Mexico.)

Bassett Healthcare

"The mission of Bassett Healthcare is to provide excellent patient care services, to educate physicians and other health care professionals and to pursue health research." (Bassett Healthcare is headquartered in Cooperstown, New York.)

Scott & White

Scott & White's vision is to "[p]rovide personalized, comprehensive high-quality health care enhanced by medical education and research." (Scott & White is based in Temple, Texas.)

Baptist Health System

"As a witness to the love of God, revealed through Jesus Christ, the Baptist Health System is committed to enhance the health, dignity and wholeness of those we serve through compassionate care, innovation and performance, education and research." (Baptist Health System is headquartered in Birmingham, Alabama.)

HealthSystem Minnesota

"The mission of HealthSystem Minnesota is to be the premier comprehensive regional health care system in the nation." (HealthSystem Minnesota [recently renamed Park Nicollet Health Services], the result of a merger between Methodist Hospital and Park Nicollet Clinic, is based in Minneapolis.)

Source: Coddington, Chapman, and Pokoski, 1996, pp. 3, 50, 75, 100, 125.

Small Steps and Sustained Effort

Do not stop the strategy process to "get it right." We believe that the definition or development of core values, a vision, and a mission statement should be accomplished in small steps over the entire period of strategy development, and longer if necessary. However, for many organizations it may be a matter of assessing the relevance of previous vision and mission statements and attempts to identify core competencies. We suspect that with the kinds of changes anticipated in the new health care marketplace, a serious look at core values, vision, and mission may be timely.

Step 2: Environmental, Consumerism, and Technology Assessment

With the growth in technology and concerns over how it will affect the organization (both potential adverse effects and opportunities), an environmental, consumerism, and technology assessment is a key aspect of strategy development in the twenty-first century. Plenty of energy, research, and hard thinking need to go into consideration of the impact on the local market of the Internet, telehealth, telemedicine, and clinical information systems. This part of the strategy process should also consider likely development of new drugs and advances in medical technology and how these important factors are likely to affect the future of the organization. Exhibit A.3 is our checklist of questions to ask about possible changes in the external environment, consumerism, and technology (from a hospital perspective) as part of an assessment of these three forces. Exhibit A.3 is not intended to be a complete checklist of the information needed to perform such an assessment, and it does not take into account special local circumstances.

Step 3: Market Analysis, Including Market Segmentation and Competitive Assessment

Market analysis often requires original research (such as surveys of community residents or focus group interviews with seniors, women, or other key customer groups) and a substantial amount of data collection from secondary sources. The data collection is hard

Exhibit A.3. Checklist of Questions About the Potential Impact of the External Environment, Consumerism, and Technology.

- How fast will increased Internet use and high-speed Internet access affect the residents of our service area?

- What are local physicians doing to prepare themselves for the quantum leap in e-mail communication with better-educated and more prepared consumers, health plans, and other physicians?

- Does our organization need to invest in a substantial upgrade of our business systems so that we can use instantaneous information in management? What difference would this make in patient care and overall profitability?

- Given the medical specialties most dominant in our service area, what kinds of investments do we need to make in new medical technology?

- What are the demographics of our service area, and how will they change over the next three to five years? (The focus should be on Medicare eligibility, income levels, and net worth—in other words, the ability to pay for health care services.)

- What are employers in our service area likely to do when faced with substantial year-to-year increases in their health care costs? Will some drop benefits entirely? How many will move to some form of defined-contribution arrangement?

- What assumptions should we make about federal payment and the impact of rules and regulations? (The impact of the BBA, possible changes in gain-sharing arrangements, and continued efforts to reduce fraud and abuse, leading to high investment in corporate compliance, are examples.)

- What can we expect in the way of increased competition from for-profit niche players, such as those who establish ambulatory surgery centers or rehabilitation facilities or who provide other specialized services?

work, and the analysis of the information is even more important. A sample focus group leader's interview guide for use with seniors is shown in Exhibit A.4.

Market Segmentation

Many of the physician leaders and health care executives interviewed for this book stressed the importance of obtaining sufficiently detailed market information to be able to segment the market into various categories of customers. One individual told us, "By definition, if consumers are going to call the shots, we have to segment individuals and households into relevant groups for marketing and product development." (Market segmentation is discussed in Chapter Fifteen.)

Competitive Assessment

The competitive assessment should include existing and potential competitors. One health care association executive told us he was especially concerned about e-commerce firms as competitors. Another individual told us, "The competitor we really worry about is the one we can't identify." We agree; the competitors of the new era in health care will show up in unexpected places. However, we believe that with more effort, organizations can detect at least some of these difficult-to-identify competitors.

Step 4: Internal Business Assessment

By "internal business assessment" we mean a careful analysis of historical data on a variety of key indicators for the organization. The data should be assembled and presented in easy-to-understand charts and graphs and interpreted in the context of what it means for the future of the organization.

Here are examples of the kinds of historical data (covering the past three years) that might be collected and analyzed:

- *For hospitals:* data on inpatient admissions and patient days, outpatient visits, net revenues from both inpatient and outpatient sources, average length of stay, severity of illness of patients, payer mix, primary physician admitters (by specialty),

Exhibit A.4. Seniors Focus Group Discussion Leader's Guide.

1. *Make introductions. Present rules of the discussion.*
2. *Ask the following questions. Make sure everyone responds.*
   - What kind of health care coverage do you have now?
   - Do you have Medicare? If so, what type?
   - Do you have supplemental insurance?
3. *Ask the following questions and discuss.*
   - Do you have a primary care physician?
   - If not, why not?
   - If so, how long have you been with this individual?
   - What do you like best about your physician?
4. *Ask the following question. Probe to elicit relevant details.*
   - Could you talk about how you evaluate the quality of care you receive from your physicians?
5. *Ask the following questions and discuss.*
   - How many different prescription drugs do you take?
   - How much does this cost you a month?
   - Do you have any help with these costs, such as from supplemental insurance, retiree coverage, or a Medicare HMO?
6. *Ask the following question and discuss.*
   - How much of a hassle is the paperwork associated with your health care coverage?
7. *Ask the following questions. Probe to elicit relevant details.*
   - Do you have access to the Internet?
   - If so, how often do you use it, and what do you use it for?
8. *Ask the following question. Probe to elicit relevant details.*
   - Based on your personal experience, what changes would you like to see to make health care better for you and your spouse?
9. *Ask the following question. Probe to elicit relevant details.*
   - What could be done in your local area by your physician or hospital to make health care more convenient and affordable for you?
10. *Ask the following question and discuss.*
    - Do you have any problems that affect your ability to receive health care, such as unavailability of transportation to physicians' offices, adult day care, or long-term care services?
11. *Ask the following question and discuss.*
    - Do you have any additional comments or suggestions?

number of uninsured patients served, and the impact of Medicare and Medicaid

- *For medical groups:* data on the number of patients, patient encounters, gross revenues, discounts, net revenues, overhead as a percentage of revenues, payer mix (including managed care, private pay, Medicare, Medicaid, and others), productivity of individual physicians, ancillary income, patient origin, and results of patient satisfaction surveys

- *For health plans:* data on the number of subscribers by type of product and by geographical location, number and size of employers, penetration of major employers (percentage of employees who sign up), overhead and medical loss ratio as a percentage of revenues, marketing expenses, moneys paid to various medical groups and hospitals, quality and patient service indicators, and the nature of payment models used and how these are changing over time

Among the first tasks in the strategy process are preparing one- or two-page checklists of data needs, deciding who will be responsible for assembling the data, and establishing deadlines. Our experience is that the presentation of this type of information at interim strategy meetings is valuable in keeping the process productive, interesting, and moving forward.

Step 5: Development of a Financial Model

We find that developing a financial model is often omitted in the strategy process. With the ready availability of spreadsheet financial models, it is difficult to understand why "what if" financial analysis is not being done on a regular basis. In fact, if such a model does not already exist, one of the first assignments in the strategy process would be to have the chief financial officer prepare a model that can be used to test the impact of various courses of action, or "futures," for the organization. Financial models should be part of every interim meeting. Their proper use helps keep the strategy process on track by identifying those actions that will have significant financial impact and those that will not. In other words, a good financial model helps prioritize the process right from the start by clearly identifying the real driving forces of the organization.

Step 6: Identification of Key Issues and Opportunities

The identification of key issues and opportunities is ongoing throughout the strategy process. We often use the core group—the CEO and management team—to help identify the key issues facing the organization over the upcoming three years and the major opportunities that need to be evaluated.

Step 7: Development of a List of Strategic Initiatives

In going through step 6 and continually feeding in new ideas, it is not unusual to end up with fifteen to twenty-five items that are of strategic importance to the organization. Given the anticipated changes in the health care marketplace, there should not be any shortage of new strategic opportunities to be considered. Again, the financial model can help in quickly identifying those that are most important to the future financial viability of the organization. In developing strategies when there are multiple scenarios of the type we propose, it is helpful to use the type of matrix shown in Table 10.1 (see Chapter Ten). William Corley, CEO of Methodist Community Hospitals in Indianapolis, developed this matrix to show how strategies would change based on our four scenarios for the future.

Step 8: Prioritization of Strategies

Prioritization of strategies is usually not difficult. At this stage of the process, where the internal business assessment has been completed and the financial model is up and running, those strategic initiatives that deserve a top priority should stand out. Those strategies that work well with any scenario should be given special consideration. If it is more complicated than this, the core group needs to develop a list of criteria, or weighting factors, to use in prioritizing the potential strategic initiatives. These factors might include financial implications, competitive considerations, the needs of customers, impact on physician relationships (for a hospital), relevance to positioning for the future, and consistency with overall vision and core values. The criteria might also include a rating of the likelihood of a particular scenario coming to fruition.

Step 9: "What If" Scenarios

The implementation of the various strategic initiatives will require capital investment and possible increases in operating expenses and will have an impact on the bottom line. All of this needs to be modeled, and the core strategy group needs to be able to ask "what if" questions and get almost instantaneous responses. At this stage many of the strategic initiatives will be combined, and the financial modeling needs to be able to predict the financial implications of specific initiatives as well as the implications of all initiatives as a group.

Step 10: Finalization of Strategies

At this point in the process, the next step is to finalize strategies, usually by preparing a series of transparencies or other presentation materials. Parts of the plan may be documented in written reports. Data from consumer surveys and from the internal business assessment should be packaged in a report.

Step 11: Presentations and Stakeholder Buy-In

It is important that presentations of data, analysis, and initial ideas take place throughout the strategy development process. For example, if there are focus groups with physicians, the participating physicians and medical leadership need to have access to the results as soon as possible. The key to a successful strategy process is the absence of surprises. Well before the final presentation, all participants should have a fairly good idea of how the plan is coming together. We have not said much about how to accomplish this part of the process—this is up to the individual organization, which must decide on the best way to communicate with physicians, the board, and the management team.

Step 12: Implementation

It goes without saying that the final plan will include assignment of responsibilities and deadlines for implementation. It should also include a recommended system for monitoring progress in achieving the objectives of the new strategies.

Tips for Hospitals, Medical Groups, Integrated Systems, and Health Plans

This part of the Appendix identifies special strategy development considerations—key issues to consider—for various groups in health care.

Hospitals and Multihospital Systems

Hospitals tend to make longer-term investments in "bricks and mortar" (and in the new millennium, in information systems) and to use more long-term debt to finance their needs. Therefore hospital strategy development generally has a longer time perspective than that of medical groups or health plans—three to five years or more. Most hospital strategies succeed or fail based on physician participation and buy-in, which hospitals must make a special effort to ensure. Conducting focus group interviews with physicians is an excellent way to obtain their initial ideas about issues and opportunities for the hospital.

Medical Groups and Physician Networks

Our experience in working with physicians is that they want to bypass the process stage and move directly into the results and decision-making phases of a strategic plan. Therefore it is especially important to do a careful job on the internal business assessment and the assessment of the external environment, consumerism, and technology in order to establish a factual base that physicians will consider in making their decisions. The financial modeling is also important because potential strategies affect each physician financially, and they are vitally interested in these effects. If more medical groups had undertaken this type of strategy development when they decided to join a PPM, the results might have been dramatically different.

If possible, it is important to interview a large number of physicians and key administrative staff. Almost every physician will have ideas on where the group should be going in the future, and these thoughts need to be considered (and possibly rejected) during the strategy process. Physicians almost always have a direct professional and financial interest in the group's strategy, and they are not afraid to make decisions. However, they sometimes have difficulty sticking to these decisions. With medical groups the follow-through from strategy development is often not as strong as with hospitals. In other words, implementation often falls between the cracks. Therefore the group practice administrator or board chairperson has a special responsibility to ensure that the medical group is moving in the agreed-on directions.

Integrated Systems

Strategy development for integrated systems is the most complex because of the variety of activities included in the scope of services offered—hospitals, primary care satellite offices, care centers, the specialist core group, and sometimes a health plan. Nevertheless, the results of the strategy process can be more valuable; the chances of implementation are higher because most of the key elements of a health care system are present and under single governance and leadership. Because of the complexity of large integrated systems and the various constituencies, it is difficult to think of a health care organization that can benefit more from a coordinated approach to the market. Key issues often include clinical integration, coordination, compensation, meeting customer needs, information systems, health plan financial viability, and overall system financial performance.

Health Plans

Clearly, health plans are in trouble for a variety of reasons: consumers' concern over quality of care and financial incentives, physicians' antagonism, employers' negative reactions to escalating costs, and public policy pressures regarding consumer protection. The desire of consumers for more choice at lower costs poses an almost intractable problem for many health plans; it is difficult to offer both.

Strategy development for health plans also must take into account the growth in consumerism. In scenario 4 (see Chapter One for an explanation of this scenario), a substantial number of consumers would have individual insurance not directly connected with their employer. This, of course, would lead to a complete change in the marketing efforts of health plans; these efforts would also become substantially more expensive. We believe that the first five years of the new century are a critical time for health plans and a time to very carefully consider strategic options. We also note that many health plan leaders are taking an incremental-change view of the future. In our opinion this is a particularly dangerous course of action.

Evaluation of a Strategy Development Effort

By its very nature, the effectiveness of strategy development is difficult to measure. Furthermore, the results are not evident for several years, and by then most of those involved in developing strategies may be gone. Despite these problems with evaluating how well the process was carried out, we believe there are several measures that can be taken to assess the quality of the effort. These include the items discussed in the following paragraphs.

Strategy Development Converted from a Sporadic Effort to a Regular Endeavor

Anyone associated with developing strategy at even the most elementary level knows that to be effective, plans need to be periodically evaluated and updated. Many organizations do this annually. One way to keep the strategy process from becoming routine is to identify themes, or major issues, to be discussed each year: What are the key challenges and opportunities facing the organization over the next two or three years? Also, if strategies are based on scenarios, the scenarios for the future need to be revisited annually and perhaps restated. We certainly do not anticipate any shortage of new topics for health care strategy retreats.

Strategy Development Bringing Disparate Elements of the Medical Community Together

The strategy process, if carried out properly, should be a unifying force for the medical staff, board, and management team. Even though controversial issues may be analyzed and discussed, the process itself should generate respect, credibility, and an understanding of the issues. We know from experience that it can work this way.

Strategies Referred to on a Regular Basis During Formal and Informal Meetings

If no one ever talks about the plan once a strategy review and development cycle has been completed, the plan's relevance is in question. It is up to management to ensure that the results of the most recent process are included in reports of monthly meetings and that discussion of these results is on the agenda; this may not take place without a deliberate effort to make it happen.

Identifiable Strategic Initiatives Put into Motion

In looking back, it is usually possible to identify specific strategies that were initiated or received a boost as a result of the strategy process. Leadership needs to remind the group—board members, management, and physicians—that certain initiatives that have had long-term benefits came out of a previous strategy effort. If the board of directors or trustees shows continuing interest in the strategy process, this is a strong indication of a job well done. After all, the board has the staying power to bridge management changes. Management's performance should be evaluated against strategies. Hospital boards should consider the CEO's performance in moving the organization toward meeting its strategic objectives. How well these objectives have been met should be reflected in bonuses and compensation.

Conclusions

Strategy development in health care is not passé. If anything, the need for careful development of strategies and anticipation of the future is greater than at any time over the past two decades. Who can argue against research into and discussion of the potential impact of consumerism and technology on an organization? *The assertion that management is too busy with immediate crises to consider future strategy is not a valid excuse.*

We anticipate a resurgence of interest in strategy over the next few years and substantial improvements in the sophistication of strategy efforts. The tools to improve the strategy process are readily available—spreadsheet financial analysis, new types of market research techniques, databases on consumers, advances in presentation techniques—and this should contribute to significantly better results. The primary factor, however, will be an increased interest among physicians and health care executives in the development of strategies under conditions of extreme uncertainty. The uncertainty will be driven by changes in technology and continuously growing consumer expectations.

References

Advisory Board Company. *Run to Rigor: Competing on Cost and Discipline.* Washington, D.C.: Advisory Board Company, 1997.

American Health Care Association. *The 1998 Nursing Facility Sourcebook.* Facts and Trends Series. Washington, D.C.: American Health Care Association, 1998.

Annison, M. H., and Wilford, D. S. *Trust Matters: New Directions in Health Care Leadership.* San Francisco: Jossey-Bass, 1998.

Appleby, J. "Want a CAT Scan? Step Right Up." *USA Today,* May 25, 2000, pp. 1B–2B.

Austin, M. "Patients Test Card." *Denver Business Journal,* Aug. 20–26, 1999a, p. B8.

Austin, M. "Schonbrun's Back, and He's Thinking Ahead." *Denver Business Journal,* May 21–27, 1999b, p. A12.

Baldwin, G. "Mind-Body Economics." *American Medical News,* Oct. 26, 1998, pp. 23–24.

BBC Research & Consulting. *The Economic and Social Contributions of Health Care in Maine: Farmington Case Study.* Denver, Colo.: BBC Research & Consulting, 1997.

Beckham, J. D. "Part 2: A Solid Competitive Strategy, Bricks & Mortar." *Health Forum Journal,* Nov.–Dec. 1999, pp. 48–51.

Beer, M., and Nohria, N. "Cracking the Code of Change." *Harvard Business Review,* May–June 2000, pp. 133–141.

Bellandi, D. "Searching for Better Bait: Systems Struggling to Lure Docs, Trustees to Integration." *Modern Healthcare,* Oct. 5, 1998, pp. 28, 30.

Berwick, D. "The Total Customer Relationship in Health Care: Broadening the Bandwidth." *Journal on Quality Improvement,* 1997, *23*(5), 245–249.

Bickert, J. "Cohorts: A New Approach to Market Segmentation." *Journal of Consumer Marketing,* 1997, *14*(5), 362–377.

Blumenthal, D. "Part 1: Quality of Care—What Is It?" *New England Journal of Medicine,* 1996, *335*, 891–894.

Bodenheimer, T. "The American Health Care System: The Movement for Improved Quality in Health Care." *New England Journal of Medicine*, 1999a, *340*, 488–492.

Bodenheimer, T. "The American Health Care System: Physicians and the Changing Medical Marketplace." *New England Journal of Medicine*, 1999b, *340*, 584–588.

Bodenheimer, T. "Disease Management—Promises and Pitfalls." *New England Journal of Medicine*, 1999c, *340*, 1202–1205.

Burda, D. "S.C. Systems Shutting Down Joint HMO." *Modern Healthcare*, Oct. 11, 1999, p. 3.

Burton, T. M. "UnitedHealth Gets Physicians to Improve Medical Care." *Wall Street Journal*, Aug. 19, 1999, p. B4.

"Business and the Internet." *The Economist*, June 26, 1999, pp. 6–40.

Butler, S. M., and others. "Crisis Facing HCFA & Millions of Americans." *Health Affairs*, Jan.–Feb. 1999, pp. 8–10.

Center for the Evaluative Clinical Sciences, The. *The Dartmouth Atlas of Health Care 1999*. Lebanon, N.H.: Dartmouth Medical School, 1999.

Chassin, M. R., Hannan, E. L., and DeBuono, B. A. "Benefits and Hazards of Reporting Medical Outcomes Publicly." *New England Journal of Medicine*, 1996, *334*, 394–398.

Cochrane, J. D. "The Summer Meltdown." *Integrated Healthcare Report*, June 1999, pp. 1–7.

Coddington, D. C., Ackerman, F. K., Fischer, E. A., and Moore, K. D., *The Changing Dynamics of Integrated Health Care: Success Factors for the Future*. Englewood, Colo.: Medical Group Management Association, 2001.

Coddington, D. C., and Bendrick, B. J. *Integrated Health Care: Case Studies*. Englewood, Colo.: Center for Research in Ambulatory Health Care Administration, 1994.

Coddington, D. C., Chapman, C. R., and Pokoski, K. M. *Making Integrated Health Care Work: Case Studies*. Englewood, Colo.: Center for Research in Ambulatory Health Care Administration, 1996.

Coddington, D. C., Fischer, E. A., Moore, K. D., and Clarke, R. L. *Beyond Managed Care: How Consumers and Technology Are Changing the Future of Health Care*. San Francisco: Jossey-Bass, 2000.

Coddington, D. C., Moore, K. D., and Clarke, R. L. *Capitalizing Medical Groups: Positioning Physicians for the Future*. New York: McGraw-Hill, 1998.

Coddington, D. C., Moore, K. D., and Fischer, E. A. *Integrated Health Care: Reorganizing the Physician, Hospital and Health Plan Relationship*. Englewood, Colo.: Center for Research in Ambulatory Health Care Administration, 1994.

Coddington, D. C., Moore, K. D., and Fischer, E. A. *Making Integrated Health Care Work.* Englewood, Colo.: Center for Research in Ambulatory Health Care Administration, 1996.

Collins, J. C., and Porras, J. I. "Building Your Company's Vision." *Harvard Business Review,* Sept.–Oct. 1996, pp. 65–77.

Coy, P., and Gross, N. "21 Ideas for the 21st Century: Introduction." *Business Week,* Aug. 30, 1999, pp. 81–82.

Daily, L. "More HMO's Covering Alternative Treatments and Complementary Care." *Physician's Financial News,* June 20, 1999, pp. S1, S6.

Dartmouth Medical School. *The Dartmouth Atlas of Health Care.* Chicago: American Hospital Publishing, 1996.

de Geus, A. P. "Planning as Learning." *Harvard Business Review,* Mar.–Apr. 1988, pp. 1–6.

de Geus, A. P. "The Living Company." *Harvard Business Review,* Mar.–Apr. 1997, pp. 51–59.

de Graffenried Ruffin, M. *Digital Doctors.* Tampa, Fla.: American College of Physician Executives, 1999.

Dewey, L. R. "Consumer Marketing Comes to Eye Surgery." *Marketing Health Services,* Fall 1999, pp. 47–49.

"Does Alternative Medicine Fit into Your Practice?" *Practice Marketing and Management,* Feb. 1999, pp. 15–17.

Drucker, P. F. *Innovation and Entrepreneurship.* New York: HarperCollins, 1993.

Egger, E. "Capitated Physicians Aren't Controlling Utilization, PacifiCare CEO Says." *Health Care Strategic Management,* Nov. 1999a, p. 4.

Egger, E. "Physician Buy-In, Scientific Data Crucial to CAM Programs." *Health Care Strategic Management,* Aug. 1999b, pp. 1, 21–23.

Feorene, B. T. "Physician Practice Management Companies: Industry Overview & Status." In *1999 Directory of Physician Groups & Networks.* Irvine, Calif.: Center for Healthcare Information, 1999.

"Financial Brands: Round 'Em Up." *The Economist,* July 31, 1999, p. 65.

Fischman, J. "The New Chicago Hope: Can Northwestern Pamper Patients—and Cut Costs?" *U.S. News & World Report,* July 19, 1999, pp. 68–69.

Flower, J. "What Experience Are You Selling?" *Health Forum Journal,* Jan.–Feb. 2000, pp. 12–17.

Galbraith, J. K. *The Affluent Society.* Boston: Houghton Mifflin, 1958.

Gates, B. *Business @ the Speed of Thought.* New York: Warner Books, 1999.

Gentry, C. "Seeing the Body Electric, in 3-D." *Wall Street Journal,* Jan. 24, 2000, pp. B1, B4.

Goodman, D., Symposium on E-Healthcare Strategies for Physicians, Hospitals & Integrated Systems, Scottsdale, Arizona. Speech, Feb. 8, 2000.

Gorey, T. M. *Case Study Analysis of Physician Hospital Organizations.* Sponsored by the American Medical Association, Illinois State Medical Society, Indiana State Medical Association, and Michigan State Medical Society. Crystal Lake, Ill.: T. M. Gorey, 1994.

Gorey, T. M. *Management Services Organizations: Cases and Analysis.* Chicago: Health Administration Press, 1997.

Gorey, T. M., and Bannon, N. K. *Case Study Analysis of Single Specialty Physician Networks.* Crystal Lake, Ill.: T. M. Gorey and N. K. Bannon, 1997.

Grandinetti, D. A. "Your Newest Competitors: Alternative-Medicine Networks." *Medical Economics,* May 24, 1999, pp. 44, 46, 51.

Hamel, G. "Bringing Silicon Valley Inside." *Harvard Business Review,* Sept.–Oct. 1999, pp. 70–84.

Hassett, M., and Rybarski, M. "Transforming and Repositioning Healthcare for the Boomers." *The Healthcare Strategist,* Feb. 1999, p. 2.

HCIA. *A Comprehensive Review of Hospital Finances in the Aftermath of the Balanced Budget Act of 1997.* Baltimore: HCIA, 1999.

Health Care Advisory Board. *Network Advantage: Scale Economies and Cost Savings.* Washington, D.C.: Health Care Advisory Board, 1994.

Health Care Advisory Board, Nursing Executive Center. *Hardwiring for Service Excellence.* Washington, D.C.: The Health Care Advisory Board, 1999.

Health Care Financing Administration. "Medicare Enrollment Trends, 1996–1998." [www.hcfa.gov/stats/enrltrnd.htm]. June 30, 1999.

Heimoff, S. "3 Health Care Startups Refuse to Be Boxed In." *Managed Care,* Dec. 1999, pp. 1–7.

Herzlinger, R. *Market Driven Health Care.* Reading, Mass.: Addison-Wesley, 1997.

Hoechst, M. R. "Home Care Industry Summary." *Managed Care Digest Series,* 1999, p. 32.

Hofgard, M. W., and Zipin, M. L. "Complementary and Alternative Medicine: A Business Opportunity?" *MGM Journal,* May–June 1999, pp. 16–27.

Hopkins, M. S. "Physician Hospital Organizations: Evolution or Extinction?" In *1999 Directory of Physician Groups & Networks.* Irvine, Calif.: Center for Healthcare Information, 1999.

"How Does Your HMO Stack Up?" *Consumer Reports,* Aug. 1999, pp. 23–29.

Howgill, M.W.C. "Health Care Consumerism, the Information Explosion, and Branding: Why 'Tis Better to Be the Cowboy Than the Cow." *Managed Care Quarterly,* Fall 1998, pp. 33–43.

Huber, R. "Managed Care Gets a Bum Rap." *Business Week,* Jan. 25, 1999, p. 12.

Hubler, E. "Physicians Finding Pain in Bid to Heal Themselves." *Denver Post,* Jan. 16, 2000, pp. L1, L8.

Humana. "Humana Adopts TriZetto's HealthWeb as E-Business Portal; Humana's 6.1 Million Members and 330,000 Physicians to Benefit." Press release, Oct. 18, 1999a.

Humana. "Humana Introduces Nationwide Disease Management Program for Members with Coronary Artery Disease; Health Plan Teams with Cardiac Solutions to Deliver Proactive Program." Press release, Sept. 2, 1999b.

Institute for the Future. "Executive Summary: 'New' Health Care Consumer." [www.iftf.org]. May 1998.

Jaklevic, M. C. "Millennial Ends with the Millennium." *Modern Healthcare,* Dec. 20–27, 1999, p. 22.

Jeffrey, N. A. "Internet Medicine: Doctors Are Suddenly Swamped with Patients Who Think They Know a Lot More Than They Actually Do." *Wall Street Journal,* Oct. 19, 1998.

Jensen, K. H. *Assisted Living Industry Analysis.* Baltimore: Legg Mason Wood Walker, 1999.

Johnson, D.E.L. "Pointer and Orlikoff Score with 'Board Work.'" *Health Care Strategic Management,* Sept. 1999, pp. 2–3.

Kane, L. "Collect Premium Fees for Premium Care?" *Medical Economics,* Jan. 11, 1999, pp. 127–130.

Kassirer, J. P., and Angell, M. "Quality of Care." Selections from the *New England Journal of Medicine:* Boston, Massachusetts Medical Society, 1997.

Keller, K. L. "The Brand Report Card." *Harvard Business Review,* Jan.–Feb. 2000, pp. 147–157.

Kilborn, P. T. "Health Care System Under Scrutiny." *Denver Rocky Mountain News,* Dec. 26, 1999, p. A52.

Kohn, L. T., Corrigan, J. M., and Donaldson, M. S. (eds.). *To Err Is Human: Building a Safer Health System.* Washington, D.C.: National Academy Press, 2000.

KPMG. *Equal Footing: The Hospital CEO Perspective on Balancing Market Power.* Brochure. KPMG Peat Marwick LLP, October 1998.

"KPMG Study Reveals Need for 'Balance of Power' in Health Care Industry: Next-Generation Business Model Offers Consumer-Focused Solution to Level Market Influence." *Business Wire,* Oct. 21, 1998.

Krohn, R. *Physician Networks: Strategy, Start-Up, and Operation.* ACHE Management Series. Chicago: Health Administration Press, 1998.

Kuttner, R. "Must Good HMOs Go Bad? The Search for Checks and Balances." *New England Journal of Medicine,* 1998, *338,* 1635–1639.

Kuttner, R. "Managed Care and Medical Education." *New England Journal of Medicine,* 1999, *341,* 1092–1096.

Lagnado, L. "Squeezed by HMOs, a Revered Hospital Muscles the Legislature." *Wall Street Journal,* Feb. 17, 2000, pp. A1, A6.

Larson, L. "Take a Deep, Cleansing Breath—and Feel 21st Century Medicine." *Trustee,* June 1998, pp. 14–17.

Levinson, W., and Rubenstein, A. "Mission Critical—Integrating Clinician-Educators into Academic Medical Centers." *New England Journal of Medicine,* 1999, *341,* 840–843.

Lundberg, G., Symposium on E-Healthcare Strategies for Physicians, Hospitals & Integrated Systems, Scottsdale, Ariz., Feb. 8, 2000.

MacStravic, S. "Market Memo: Seven Approaches to Branding: Take Your Pick." *Health Care Strategic Management,* Apr. 1999, pp. 1, 20–23.

Masciantonio, A. "Healthcare Like Home, Away from Home." *HealthcareBusiness,* May–June 1999, p. 94.

McDermott, S. "Betting the Farm: The Internet as a Survival Strategy for Managed Care Organizations." Speech presented at Symposium on E-Healthcare Strategies for Physicians, Hospitals & Integrated Systems, Scottsdale, Ariz., Feb. 8, 2000.

McGinley, L. "Joint Venture Displays New American Export: High-Tech Medicine." *Wall Street Journal,* Feb. 14, 2000, pp. A1, A11.

Mechanic, D., and McAlpine, D. D. "Mission Unfulfilled: Potholes on the Road to Mental Health Parity." *Health Affairs,* Sept.–Oct. 1999, pp. 7–21.

Miller, K. "Healthcare Intentions: Seeing Demand as Consumers Do." *Healthcare Strategist,* Feb. 1999, pp. 7–10.

Moore, J. D. "Study: HMOs Moving Toward Quality; NCQA Finds Links Between Quality of Care and Member Satisfaction, Disclosure and Performance." *Modern Healthcare,* Sept. 13, 1999, p. 66.

Moore, J. D. "One Thing Leads to Another: Medical Errors Report Means Money for Medical-Outcomes Research." *Modern Healthcare,* Jan. 24, 2000, p. 2.

Morrissey, J. "Internet Company Rates Hospitals." *Modern Healthcare,* Aug. 16, 1999, p. 24.

Nakhnikian, E. "Not-for-Profits' New Role." *Contemporary Long Term Care,* Dec. 1999, p. 76.

National Association of Children's Hospitals and Related Institutions. *Serving the Nation's Children: 1999 Chart Book of Children's Hospitals.* Alexandria, Va.: National Association of Children's Hospitals and Related Institutions, 1999.

O'Leary, D. "Medical Errors Editorial Goofs." *Modern Healthcare,* Jan. 3, 2000, p. 23.

Pappelbaum, S., Symposium on E-Healthcare Strategies for Physicians, Hospitals & Integrated Systems, Scottsdale, Ariz., Feb. 8, 2000.

Pennyslvania Health Care Cost Containment Council. *Pennsylvania's Guide to Coronary Artery Bypass 1992.*

"Philadelphia International Medicine." Brochure. Philadelphia: Philadelphia International Medicine, 1999.

Philipson, K., and Stifler, J. "Can a Provider-Owned HMO Model Really Work?" *Towers Perrin Integration Advisor,* Sept. 1999, pp. 1–6.

Pine, B. J., II, and Gilmore, J. H. *The Experience Economy: Work Is Theatre & Every Business a Stage.* Boston: Harvard Business School Press, 1999.

Ricci, R. Symposium on E-Healthcare Strategies for Physicians, Hospitals & Integrated Systems, Scottsdale, Ariz., Feb. 7, 2000.

Robinson, J. C. "At the Helm of an Insurance Giant: Aetna's Richard L. Huber." *Health Affairs,* Nov.–Dec. 1999, pp. 89–99.

Robinson, S. "Hearty Health Care." *Albuquerque Tribune,* Feb. 24, 2000, http://www.abqtrib.com.

Rowley, R. Symposium on E-Healthcare Strategies for Physicians, Hospitals & Integrated Systems, Scottsdale, Ariz., Feb. 7, 2000.

Sadowy, H. "IPAS: Industry Overview & Current Status." In *1999 Directory of Physician Groups & Networks.* Irvine, Calif.: Center for Healthcare Information, 1999.

Saphir, A. "For-Profit Outpatient Centers Playing Bigger Role in Treatment, Clinical Trials." *Modern Healthcare,* May 31, 1999, p. 28.

Schlesinger, M., and others. "A Broader Vision for Managed Care, Part 2: A Typology of Community Benefits." *Health Affairs,* Sept.–Oct. 1998, pp. 26–49.

Schneider, E. C., and Epstein, A. M. "Influence of Cardiac-Surgery Performance Reports on Referral Practices and Access to Care: A Survey of Cardiovascular Specialists." *New England Journal of Medicine,* 1996, *335,* 251–256.

Schroeder, S. A. "A Saga of 'Paradise Lost.'" Review of *Time to Heal: American Medical Education from the Turn of the Century to the Managed Care Era,* by Kenneth M. Ludmerer. *Health Affairs,* Jan.–Feb. 2000, p. 256.

Senge, P., and others. *The Dance of Change: The Challenges of Sustaining Momentum in Learning Organizations.* New York: Doubleday, 1999.

Serb, C. "Branding: The Key to Luring New Consumers." *Hospitals & Health Networks,* Dec. 1999, p. 33.

Shalala, D. E., and Reinhardt, U. E. "Viewing the U.S. Health Care System from Within: Candid Talk from HHS." *Health Affairs,* May–June 1999, pp. 47–55.

Solovy, A. "The Future of the Future." *Hospitals & Health Networks,* Aug. 1999, p. 36.

Spurgeon, D., and Burton, T. M. "For the Very Cautious, a Physical Exam Now Includes a CAT Scan." *Wall Street Journal,* Mar. 23, 2000, pp. A1, A12.

Stevens, S. "Many Hospitals Merge Alternative Therapies with Standard Methods." *Physicians Financial News,* Oct. 15, 1999, p. 31.

Taylor, B. E., Chait, R. D., and Holland, T. P. "The New Work of the Non Profit Board." *Harvard Business Review,* Sept.–Oct. 1996, pp. 36–46.

Taylor, M. "End of the Line for Fla. System's HMO." *Modern Healthcare,* Oct. 11, 1999, p. 3.

Thompson, E. "The Power of Group Visits: Improved Quality of Care, Increased Productivity Entice Physicians to See up to 15 Patients at a Time." *Modern Healthcare,* June 5, 2000, pp. 54–62.

Tokarski, C. "Health Systems See Mission and Strategic Gain in Alternative Therapies." *Medical Network Strategy Report,* June 1998, pp. 1–3.

Towers Perrin. "Do Health Systems Pay Primary Care Physicians More for Less?" *Health Industry Research Report,* First Quarter 1999a.

Towers Perrin. "1999 Market Forecast." *Integration Advisor,* Jan. 1999b, pp. 1–8.

Trout, J. *The Power of Simplicity.* New York: McGraw-Hill, 1999.

VHA/Tiber Group. *The New Playbook: Transforming Health System-Physician Relationships.* Dallas, Tex.: VHA/Tiber Group, 1999.

Walker. L. W. "Governing Board, Know Thyself." *Trustee,* Sept. 1999, pp. 15–19.

Waterman, R. H., Jr. *The Renewal Factor: How the Best Get and Keep the Competitive Edge.* New York: Bantam Books, 1987.

Weber, D. O. "Saddleback Memorial Issues Annual 'Quality Report Card' to Grade Itself in Private—and in Public." *Strategic Healthcare Excellence,* May 1997, pp. 1–6.

Weber, T. E. "A Doctor, 700 Patients and the Net: Inventing the Virtual House Call." *Wall Street Journal,* Jan. 17, 2000, p. B1.

Whitelaw, N., and Warden, G. "Reexamining the Delivery System as Part of Medicare Reform." *Health Affairs,* Jan.–Feb. 1999, pp. 132–143.

Wolper, L. F. "Turning Around a Financially and Operationally Distressed Ophthalmology Practice." *Administrative Eyecare,* Spring 1999, pp. 11–15.

Young, D. W., and McCarthy, S. M. *Managing Integrated Delivery Systems: A Framework for Action.* Washington, D.C.: AUPHA Press, 1999.

Zablocki, E. "When East Meets West." *HealthcareBusiness,* Nov.–Dec. 1999, pp. 66–77.

Index

A

Ability to pay, growth in, 68

Academic medical centers, 171–179, 192, 363, 369

Access Health, 226, 229

Access, defined, 55–56. *See also Service entries*

Access to care, 5, 21; debate over, 368–369

Accountability: assigning, 339; of boards, 284, 291; of consumers, 66

Ackerman, F. K., Jr., 207–208

Acquisitions. *See* Consolidation

Action-oriented agendas, 284, *285*

Action plans, producing, 272, *273*

Action, taking, considerations in, 270

Adapters, early and defensive, 88–89

Administration simplification, health plans and, 240–241

Administrative overhead, 11, 113, 124, 346, 347

Administrative tasks, automating, 106–107, *108*, 113

Advertising claims, 315–316

Advertising to consumers. *See* Direct-to-consumer marketing

Advice nurses, centralizing, problem with, 61

Advisory Board Company, 157

Advocate Medical Group, 196, 231

Aetna U.S. Healthcare, 236, 346, 361

Affluent customers, 309–310

Affordability, 6, 67–68, 71–73, 77

After-hours care, 56

A.G. Edwards, 251

Age factor, *19*

Agendas, 284, *285*, 388

Aging population, 84, 101; as a driver of spending, 10–11, 357

Albert Einstein Healthcare Network, 186

Allegheny Health, Education and Research Foundation (AHERF), 291, 355

Allina, 202

Alzheimer's care, 216, 218

American Association of Homes and Services for the Aging, 217

American Express, 314

American Health Care Association, 214

American Medical Association board, 119

American Oncology Resources, 134

Ancillary income, *100*, 114, 131

Ancillary services, 123–124, 149, 151

Anderson Consulting, 52

Angell, M., 29

Annison, M. H., 148, 292

Antitrust laws, fear of violating, 159

Aon Managed Care, 235

Appleby, J., 70

Application service providers, 118, 139

Arizona Centers for Health and Medicine, 232

Arnwine, D., 145, 161–162, 278, 279–280, 280–281, 288–289

Assisted living, *215*, *216*, 217–219, 234, 308

Association of American Medical Colleges, 171, 174

Asthma, managing, 225, 226

Attitude factor, *19*, 268

Attitude of providers, overall. *See* Morale

Aurora Associated Physicians, 137

Aurora HealthCare, 196, 202, 233

Aurora Pharmacy, 233

Austin, M., 84, 85, 105

Automation of tasks, 106–107, *108*, 113

Aycox, R., 70

B

Babies and Children's Hospital, 183

Baby boomers, 5, 76, 87, 111, 233; increasing importance of, 52–53, 73–74; and market segmentation, 309, 310

Hospital market share, 15–16, *17*, 145, 147–148, 168, 363
Hospital networking, 158, 159–160, 169
Hospital-affiliated medical groups, 103
Hospital-led integrated systems, 196, 197–198, 202; versus clinic-led systems, 195, 349; strategic emphasis of, *199*
Hospital-owned primary care practices, 150–153, 169
Hospitals & Health Networks, 371
Hospitals and multihospital systems: strategic emphasis of, *146*; struggles of, 144–145. *See also specific issues and strategies*
Hospitals, as partners, 212, 262, 333
Howe, R., 226
Howgill, M.W.C., 314, 315
Huber, R., 236, 238, 249, 346
Hubler, E., 138
Human Genome Project, 20, 369
Human resource issues, 264–265
Humana, 228, 249–250
Humor, using, 258, 267
Hunter Group, 175
Hutts, J., 90

I

IBM, 205
IDX basic platform, use of, 129
Income factor, *19*
Incongruities, *82*, 85–86
Incremental change (scenario 1): and ancillary income, 114; characteristics of, *26–27*; factors defining, *25*; growth of uninsured in, 67; health plans and, 237, 387; hospitals and, *146*; integrated systems and, *199*, 206, 211–212; medical groups and, *100*; outpatient services and, 101
Indemnity plans, drug coverage in, 248
Independent Health, 238, 240, 246
Independent living, *215*, *216*
Independent practice associations (IPAs): and capitation, 244; conclusions on, 142; development of, 127–129; failure of, 137–138; financial reserves of, 245; future of, 139; joining, 126; and managed care contracting, 114; regulatory demands on, 253
Independent specialists: competition facing, 120; overhead of, 124
Individual insurance: and consumer

choice, 74; and decline in uninsured, 22; health plans adapting to, 239; impact of, on managed care, 119; move toward, 23, *24*
Industry decline, dispelling myth about, 357–358
Industry/market structure, changes in, *82*, 83–84
Information crossover, within organizations, 269–270
Information providers, 144; health plans as, 241–243, 250; opportunities as, 366
Information sharing, basic, 107, *108*
Information systems (IS): academic medical centers and, 176; accelerating development of, 19; acquisition of, board involvement in, 288; assessing impact of, 378; and the four scenarios, *27*; and health plans, 241, 249–250; hospitals and, 161–162; integrated systems and, *199*; for transaction processing, 106–107, *108*, 113. *See also* Electronic medical records (EMRs)
Information technology (IT): academic medical centers and, 172, 176; for cost containment, 249, 347–348; embracing, 263–264; expected developments in, 18–20; financing, options for, 118–119; and the four scenarios, *27*; hospitals and, 161–162, 168; improving service and access with, 111–112; integrated systems and, 204–206; integrating, in overall strategy, 270–271; investing in, 88; and IPAs, 129; leadership in, 328–329; outreach services and, 102–103; physicians and medical groups and, 104–108; promises of, 358; substituting, for people, 265; and value added, 107, *108*, 113. *See also Internet entries*; Telehealth; Telemedicine
Information technology (IT) readiness, assessing, 272, *273*
Informed consumers. *See* Consumer empowerment
Infrastructure issues, of physician networks, 128, 130, 139, 140
Initiatives, portfolio of, selecting, 272
Innovation and entrepreneurship, 8, 89; best practices for, 90–92; connection between, 80–81; dormant period of, 78; key trends impacting, 87–88; leaders